Spinal Manipulations and Mobilization Techniques

Spinal Manipulations and Mobilization Techniques

Theory and Practice

John Gibbons

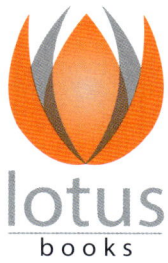

lotus
books

Library of Congress Cataloging-in-Publication Data

Library of Congress Cataloging-in-Publication information is available. LCCN 2025003765 (print)

ISBN: 978-1-7182-4496-2 (print)

This publication is written and published to provide accurate and authoritative information relevant to the subject matter presented. It is published and sold with the understanding that the author and publisher are not engaged in rendering legal, medical, or other professional services by reason of their authorship or publication of this work. If medical or other expert assistance is required, the services of a competent professional person should be sought.

The web addresses cited in this text were current as of March 2025, unless otherwise noted.

Illustrations Amanda Williams
Photographs Ian Taylor
Text Design Medlar Publishing Solutions Pvt Ltd., India
Cover Design Keri Evans
Cover Illustration Science Photo Library/Getty Images
Printed By Versa Press

Books from Lotus Books are available at special discounts for bulk purchase. Special editions or book excerpts can also be created to specification. For details, contact the Special Sales Manager at Human Kinetics.

Printed in the United States of America   10   9   8   7   6   5   4   3   2   1

The paper in this book is certified under a sustainable forestry program.

Lotus Books
An Imprint of Human Kinetics
1607 N. Market Street
Champaign, IL 61820
USA

United States and International
Website: **US.HumanKinetics.com/pages/lotus-books**
Email: info@hkusa.com
Phone: 1-800-747-4457

Canada
Website: **Canada.HumanKinetics.com**
Email: info@hkcanada.com

Human Kinetics' authorized representative for product safety in the EU is Mare Nostrum Group B.V., Mauritskade 21D, 1091 GC Amsterdam, The Netherlands.
Email: gpsr@mare-nostrum.co.uk

L1293

Contents

Acknowledgments

I like to think that the professional relationship I have with my publisher, Jon Hutchings, is going from strength to strength. After writing for many years, I still feel honored to have the privilege of being asked again to continue my dream of writing and influencing therapists throughout the world. Without his input and guidance, none of this would be achievable, and, Jon, I truly thank you for allowing me the opportunity. Jon has now sold the business to Human Kinetics, so I look forward to establishing a similar relationship with them.

My photographer, Ian Taylor, has become a good friend over the years, and with my hand on my heart I honestly believe he completely understands what being an outstanding photographer is all about. He achieves amazing results with the photographs because he is a true professional, and it's all about the finer details to get the best results.

I must give my medical illustrator, Amanda Williams, a headache when I am in constant contact with her regarding the illustrations. I'm sure she doesn't know exactly what it is I want to be drawn sometimes, as I can be a bit vague … I hope that, after many years of being involved with the way I work, she now understands me. I must say, Amanda, you are an amazing medical illustrator, and I truly thank you for all your hard work.

Thanks a million to Jatinder Gill and Lee Thomas; they have both been instrumental in the filming and editing of all the educational videos that are linked via QR codes in this book. You are both true professionals in your field and for that I genuinely thank you.

To the models Nicki Purchase and Tom Miller, who painstakingly spent hours taking it in turns to get the right pose. Hopefully, you will be both be happy with the final outcome.

To my mother, Margaret Gibbons, who sadly passed away while I was writing this book on June 9, 2021. I also extend my wishes for a happy and prosperous life to my sister, Amanda Williams, to her husband, Philip, and to her son James and daughter Victoria, who are both doing exceptionally well on their own career pathways.

Lastly, I wanted to say that not a day goes by without me thinking about my son, Thomas Rhys Gibbons, who left my world on February 28, 2017. I would like to think he is looking down on me, feeling proud of what his dad has achieved in his life and knowing that through his teachings and books he is changing lives throughout the world. I miss you so much, Tom-Tom—one day, we will be together again, but not yet!

Of all my books, this has taken me the longest to write, so I would like to dedicate this book to the family I have lost, which is in the past and for the present and future. Life is always full of surprises; for example, on September 15th, 2024, at 7.41 pm, a new family member arrived: we now have a baby girl called Yasmin in our lives, and her name means "gift from God," so seeing her growing up is going to be a completely new chapter in my life!

Introduction

This book has literally been a draft on my computer for many years and it has taken me the longest time to bring it all together. I simply say this has been partly due to life's exciting distractions and partly to the pandemic, which had a big part in all that as well, even though that time would have been the perfect time to write a book, especially as most of us were at home twiddling our thumbs!

Spinal courses are particularly popular because there are an exceptional number of physical therapists who would like to learn how to perform some, if not all, of these spinal manipulative techniques. However, while most would like to learn these advanced spinal techniques within a very short period, as with any professional skill, it will take many years of training, including thousands of hours of theoretical and practical study.

My initial basic training (due to my military background) to learn the techniques of spinal manipulation was to undertake a five-year osteopathy degree in Oxford between 1999 and 2003. During the degree program, the focus of the first couple of years was to study in depth subjects like human anatomy, physiology, histology, and pathology, to name just a few. Eventually, in years two and three, they finally started to teach us spinal mobilization techniques. I tried to learn these skills early on, and this naturally allowed me to progress in a very controlled way. I would take my time to learn the spinal mobilization techniques, one step at a time, before eventually learning how to perform the actual spinal manipulative techniques, which were structured to be taught in year three of the degree syllabus.

However, because I was a little frustrated with the training curriculum, I enrolled in a five-day spinal manipulative course in my first year of my osteopathic studies, because I wanted to learn the manipulative techniques sooner rather than later and didn't want to wait until the third year.

Students who have previously attended my spinal courses will be smiling when they read this paragraph, because I tell this story often. There were 10 students enrolled on the course in Cardiff, and although I was a first-year student with relatively basic knowledge, because I was also a sports therapy lecturer, my familiarity with anatomy and muscle origins and insertions was above average. The problem was that the other students had only just finished their basic massage course a week or two before, but had decided to continue with their studies and attend an intensive spinal manipulative course. Nothing like jumping in at the deep end! However, it was by far the wrong thing to do, and was akin to having only *one* flying lesson and then being expected to fly a commercial aircraft solo.

By the midmorning break on the first day, we were being shown how to manipulate the upper cervical complex at the specific level of C1 and C2 (go back 30 minutes and the tutor was discussing anatomy of the cervical spine, bony landmarks, vertebral arteries, etc.). When I looked around the room, I could see the other students glancing at each other, looking rather bemused. They had no idea at all what the tutor was talking about, because they had never been taught any of the functional in-depth anatomy he was teaching during this five-day intensive course. The massage course that they had attended only a week before covered simple anatomy components—the names of the major muscles, and traditional massage techniques like effleurage and petrissage—nothing about the nitty gritty components of spinal motion and the safety concerns regarding the vertebral

artery and pathologies affecting the spinal column, and so on.

A few hours passed, and it was time for the students to practice some of the techniques they had been shown by the tutor. A fellow student looked at me and while palpating my neck simply said, "John, I have got no idea what I am doing! I am not even sure what the tutor was saying earlier to us about the anatomy of the cervical spine. I can only feel the skin of your neck but I'm not sure what the facet joints are, where they are, how to feel them, or anything else, come to that."

You can imagine how confident I felt at this point. When he said, "Can I have a go?" this naturally meant he wanted to practice the actual cervical manipulation. It was hard to say no, so I said, "Ok, but please be careful." Clumsily he held my neck and tried to "have a go" by turning my neck quickly to one side and asking if I had felt a click. I said I hadn't, so he asked if he could have another go. He proceeded to try again and asked again if I had heard a click. Again, I hadn't.

After a few tries he said he couldn't do this technique, but by now was getting agitated and starting to sweat, and kept rubbing his forehead to wipe it away. His hands were also sweaty, and a few minutes later before trying again, he was holding my neck and looking down at me to check his technique. By now, the sweat droplets were dripping onto my face, so I said, "Can you please wipe yourself dry before continuing as you are sweating profusely, and the sweat droplets are falling all over my face …"

At that moment, I thought that if I ever had the opportunity to teach spinal manipulation techniques, I would do things completely differently. For example, I would insist that the students attending the courses were appropriately qualified, with experience of treating patients. If I decided to teach the cervical spine, the therapists attending would need to be either qualified or at least approaching the end of their studies, and would be mainly students of osteopathy, chiropractic, or physiotherapy.

When I woke up the next morning I couldn't move my neck without pain, so we can safely say that I didn't let anybody else "have a go" at neck manipulation during the remainder of the course …

I have been teaching spinal manipulation and mobilization techniques for many years. Almost every other month I lecture this course somewhere in the world, and most students only want to learn the *manipulative* component of the course. However, by the end of the course most of them will only be using the *mobilization* techniques, because they soon realize that to be able to manipulate an area of the body is a very difficult technique to master and cannot be learnt in a short period of time.

Manual therapy techniques for the spine, thorax, and pelvis are commonly performed for the treatment of pain and dysfunctional movement patterns. The purpose of this text is to introduce qualified and experienced manual therapists to techniques to mobilize and manipulate the cervical, thoracic, and lumbar spine, as well as the pelvic girdle. The techniques demonstrated throughout are very safe and effective as long as they are performed correctly. Proficiency in their use requires training and practice on a continual basis. The term "manipulation" is often used to describe a range of physical therapy techniques. The manipulative techniques that will be demonstrated within this text are known as a high-velocity thrust (HVT), and we do these techniques to achieve a joint cavitation that is accompanied by an audible cracking sound.

Naturally, these techniques are easier to show you in person than to explain through a textbook, and the online YouTube videos that you can find through the QR codes are there to assist you to learn these specialized techniques, as well as watch the face-to-face spinal courses that I offer.

I truly hope you enjoy reading the book, and maybe one day you will attend a course with me in person, so that I can help you fine-tune your spinal techniques.

John Gibbons
Oxford, 2025

If you have any difficulty viewing the videos on YouTube, you can also find them at https://ancillaries.humankinetics.com/ SpinalManipulationsAndMobilizationTechniques1E

PART I

THEORY

Anatomy of the Vertebral Column

It makes perfect sense to briefly discuss the anatomy of the vertebral column, but also to include the pelvic girdle (see chapter 2). The focus of this book will be to specifically mobilize and manipulate the vertebral structures located within the spinal column, including the sacroiliac joint (SIJ), plus other anatomical areas of the pelvic girdle.

In chapter 1, I will briefly introduce you to the major components of the vertebral column, and I will discuss each of these specific spinal areas in far more detail in the subsequent chapters. It's more logical to demonstrate the mobilizing and manipulative techniques after you have read more about the specific functional anatomy of each region of the spine.

The vertebral column, also known as the spinal column, consists of five segmented areas, known as the cervical, thoracic, and lumbar spine, the sacrum, and the coccyx (figure 1.1).

There are 33 individual vertebrae that make up the vertebral column (see figure 1.1):

- 7 cervical vertebrae (C1–C7)
- 12 thoracic vertebrae (T1–T12)
- 5 lumbar vertebrae (L1–L5)
- 5 sacral vertebrae (S1–S5; the sacrum)
- 4 coccygeal vertebrae (C1–C4; the coccyx)

However, we consider that there are only 24 vertebrae that are capable of motion, because the vertebrae of the sacrum and coccyx start to fuse around 16–18 years of age and become completely fused around 30–32 years of age. By then, no individual vertebral motion is possible at either the sacral or coccygeal level.

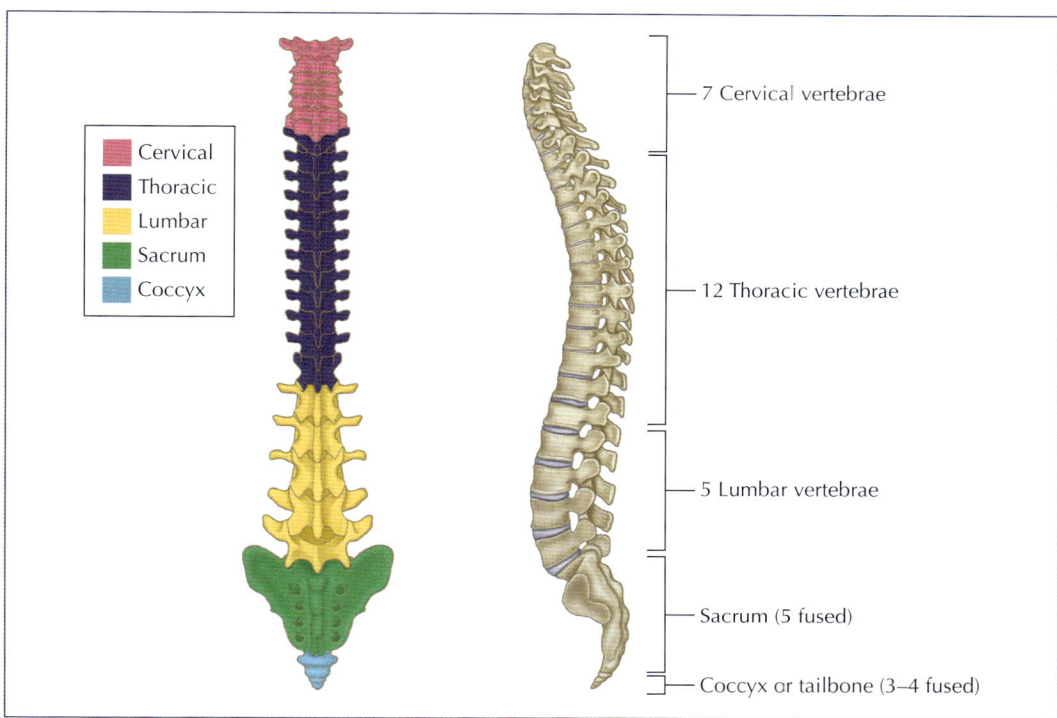

Figure 1.1. The vertebral or spinal column and its five segments.

Functions of the Vertebral Column

There are four functions of the vertebral column:

- **To provide a safe environment for the spinal cord and nerve roots:** The spinal cord and associated nerve roots send messages up and down the body and affect some of the most important structures we have within our body. Naturally, we need these delicate structures protected, and the spinal column provides an armored coating to the soft tissue within—a bit like being in a military tank with a six-inch metal shield around you.

- **To maintain and allow the upright posture:** Without the spinal column, you simply wouldn't be able to stand upright and maintain what we perceive as the perfect posture. It is the role of the spinal column to allow this unique position.

- **To be a flexible adapter:** The spinal column is a truly amazing structure as well as a superb feat of engineering, because it not only moves in various planes of motion but allows your whole body to move: to bend forward, backward, and to the side, and to rotate.

- **To provide a base of attachment:** There are an abundance of ligaments, muscles, and tendons that directly attach to the spinal column, and these soft-tissue attachments utilize its solid bony structure through anchor points. Some muscles like the quadratus lumborum and even the iliolumbar ligament act much like the guy ropes that help keep the tent up when you go camping.

Spinal Curvatures

Developing as a fetus within our mother's womb, we have only one flexion curvature (a *kyphosis* curve), and this is known as a *primary curve*. When as a child we learn how to sit, stand, and walk, this assists the spinal column to develop our two *secondary curves*. However, the primary curvature is still maintained within the thoracic and sacral regions.

The first of these secondary curves develops from the cervical spine as the child learns to hold their head upright, and then the second, lumbar spine curvature forms as the child learns how to stand and walk. The lumbar and cervical spine exhibit a *lordosis* curvature, which develops into extension curves.

So, to recap: the vertebral column has four curves in total: two primary flexion curves of the thoracic and sacral spine regions and two secondary extension curves of the lumbar and cervical spine regions (figure 1.2).

The Facet Joints

There are over 100 facet joints, also known as zygapophyseal, apophyseal, or Z-joints, that are formed within the vertebral column. They form as a set of synovial joints located between the articular processes of two adjacent vertebrae. The facet joint is a unique and crucial anatomical part of the spine, which allows articulation between vertebrae as well as helping to transfer the load that the column experiences each day of our busy lives (figure 1.3).

The facet joint is a diarthrodial (synovial) joint, has opposing articular cartilage, and is surrounded by a ligamentous capsule that protects and encases the joint space. The facet joints, in a nutshell, allow the vertebral column to move in all planes of motion. However, depending on their

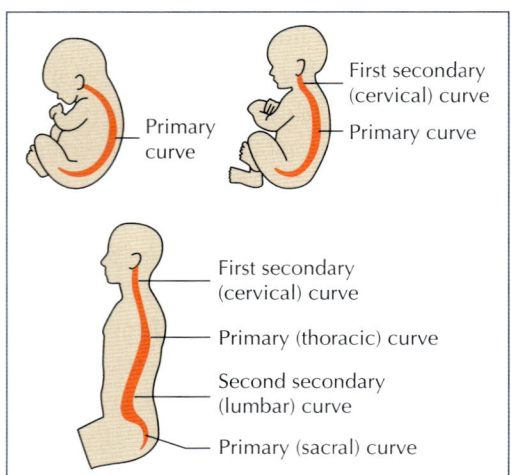

Figure 1.2. Spinal curvatures.

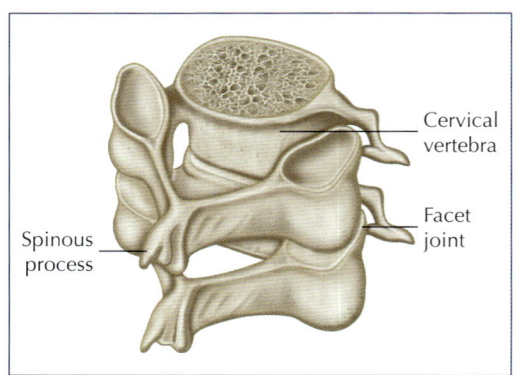

Figure 1.3. Anatomy of a cervical facet joint.

location, the facet joints will also restrict motion because of their orientation, and so act as a type of active ligament. For example, within the lumbar spine we can perform flexion and extension with relative ease and without too much restriction, because the facet joints there will relatively open and close to allow these movements. However, because the facet is more vertically orientated within the lumbar spine, rotation is limited—there is only around 1°–2° of segmental rotation possible within the lumbar spine. The cervical spine has substantially more rotation, and again, this is simply because of the way the facet joints are orientated.

The facet joint is formed by two adjacent vertebrae, with the inferior facet of the vertebra above articulating with the superior facet of the vertebra below. Within the cervical spine, the facet joints are orientated more within a horizontal plane, allowing the increased rotation. As we travel down to the lower thoracic and lumbar spine, the facet joints gradually become more vertically orientated, which is why rotation in the lumbar spine is limited. This change of facet orientation, which restricts motion in certain planes, is simply to protect the intervertebral discs and spinal cord from undue and excessive motion.

It is important that the reader understands the orientation of facet joints at each level of the vertebral column (see table 1.1), especially when it comes to applying manual therapy techniques. For example, it is common to use a rotation thrust to the cervical spine to cavitate the joint space; however, in the lumbar spine, we might apply a side-bending type of thrust through the direction of the femur because

of the limited rotation caused by the facet orientation. If we decided to apply more of a rotatory rather than a side-bending thrust within the lumbar spine, the facet joints might become *impacted* and potentially cause more pain to the patient. Furthermore, a cavitation would now not be possible because you are forcibly closing the joint rather than physically trying to open the joint, which is what typically causes the cavitation noise (explained in detail later).

Cervical Facet Joints

All movements are possible within the cervical region: flexion, extension, rotation, and lateral flexion (table 1.2). This is because the facet joints are oriented around 45° to the transverse plane; however, they are parallel to the frontal plane (figure 1.4a). The superior articulating surface will face posteriorly, superiorly, and medially, and the inferior articulating facet will face anteriorly, inferiorly, and laterally.

Thoracic Facet Joints

The thoracic spine has a smaller range of motion in all planes (table 1.2), especially flexion and extension, compared with the cervical spine (figure 1.4b). This is partly due to the associated ribcage and partly because the facet joints between adjacent thoracic vertebrae are angled approximately 60° to the transverse plane and 20° to the frontal plane, with the superior facets facing posteriorly, superiorly, and laterally, and the inferior facets facing anteriorly, inferiorly, and medially.

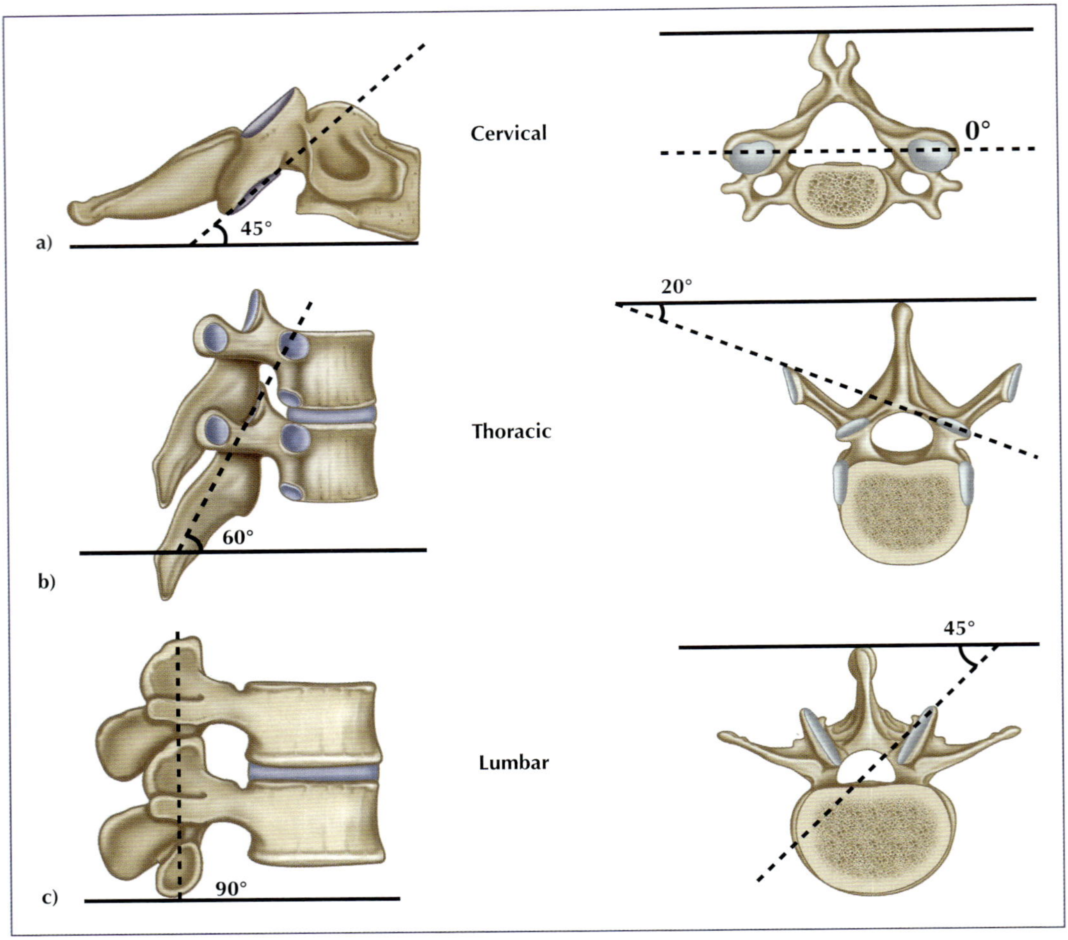

Cervical

0°

a) 45°

20°

Thoracic

b) 60°

45°

Lumbar

c) 90°

Figure 1.4. Facet joint orientation. (a) Cervical; (b) thoracic; (c) lumbar.

Lumbar Facet Joints

The facet joints in the lumbar region lie 90° to the transverse plane and 45° to the frontal plane, with the superior articular facets facing medially, and the inferior articular facets facing laterally. However, there is a slight change of the orientation at the lumbosacral (LS) junction, and this modification keeps the vertebral column from sliding anteriorly in relation to the first sacral vertebra (S1), which is located directly below (figure 1.4c).

Table 1.1. Facet Joint Orientation for Each Spinal Region.

Region	Facet Joint Orientation
Cervical	45° transverse plane, 0° frontal plane
Thoracic	60° transverse plane, 20° frontal plane
Lumbar	90° transverse plane, 45° frontal plane

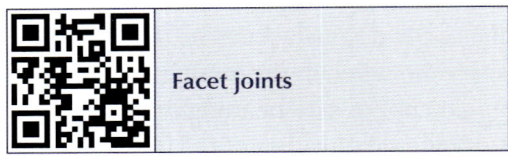

Facet joints

Table 1.2. Vertebral Motion for Each Spinal Region.

Motion	Cervical	Thoracic	Lumbar
Flexion	0°–60°	0°–50°	0°–60°
Extension	0°–75°	0°–45°	0°–25°
Rotation	0°–80°	0°–30°	0°–12°
Lateral flexion	0°–60°	0°–40°	0°–25°

Ligaments of the Vertebral Column

In the list below are some of the ligaments of the vertebral column; some are mentioned in chapter 2 because they relate in particular to the lumbar spine and pelvis. Figure 1.5 shows the cervical spine ligaments.

- Posterior and anterior longitudinal ligaments
- Ligamentum flavum
- Interspinous ligament
- Supraspinous ligament
- Ligamentum nuchae
- Alar ligament
- Transverse ligament of atlas
- Cruciform ligament

Posterior and Anterior Longitudinal Ligaments

These two ligaments—as the name suggests—are long ligaments that attach to the vertebral bodies from the cervical spine all the way down to the sacrum. They limit the amount of flexion (posterior longitudinal ligament) and extension motion (anterior longitudinal ligament) of the vertebral column, as well as assisting the stability of the intervertebral discs.

Ligamentum Flavum

The ligamentum flavum is very different to the longitudinal ligaments because it

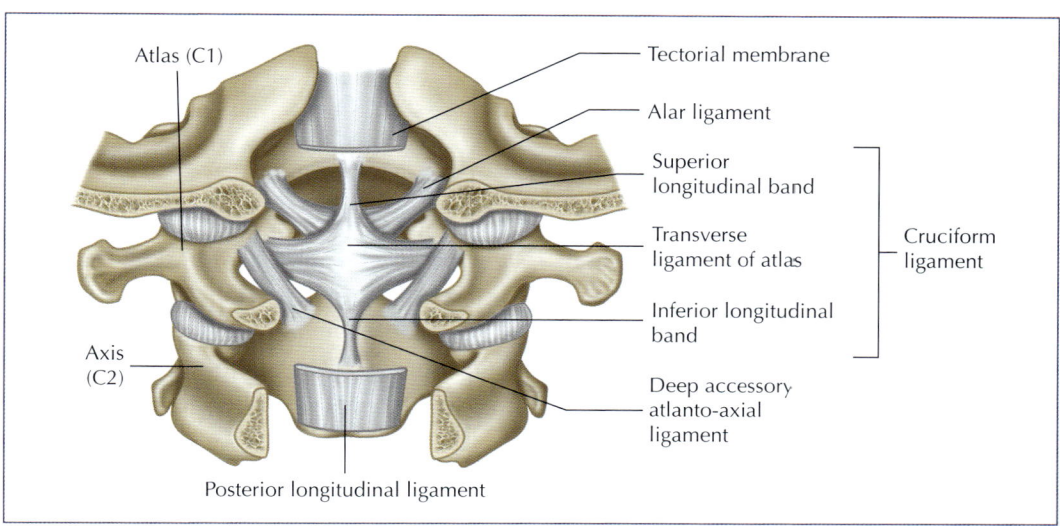

Figure 1.5. Cervical spine ligaments: atlanto-axial joint.

is both very short and thick—especially in the lumbar spine—and connects the laminae of adjacent vertebrae, from C2 all the way down to S1. This unique ligament is very interesting because it contains approximately 80% elastin fibers, which provide the flexible motion and give the ligament its yellow appearance. The remaining 20% is collagen. Because of the increased number of elastic fibers, this ligament provides a kind of recoil to maintain the column's shape after flexion. Ligamentum flavum also prevents the capsules of the facet joints being pinched during spinal movements.

Interspinous Ligament

As the word suggests, these ligaments connect the spinous processes of adjacent vertebrae—one segment at a time—from C1 all the way down to S1. Their role is to limit flexion of the spinal column by restricting the separation motion of the spinous processes.

Supraspinous Ligament

This strong fibrous connection links the spinous processes of vertebrae from C7 to the sacral spine. The supraspinous ligament becomes progressively wider as it travels from the thoracic to the lumbar spine and also merges with a fascial structure called the thoracolumbar fascia. Its main role is to limit flexion of the spinal column and provide an attachment for certain muscles.

Ligamentum Nuchae

Also known as the nuchal ligament, this is continuous with the supraspinous ligament and attaches to the occipital protuberance (so-called "bump of knowledge") located at the base of the occipital bone (spinous process of C2) and the nuchal line and connects with the spinous process of C7. There is also a small attachment directly to the posterior tubercle (no spinous process present here) of the atlas (C1) vertebra.

This ligament will limit flexion of the cervical spine and allows the attachment of two important muscles, the trapezius and splenius capitis.

Alar Ligaments

These are two rounded structures that stabilize the level of C1 and C2, especially for rotation, and become taut in cervical flexion. They attach from either side of the odontoid process to the occipital condyles.

Transverse Ligament of Atlas

This small but very thick, strong ligament stabilizes the odontoid process. Interestingly, the anterior part of this ligament is covered with articular cartilage because of the articulation it serves with the odontoid process for rotation of the cervical spine. The attachment of this ligament separates the atlas (C1) ring into two distinct parts of unequal size. The smaller space allows for the odontoid process, and the larger space accommodates the spinal cord and its membranes.

Cruciform Ligament

As the name suggests, this ligament is similar in shape to a cross, and is also commonly called the cruciate ligament of the atlas. It serves to stabilize the atlanto-axial joint (AAJ) joint (C1/C2) by maintaining the posterior part of the dens (odontoid process) of C2 in place within the AAJ.

The cruciform ligament has two individual bands: the longitudinal band, which has a superior and inferior part, and the transverse ligament of atlas (explained above). Together they form this unique structure.

Anatomy of the Pelvic Girdle and Sacroiliac Joint

2

This book is primarily about spinal manipulation and mobilization techniques; however, I believe it is also necessary to discuss the anatomy and function of the pelvis and the sacroiliac joint (SIJ), especially as many of the techniques throughout the later chapters are focused specifically on this complex region of the body.

The pelvic girdle is composed of the sacrum, the coccyx, and the three so-called "hipbones"—the ilium, ischium,

and pubis. The bones of the adult pelvis join to form four joints: the left and right SIJs, the sacrococcygeal joint, and the symphysis pubis joint (SPJ) (figure 2.1).

At birth, the ilium, ischium, and pubis bones are separated by hyaline cartilage; by the end of puberty, they will have naturally conjoined (fused together), with complete ossification normally occurring by the time a person has reached the age of approximately 20–25. Once fused, the three bones are collectively called the *innominate*

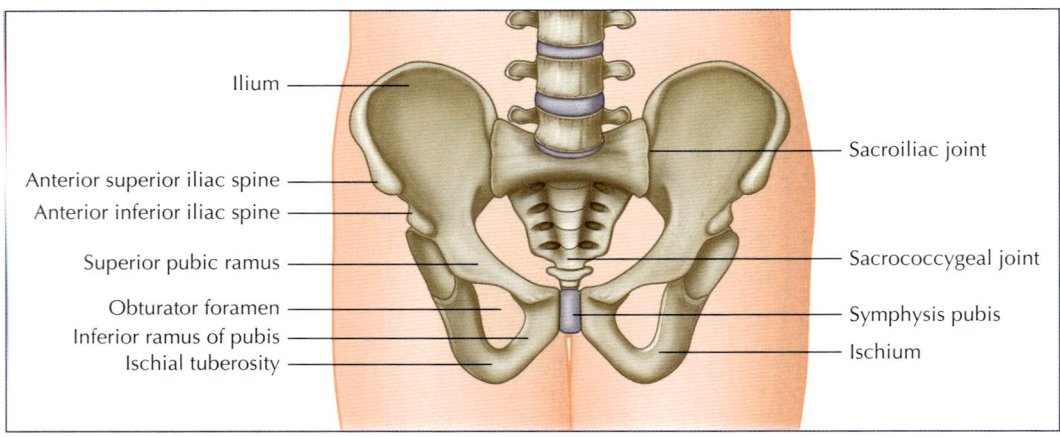

Figure 2.1. Bones of the pelvic girdle, and their associated joints.

Labels (left side, top to bottom): Ilium; Anterior superior iliac spine; Anterior inferior iliac spine; Superior pubic ramus; Obturator foramen; Inferior ramus of pubis; Ischial tuberosity

Labels (right side, top to bottom): Sacroiliac joint; Sacrococcygeal joint; Symphysis pubis; Ischium

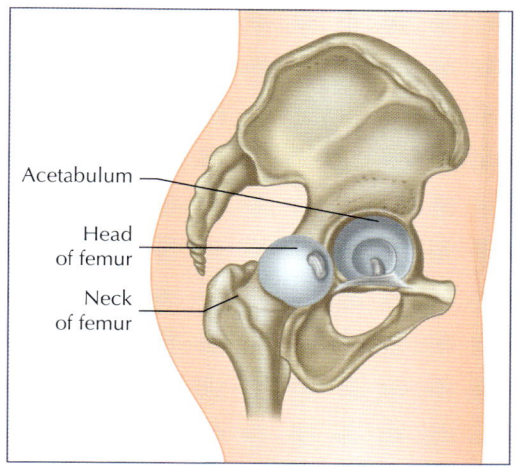

Figure 2.2. Iliofemoral (hip) joint.

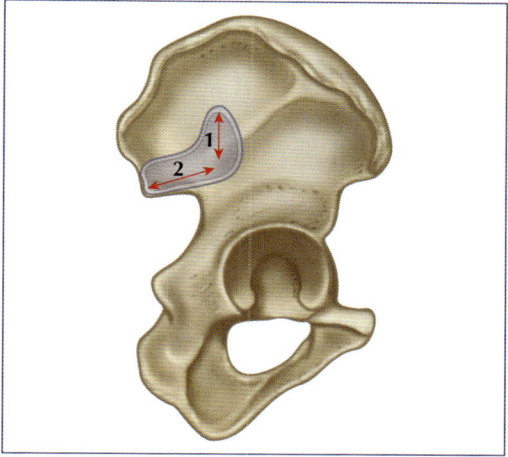

Figure 2.3. L shape formed by the short (vertical [1]) and long (horizontal [2]) arms of the ilium.

bone, or simply the "innominate." On the lateral side of the innominate is the *acetabulum*; this area forms the articulation with the head of the femur to create the iliofemoral (hip) joint (figure 2.2).

The Innominate Bones

Ilium

The ilium is fan shaped and is the most superior as well as the largest of the three hipbones, making up approximately two-fifths of the acetabulum, the deep, cuplike socket of the hip joint. The body of the ilium and the sacrum form the SIJ. This L-shaped articulation is located on the posterior superior aspect of the ilium and has a vertically (vertical plane) orientated "short arm" and a more horizontally (anteroposterior plane) positioned "long arm" (figure 2.3).

If you place one hand on your hip, you can feel the curved ridge of the superior aspect of the ilium, known as the *iliac crest*. From this crest, if you lightly move your fingers down inferior to the anterior aspect of the ilium, you should feel the bony projection known as the *anterior superior iliac spine* (ASIS), which allows for the attachment of soft tissues (e.g., the sartorius muscle).

If you continue slightly inferior to the ASIS, you will come to another bony landmark called the *anterior inferior iliac spine* (AIIS); this is where one part of rectus femoris attaches. Palpating the posterior aspect of the ilium as it curves inferiorly, you will feel the bony prominence of the *posterior superior iliac spine* (PSIS); again, this is an attachment for soft tissues. ASIS and PSIS are commonly used as palpatory landmarks when one is assessing the position of the pelvic girdle (figure 2.4).

Ischium

The ischium is narrower than the ilium and is located inferior to it and behind

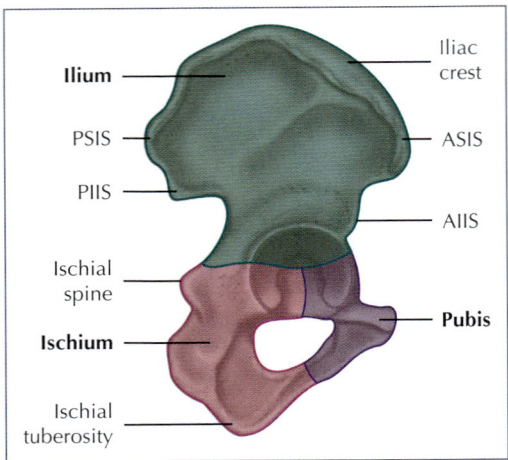

Figure 2.4. Anatomical landmarks of the iliac crest: ASIS, AIIS, and PSIS.

the pubis. The ischium has an easily palpable landmark called the *ischial tuberosity* (figure 2.5). This is commonly called the sitting bone or sit bone, and provides the necessary landmark for the attachment of the hamstrings. It is the ischial tuberosity, along with the coccyx, on which you rest your body weight when sitting. The ischium is the strongest of

the three bones and forms approximately two-fifths of the acetabulum.

Pubis

The pubis, or pubic bone, is the most anterior as well as the smallest of the three hipbones and makes up approximately one-fifth of the acetabulum. The body of the pubis is wide, strong, and flat, and together with the opposite pubic bone makes the symphysis pubis joint (SPJ). This joint is classified as an amphiarthrosis, because it is connected centrally by a broad piece of fibrocartilage (figure 2.6).

On the superior aspect of the pubis there is a bony projection called the *pubic tubercle*, which allows for the attachment of the inguinal ligament and is also used as a palpatory landmark when one is assessing the position of the pelvic girdle.

Sacrum

The sacrum ("sacred bone") is a large triangular bone located at the base of the lumbar spine and forms the back part of the pelvic cavity. The sacrum starts at birth as five individual bones, before starting to fuse between the ages of 16 and 18. It is

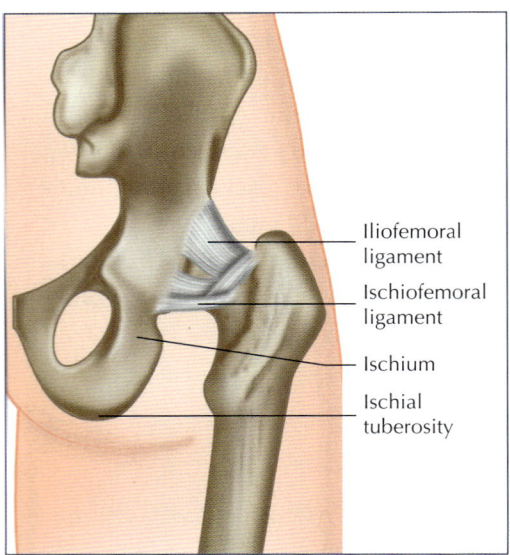

Figure 2.5. Ischium and ischial tuberosity.

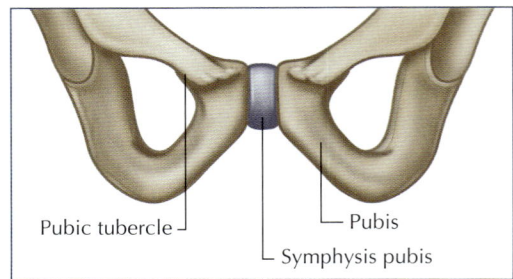

Figure 2.6. Pubis, pubic tubercle, and SPJ.

considered to have fully fused into a single bone by the age of 30.

Considerable differences in the shape of the sacrum between individuals, as well as structural differences between the left and right sides, are well documented. The connection of the sacrum to the ilium forms the SIJ.

The superior aspect of the sacrum is called the *sacral base* and is primarily made up of the first sacral segment; the base is angled in a forward direction to form a concavity. The opposite end of the sacrum is called the *sacral apex*, and this is made up of the fifth sacral segment (figure 2.7).

The natural position of the sacrum is called the *sacral angle* and is generally in the range 40°–44°, although it can be anywhere from 30° to 50°. Moreover, a specific type of motion called *nutation* (a nodding motion, which will be discussed later) can be responsible for an increase in this angle by anywhere from 6° to 8° on standing (from a sitting position). The sacral angle increases because of the change in the curvature of the lumbar spine from an

initial flexion curvature when sitting to an extension curvature (lumbar lordosis) when standing. This sacral movement allows the whole of the spinal column to adopt an upright position.

On the lateral sides of the sacrum, located between the levels of the first three sacral vertebrae (S1–S3), are the *alae* ("wings"). These auricular (earlike), L-shaped areas of the sacrum make up the articulation with the ilium—the SIJ. When discussing the ilium, I mentioned that there is a short vertical arm and a long anteroposterior (horizontal) arm (figure 2.3), and these naturally dovetail with each other, like pieces of a jigsaw puzzle.

Another way of looking at the sacrum is as a continuation of the lumbar spine, while the SIJs on either side mimic what I generally call atypical facet joints. You can think of the sacrum as a single vertebra and the left and right SIJs as the articulating facet joints, with the superior articular facet being the ilia component and the inferior articular facet being the sacral component (figure 2.8).

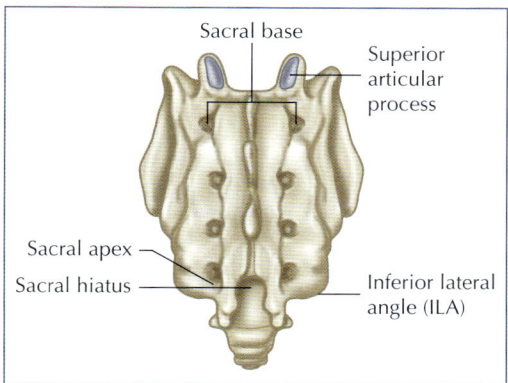

Figure 2.7. Anatomical landmarks of the sacrum, posterior view.

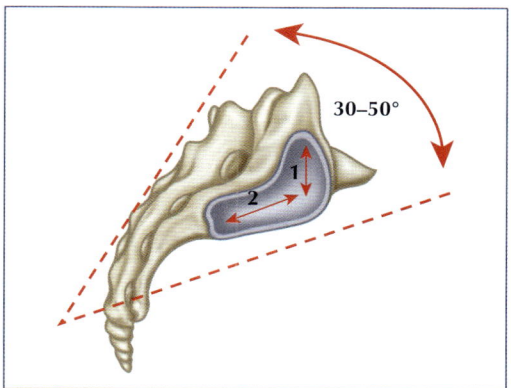

Figure 2.8. The short (vertical [1]) and long (horizontal [2]) arm of the sacrum, and the sacral angle (lateral view).

Coccyx

The coccyx is the continuation and endpoint of the vertebral column and is commonly referred to as the "tailbone." It has between three and five (normally four) vertebral segments, called the *coccygeal vertebrae*, and most textbooks state that these are actually fused; some authors, however, maintain that the coccygeal vertebrae are indeed separate and individual entities (figure 2.9).

There are many muscles with attachments directly on the coccyx. For example, the pelvic floor muscles attach to the anterior surface of the coccyx, and the gluteus maximus (Gmax) muscle and ligaments attach to the posterior surface. Likewise, some ligaments attach directly to the coccyx, such as the sacrococcygeal ligament and some of the fibers of the sacrospinous and sacrotuberous ligaments. The coccyx also plays a role in weight bearing (while sitting), forming a tripod structure with the left and right ischial tuberosities.

Symphysis Pubis Joint

The SPJ is classified as a nonsynovial fibrocartilaginous amphiarthrosis joint, and connects the left and right pubic bones. In adults, only 0.08 inches (2 mm) of movement (shift) and 1° of rotation are considered to be possible in this joint; however, these values will increase in women during pregnancy and childbirth. The available movement of the SPJ is also influenced by the natural shape of the joint, and by muscular activation from the adductor and abdominal muscles.

The ends of each pubic bone are covered by hyaline cartilage, which connects to the piece of fibrocartilage located in the center of the SPJ. The joint has strong superior and inferior ligaments and a thinner posterior ligament (figure 2.10).

One can think of the design of the symphysis pubis as being similar to the intervertebral discs of the spine, with a central disc of fibrocartilage that cushions against compressive loads, as well as providing shock absorption and contributing to passive stabilization.

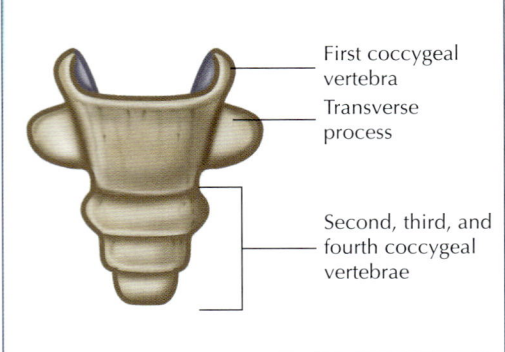

First coccygeal vertebra

Transverse process

Second, third, and fourth coccygeal vertebrae

Figure 2.9. Coccyx bone and its individual segments.

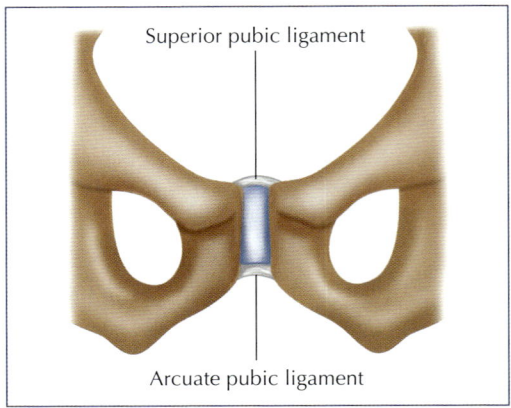

Superior pubic ligament

Arcuate pubic ligament

Figure 2.10. SPJ and associated ligaments.

Because of this similarity, the articular disc of the SPJ is also vulnerable to both degeneration and trauma, particularly when the joint is subjected to traumatic or repetitive shear forces (e.g., osteitis pubis).

Functionally, the SPJ helps to resist tension, shearing, and compression forces, and remarkably is able to widen during pregnancy. The anatomist Andreas Vesalius, who challenged the Hippocratic belief that the pubic bones separated during childbirth, was the first to recognize this joint in 1543.

Sacroiliac Joint

The link between lower back pain and the SIJ dates back to the era of Hippocrates (*c.*460–377 BCE); the medical practitioners at the time felt that under normal conditions the SIJ was immobile. Our knowledge of the role and function of the pelvic girdle has increased greatly since then, and has progressed enormously over the last few decades, particularly with respect to the SIJ.

For many years I have been teaching on the pelvic girdle, and on the SIJ in particular, which means that I have come into contact with thousands of physical therapists, ranging from osteopaths and physiotherapists to chiropractors and sports therapists, among others. I personally think that the pelvis is a relatively difficult subject to teach to my students (mainly therapists),

because I consider the SIJ to be something of a "mystery" to many therapists. It becomes especially difficult when I am trying to explain the subject to my athletes and patients.

Most physical therapists attending the course on the pelvic girdle tell me at some point that they see patients and athletes regularly with what they believe to be a presentation of SIJ dysfunction. Often, patients presenting with SIJ issues have even been referred directly to them by a local doctor or a colleague.

Vleeming et al. (2007) say that mobility of the pelvic joints is difficult to measure objectively, especially in the weight-bearing position, and that feeling motion at the SIJ during active and passive motion is difficult to prove. Bearing this in mind, you can imagine that teaching a course on this complex area of the body is not as straightforward as one might think.

Anatomy of the SIJ

The SIJ is located between the sacrum and the ilium and is classified as a true synovial arthrodial joint, as it contains a joint capsule, synovial fluid, articular cartilage, and a synovial membrane (figure 2.11).

The SIJ is unique: on the iliac side, the cartilage is mainly fibrocartilage, whereas on the sacral side, the cartilage consists of hyaline, or articular, cartilage. The articular

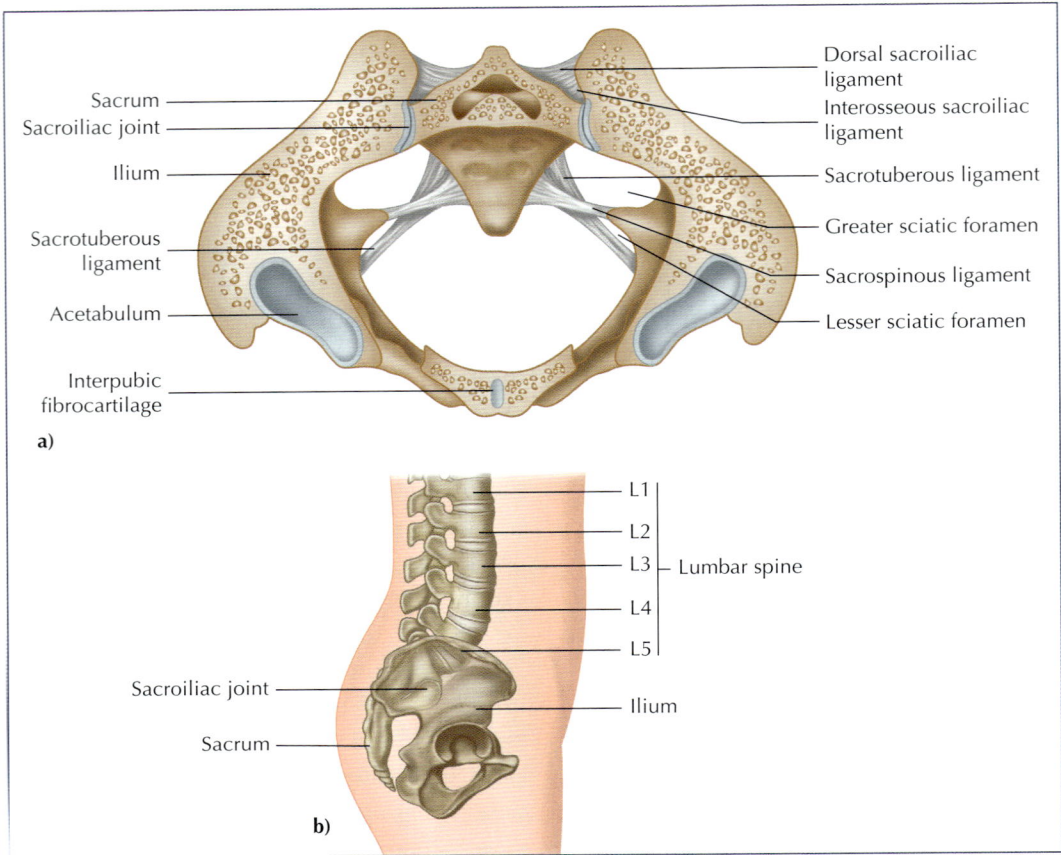

Figure 2.11. Anatomy of the SIJ: (a) transverse section; (b) lateral view.

cartilage is thicker (0.04–0.12 inches, or 1–3 mm) on the sacral side than on the iliac side. Kampen and Tillman (1998) found that in adults, the cartilage on the sacral surface of the joint can reach 0.16 inches (4 mm) in thickness, but does not exceed 0.04–0.08 inches (1–2 mm) on the iliac surface.

The reduced thickness of the cartilage on the iliac side might be one of the factors responsible for hardening (sclerosis).

The SIJ has an auricular, L-shaped appearance, similar to a kidney, with a short (vertical) upper arm and a longer (horizontal) lower arm (figure 2.3). Variation in the shape of the SIJ between individuals has been clinically proven; moreover, there can be significant structural differences between the left and right sides of the joint surfaces within the same individual. There is also clear evidence that the paired SIJs, and even the PSISs, are generally asymmetric in appearance, including in patients and athletes who present with no symptoms of pain or dysfunction (i.e., are asymptomatic).

The pelvis is able to move in all three planes of the body: flexion and extension in the sagittal plane (forward and backward bending), lateral flexion (side bending) in the frontal plane, and rotation of the trunk in the transverse plane. It used to be considered that the SIJ could move anywhere between 2° and 18°, but more recent evidence demonstrates that while movement is possible, it is only in very small amounts. Researchers such as Egund et al. (1978) and Sturesson et al. (1989, 2000a, b) have demonstrated that the motion of the SIJ is at best approximately 2°–4° in rotation and 0.04–0.08 inches (1–2 mm) in translation.

We know that during the natural aging process, the characteristics of the SIJ change. In early life, the SIJ surfaces are in general initially flat, but as we start to walk and progress through puberty, the surfaces develop distinct ridges and grooves and lose their naturally flattened appearance. These ridges and grooves fit into one another to some extent, which will potentially aid the overall stability of the SIJ, while still allowing some degree of movement.

DeStefano (2011) mentions that "during the aging process, there is an increase in the grooves on the opposing surfaces of the sacrum and ilium that appears to reduce available motion and enhance stability." Further, he says that "it is of interest to note that the age at which the incidence of disabling back pain is highest (range: 25 to 45 years) is the same age when the greatest amount of motion is available in the sacroiliac joints" (p. 328).

Because of the relationship of the three main pelvic joints (the two SIJs and the SPJ), as well as their relationship to the iliofemoral joint (hip joint), a dysfunction existing in any one of these joints can have a direct impact on the others.

Ligaments of the SIJ

The SIJ has very strong ligaments, which increase the joint's stability and make potential dislocations very rare.

The stability of the SIJ is provided partly through ligamentous attachments. These ligaments will provide joint integrity as well as resistance to shearing-type forces. The ligaments that bind the sacrum directly to the innominate are (figure 2.12):

- Sacrotuberous
- Sacrospinous
- Interosseous
- Long dorsal (posterior sacroiliac)

The iliolumbar ligament will also have a stabilizing influence on the SIJ, as well as on the lumbar spine.

Sacrotuberous Ligament

The sacrotuberous ligament attaches from the PSIS and has an attachment to the posterior sacroiliac ligaments. The ligament then continues, attaching onto the ischial tuberosity and splitting into three separate bands. The outer (lateral)

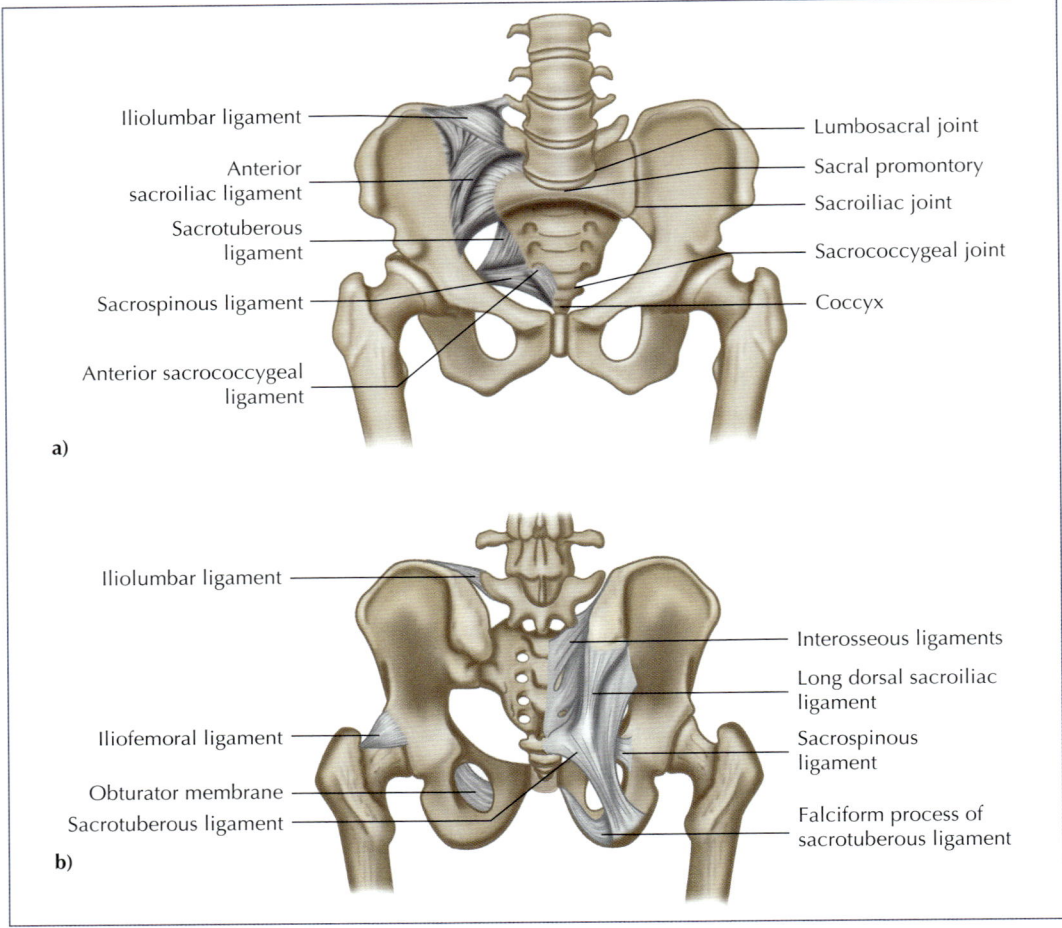

Figure 2.12. Ligaments relating to stability of the SIJ: (a) anterior view; (b) posterior view.

band attaches from the PSIS to the ischial tuberosity, the inner (medial) band attaches from the coccyx to the ischial tuberosity, and the superior band connects the PSIS to the coccyx.

Four muscles have an attachment directly to the sacrotuberous ligament and will contribute to the overall stability of the SIJ:

• Biceps femoris
• Gluteus maximus (Gmax)
• Multifidus
• Piriformis

Vleeming et al. (1989) found that in approximately 50% of subjects, the lower border of the sacrotuberous ligament was directly continuous with the tendon of the origin of the long head of biceps femoris; this muscle could therefore act to stabilize the SIJ via the sacrotuberous ligament. Part of the role of the sacrotuberous ligament is to resist the anterior nodding type of motion of the sacrum (nutation). This ligament will also prevent posterior rotation of the innominate bone with respect to the sacrum. If for some reason there is laxity in the sacrotuberous ligament (along with the sacrospinous ligament), the decreased tension can result in a posterior rotation of the innominate bone and lead to increased nutation of the sacrum.

Sacrospinous Ligament

The sacrospinous ligament has an attachment from the lateral aspect of the sacrum and coccyx and attaches to the spine of the ischium, appropriately named the *ischial spine*. The ligament has the appearance of a thin triangle and, together with the sacrotuberous ligament, modifies the greater sciatic notch in the greater sciatic foramen. The function of the sacrospinous ligament is similar to that of the sacrotuberous ligament in that it prevents the posterior rotation of the innominate bone relative to the sacrum, and also limits nutation (forward motion) of the sacrum relative to the innominate bone.

Interosseous Ligament

The interosseous ligament consists of a dense, short, thick collection of strong collagenous fibers that run in the horizontal plane and connect the sacral tuberosities to the ilium. This ligament lies deep in the narrow recess between the sacrum and the ilium, and has both deep and superficial components. Its main function is to prevent a separation or abduction of the SIJ by strongly binding the sacrum to the ilium. This will help secure the SIJ interlocking mechanism.

Long Dorsal Ligament (Posterior Sacroiliac Ligament)

The long dorsal ligament attaches from the medial and lateral crests of the sacrum to the PSIS. There is also a connection of this ligament to the thoracolumbar fascia, as well as to the multifidus and erector spinae muscles.

The long dorsal ligament mainly resists counternutation of the sacrum (posterior nutation), as well as anterior rotation of the innominate bone. Consequently, this ligament will naturally slacken when the sacrum is in a state of nutation and/ or if there is posterior rotation of the innominate bone. If sacral torsion is present (chapter 5) and the sacral base is found to be "posterior," this ligament will be under constant tension and may be tender when palpated.

Lee (2004, 22) mentions that the skin overlying the long dorsal sacroiliac ligament is a frequent area of pain in patients with lumbosacral and pelvic girdle dysfunction, and that tenderness on palpation of the ligament does not necessarily incriminate this tissue, given the nature of pain referral from both the lumbar spine and the SIJ.

Iliolumbar Ligament

The iliolumbar ligament is a very strong ligamentous structure; it attaches from the transverse processes (TPs) of L4 and L5 and travels to the inner border of the ilium. This ligament, which has five separate bands, is one of three vertebrae-pelvis ligaments responsible for stabilizing the lumbosacral spine in the pelvis, along with the sacrospinous and sacrotuberous ligaments.

Its main function essentially is to limit the motion of the lumbosacral junction by stabilizing the connection between the pelvis and L4 and L5.

Function of the SIJ

The SIJ's primary responsibility is to transfer the weight of the upper body to the lower extremities. The body weight is transferred through the vertebral column to the lumbar spine (L5), to the sacrum, and across the SIJs to the ischial tuberosities, and then out to the acetabula of the hip joints. This mechanism of bony attachments demonstrates the SIJ's role as a weight-bearing joint (figure 2.13). The SIJs are also able to transfer forces in the opposite direction when one is walking, standing, or sitting: the pressure is directed through the legs to the innominates and the sacrum, and then dissipated upward through the lumbosacral junction.

In their secondary role, the SIJs can be thought of as shock absorbers (mainly at the point of heel contact), as they help cushion the increased stress that is forced

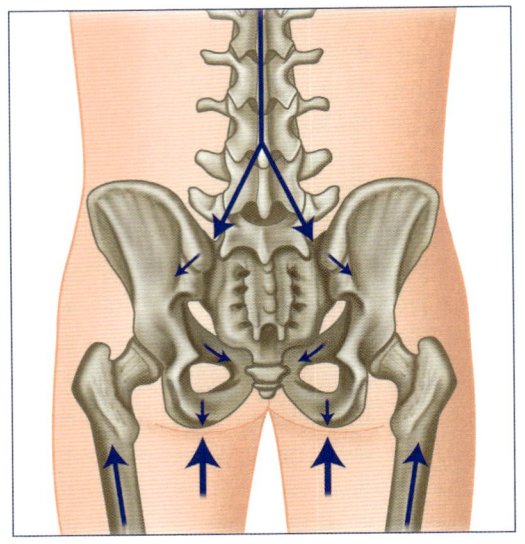

Figure 2.13. Weight transfer forces through the pelvis and the SIJs.

upon the lumbar spine and in particular upon the lower lumbar intervertebral discs. Previous authors have suggested that the incidence of lower lumbar disc disease/degeneration increases when the SIJs present with pathological changes.

Lee and Vleeming (2007) discuss the analysis of gait mechanics and demonstrate that the SIJs provide sufficient flexibility for the intrapelvic forces to be transferred effectively to and from the lumbar spine and lower extremities.

 Pelvis anatomy

Intervertebral Disc Anatomy and Spinal Pathologies

Whenever I suggest to one of my patients that I consider an intervertebral disc to be the source of their problem (especially if they are presenting with what I believe to be referred pain, such as sciatica), many of them assume that their disc has slipped or moved. (Incidentally, discs "slipping" is a myth: the disc does not slip anywhere, even though it is commonly called a slipped disc.) The problem I encounter then is that they naturally expect me, as an osteopath, to *crack* or *manipulate* the disc back into its normal position. However, you will see that this is not the case, because disc conditions can be rather complex. But, just to be clear—discs do not actually slip.

Whichever way you look at it, we will all have disc pathology at some point in our lives, and for some it will occur sooner rather than later. For patients who have referred pain (e.g., sciatica), an underlying disc condition is probably near the top of the ladder as a potential causative factor, although there are a multitude of reasons (not just disc related) why patients suffer sciatic pain. It therefore makes perfect sense to spend some time discussing disc anatomy and function, and of course conditions that can manifest within these unique structures.

I would imagine that many therapists consider disc problems to be more prevalent in those individuals who are not very active, who are overweight, and who have weak core muscles. That might be true for some patients; however, many of my patients are very fit athletes between the ages of 18 and 30. I am of the belief that it is not always "sport" in general that causes problems, but rather the continual training sessions.

For example, I was the resident osteopath for the Oxford University rowing team for over 10 years, and typically each member of the team would spend most early mornings on a rowing machine for approximately 60–90 minutes, as well as rowing on the River Thames each afternoon and at weekends. When I saw an oarsperson with back pain that I consider to be disc related, it might be that they had bent down to pick something up from the floor (even just a pen), and felt their back "go," in which case their pain was not caused by the actual rowing motion. The problem they had then, though, was that any rowing motion (bending and extending with rotation) would exacerbate the pain, whether they were using a rowing machine or rowing on the river. No doubt the continual flexion and rotation of the rowing motion had predisposed them and contributed to the overall disc condition, and the simple action of bending to pick something up (or perhaps even a bout of coughing or sneezing) ultimately caused the disc to fail and to subsequently bulge or herniate (prolapse).

When I see patients at the clinic with lower back pain, the last thing I consider as the cause would be a disc problem. However, if the patient has lower back pain with some type of pain referral pattern to the buttocks and lower limb, and they also mention that simple motions like coughing or sneezing or even sitting or bending forward increase their symptoms (mainly in the limb), then my hypothesis dramatically changes.

In this chapter, I would like to discuss the anatomy of a disc, the symptoms it can present, and the specific differences between a bulging/protruding disc and a prolapsed intervertebral disc (PID).

Even though human bodies are all very similar in structure and function, everybody is a unique individual, and symptoms will vary between patients, even when their confirmed diagnoses are similar. Nevertheless, you can use the following signs and symptoms as a type of tick-box list in establishing whether your patient might have an underlying lumbar or cervical spine intervertebral disc condition:

- There is some history of bending with a rotational component, or simply a cough or a sneeze.
- A couple of days after an initial injury, pain begins to develop in the buttock area and/or leg, as well as in the shoulder, arm, and hand (if related to a cervical disc).
- There is an aversion to sitting for long periods, which makes driving very uncomfortable.
- Standing for long periods brings on discomfort, or sleeping is difficult because of night pain.
- Stiffness is felt, and buttock/leg pain increases, when bending forward to touch the toes or simply putting on socks in the morning.
- Bending backward increases the pain (as the extension motion can potentially catch the posterior aspect of the disc bulge).
- Coughing, sneezing, or defecating (bearing down motion) increases the symptoms to the area of the lower limb (including buttocks, thigh, leg, ankle, and foot) if a lumbar disc, or can refer to the area of the upper limb—arm and hand—if a cervical disc.
- Lower back or the neck and shoulders are generally stiff and potentially painful upon waking in the morning.

- A particular discomfort is felt when sitting, with the impression of squirming in the chair seat. Adopting a position of ease is difficult.
- After lower back symptoms have eased (which typically happens), buttock/leg pain lingers. (It is worth mentioning that some individuals have no history of back pain.)
- There is an inability to plantar flex or dorsiflex the ankle on the painful leg (specific nerve dependent), as potentially the disc is contacting the tibial or common fibular nerve root, causing weakness of the related muscles.
- Slump test or straight leg raise test (SLR) is positive.
- Deep tendon reflex (DTR) of L4, L5, or S1 is reduced (1+), or C5–C7 is reduced (1+) if related to a cervical disc.

Intervertebral Disc Anatomy

Intervertebral discs lie between adjacent vertebrae, and these unique structures separate the vertebral bodies of the spine.

The disc is made up mainly of fibrocartilage, and there are 23 of these soft-tissue structures located within the human vertebral column. The disc has principally two layers—a soft inner layer known as the *nucleus pulposus* and a hard outer layer known as the *annulus fibrosus* (figure 3.1).

The inner layer of a disc, the nucleus pulposus, comprises a water-based gelatinous mass that has a direct attachment to the vertebral bodies located superiorly and inferiorly to the disc, via an area known as the *vertebral end plate* (figure 3.2). The nucleus pulposus contains

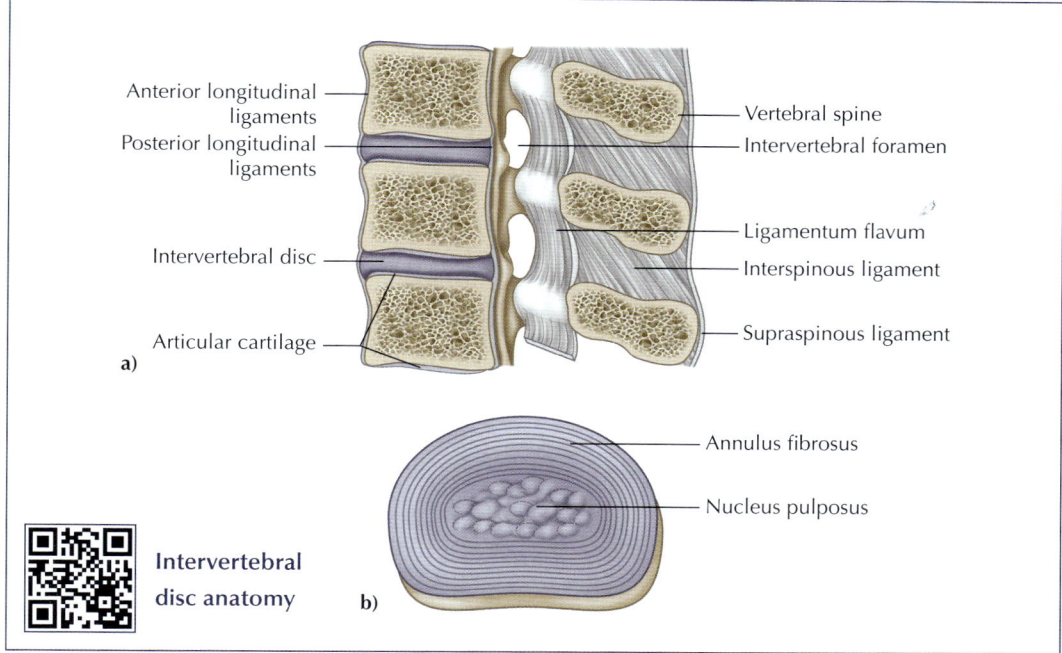

Intervertebral disc anatomy

Figure 3.1. (a) Sagittal section through the second to fourth lumbar vertebrae, (b) transverse section of a lumbar intervertebral disc.

mainly water, giving it the ability to act as a modified shock absorber every time the spinal column moves. Its water composition unfortunately decreases with age, which contributes to the progressive decrease in our height as we get older.

The outer layer of a disc consists of a tough fibrous shell known as the annulus fibrosus, and between this and the inner nucleus pulposus there are individual, ringlike fibrocartilaginous concentric layers called *lamellae*, which increase the disc's shock-absorption capability, plus allowing motion in certain planes owing to the opposing concentric rings. The lamellae assist in giving the annulus fibrosus its strength, as well as maintaining the water-based gelatinous fluid within the nucleus pulposus.

A healthy disc is very flexible; however, as we age the natural degenerative processes and other factors such as gravity and trauma will cause the disc to become compressed and hence stiffer, which makes it potentially more susceptible to injury. The nucleus at the center of the disc starts to lose its water content, a process that will naturally make the disc less elastic and less effective as a cushion or shock absorber. Furthermore, this cumulative and compressive force reduces the amount of much-needed nutrition and oxygen that can enter the disc. Nutrients are necessary for the disc to stay healthy; without an adequate supply, the disc will gradually degenerate.

Intervertebral discs are truly amazing structures, and like all living tissue, are made up of cells. A major component of the extracellular matrix of these cells, which is produced by the cells, is the protein aggrecan (a major proteoglycan). Proteoglycan aggrecans are like tiny sponges, able to carry approximately 500 times their own weight of water. Over time, these unique cells eventually die, and so less aggrecan is made, and the water content within the nucleus will reduce; this process will eventually lead to degenerative disc disease (DDD).

A disc is kept alive by its connection to the vertebral bodies through the vertebral end plates. Intervertebral discs have been likened to the parts of a tire: the inner nucleus is the air within the tire, the outer annulus is the tire's strong walls, and the tread of the tire forms the vertebral end plates. The discs are mainly avascular (lacking blood vessels) but are hydrated through diffusion from the vertebral bodies via the end plates (figure 3.2). The nerve supply derives mainly from the sinuvertebral nerves, which innervate the outer periphery of the intervertebral disc.

Nerve roots exit the spinal canal through small passageways—known as *intervertebral foramina* (sing. *foramen*)—between the vertebrae and the discs (figure 3.3). Pain and other symptoms can develop when the inner fluid from a damaged disc pushes into the spinal canal or nerve roots as they exit within the intervertebral foramina—a condition commonly referred to as a herniated intervertebral disc (HID) or a prolapsed intervertebral disc (PID).

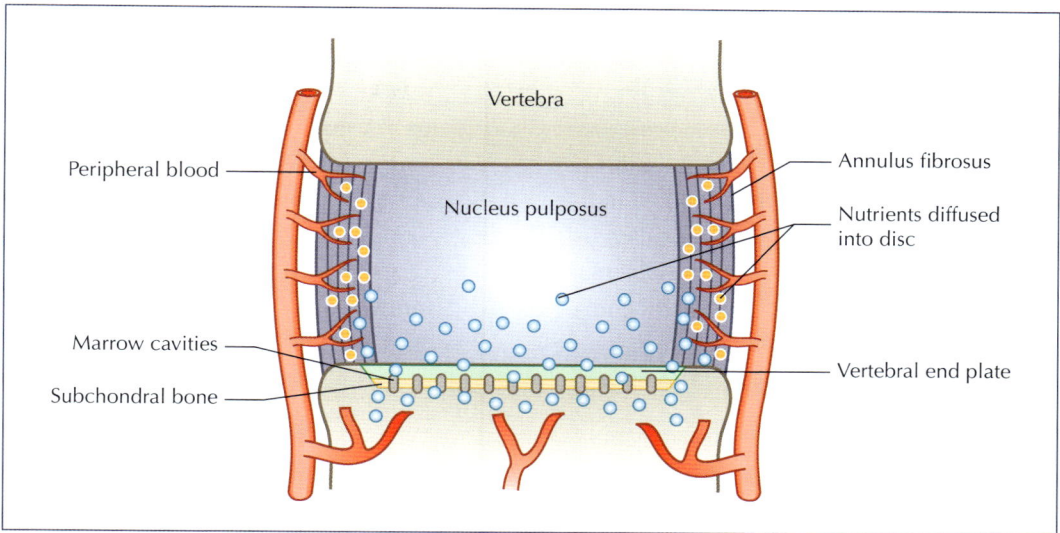

Figure 3.2. Nutrition to the intervertebral disc through the end plates.

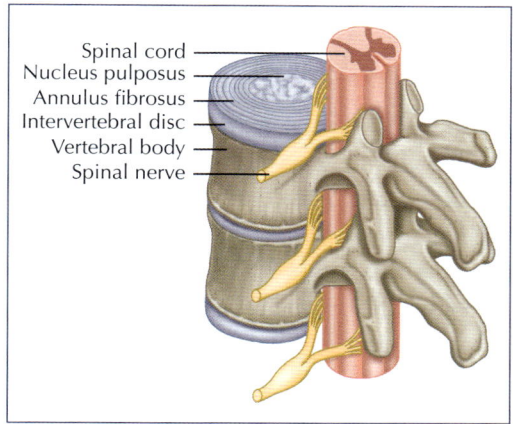

Figure 3.3. Lateral view of the lumbar spine, showing intervertebral disc and exiting spinal nerve roots.

Disc Herniation or Prolapse

One way of looking at any type of disc bulge is as a weakness in the outer covering of the shell (annulus fibrosus) that allows the soft contents inside (nucleus pulposus) to migrate outward and potentially toward the exiting spinal nerve roots. This is basically the first stage of DDD.

I regard a herniated or prolapsed disc as a natural progression from a bulge or a protrusion, where the annulus fibrosus has become weaker and can actually tear, allowing the nucleus pulposus to migrate even further toward the spinal nerves.

Some texts refer to herniated discs as bulging discs, protruding discs, prolapsed discs, or even slipped discs. These terms are derived from the action of the gel-like content of the nucleus pulposus being forced out of the center of the disc. To reiterate, the disc itself does not actually slip; however, the nucleus pulposus tissue located in the center of the disc can be placed under so much pressure that it causes the annulus fibrosus to herniate or even rupture (figure 3.4).

In a severe disc herniation the bulging tissue may press against one or more of the spinal nerves and/or the posterior longitudinal ligament, which can cause local and/or radicular pain, numbness, or weakness to the areas of the lower back,

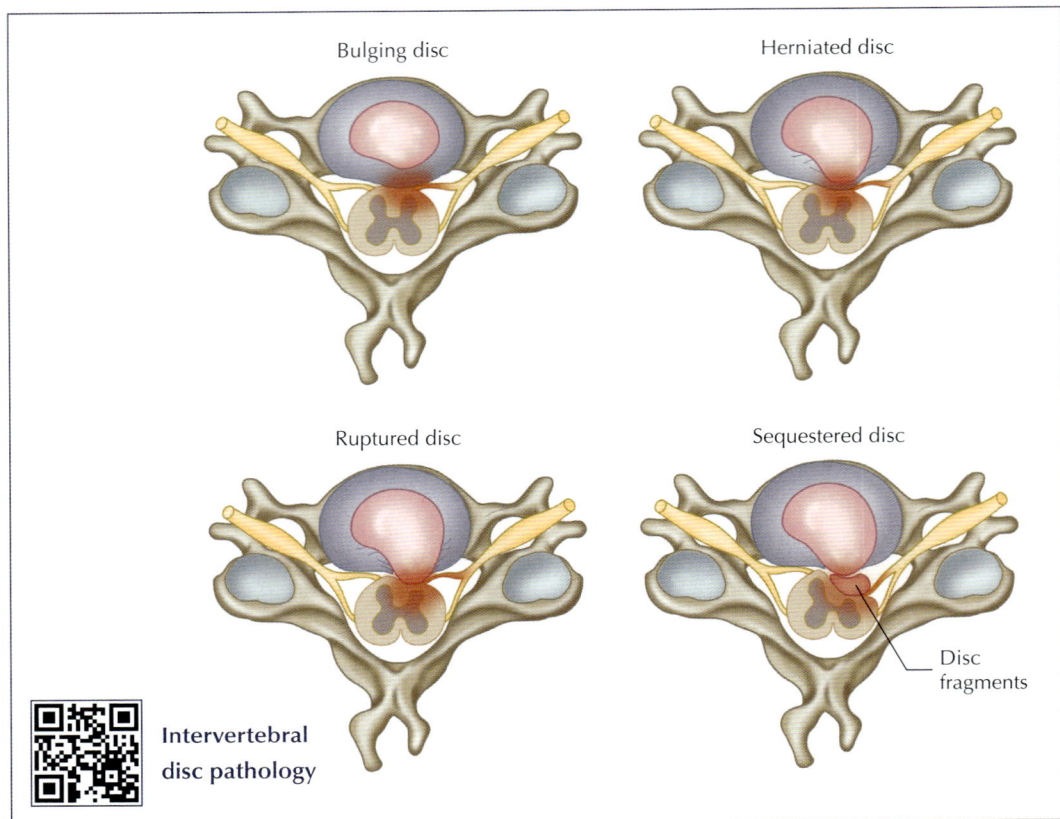

Figure 3.4. Various disc conditions and the contact with the nerve root.

buttocks, and lower limb if a lumbar disc is involved. If it is a cervical disc, the patient might perceive pain within the neck, shoulder, arm, and hand, as well as the fingers.

Discs and the Toothpaste Analogy

I like to think of a disc as a "tube of toothpaste" with the cap still tightly on. If you simply squeeze one end of the tube, the toothpaste (fluid) will migrate to the other end, and vice versa; the contents are still within the tube and there is no seepage, but you will notice a bulge at the end of the tube because you have squeezed the opposite end. Now, if you take the cap off the tube of toothpaste and squeeze the tube, the contents will obviously come out of the end.

Let us think about this concept a little bit more and relate it to the subject of this book and the nerves.

Imagine the toothpaste as the nucleus pulposus, and the outer toothpaste tube as the annulus fibrosus. Now, suppose the cap is on but almost coming off (if it takes five turns to lock the cap and five turns to lift it off, say for argument's sake that it is on two turns). If you squeeze the tube, you might notice the end bulging (as in a bulging disc). If you squeeze the tube hard enough, however, the toothpaste (fluid) might actually be seen to ooze out around the base of the cap; this might be likened to a protrusion. If the cap comes off altogether, this is what you would call a herniated or prolapsed disc, and if some of the toothpaste detaches itself, and is now separate from the rest, this would be referred to as a *sequestered disc* (see figure 3.4).

Typically, when a person starts to lift an object from the floor, due to the flexion position most of the pressure is applied to the anterior part of the disc. This will encourage the inner fluid of the nucleus pulposus to migrate posteriorly against the posterior aspect of the annulus fibrosus, which is thinner than the anterior part, and so is more susceptible to injury.

The majority of cervical spine disc herniations occur at the cervical segments C4–C5, C5–C6, or C6–C7. The nerve compression caused by the contact with the disc contents may result in perceived pain (radicular) along either the C5, C6, or C7 nerve root pathways (figure 3.5).

In the lumbar spine, the most common areas for disc herniations are lumbar segments L4–L5 and L5–S1— approximately 85%–95% will occur here. The nerve compression caused by the contact with the disc contents may result in perceived pain along the L4, L5, or S1 nerve root pathways (figure 3.6).

Note: The nerve involved is not the one emerging through the space associated with the prolapsing lumbar disc, but the next nerve down, known as the *traversing nerve*. This is because the nerve in that space emerges high in the intervertebral foramen and thus hits the nerve that is moving anteriorly to emerge through

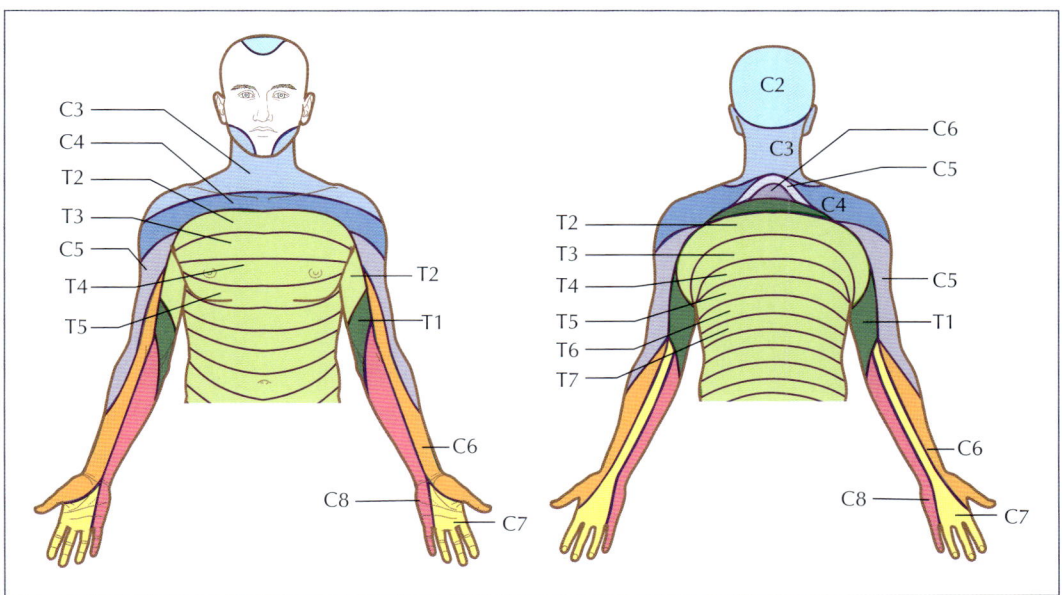

Figure 3.5. Dermatome pathways of the upper limb.

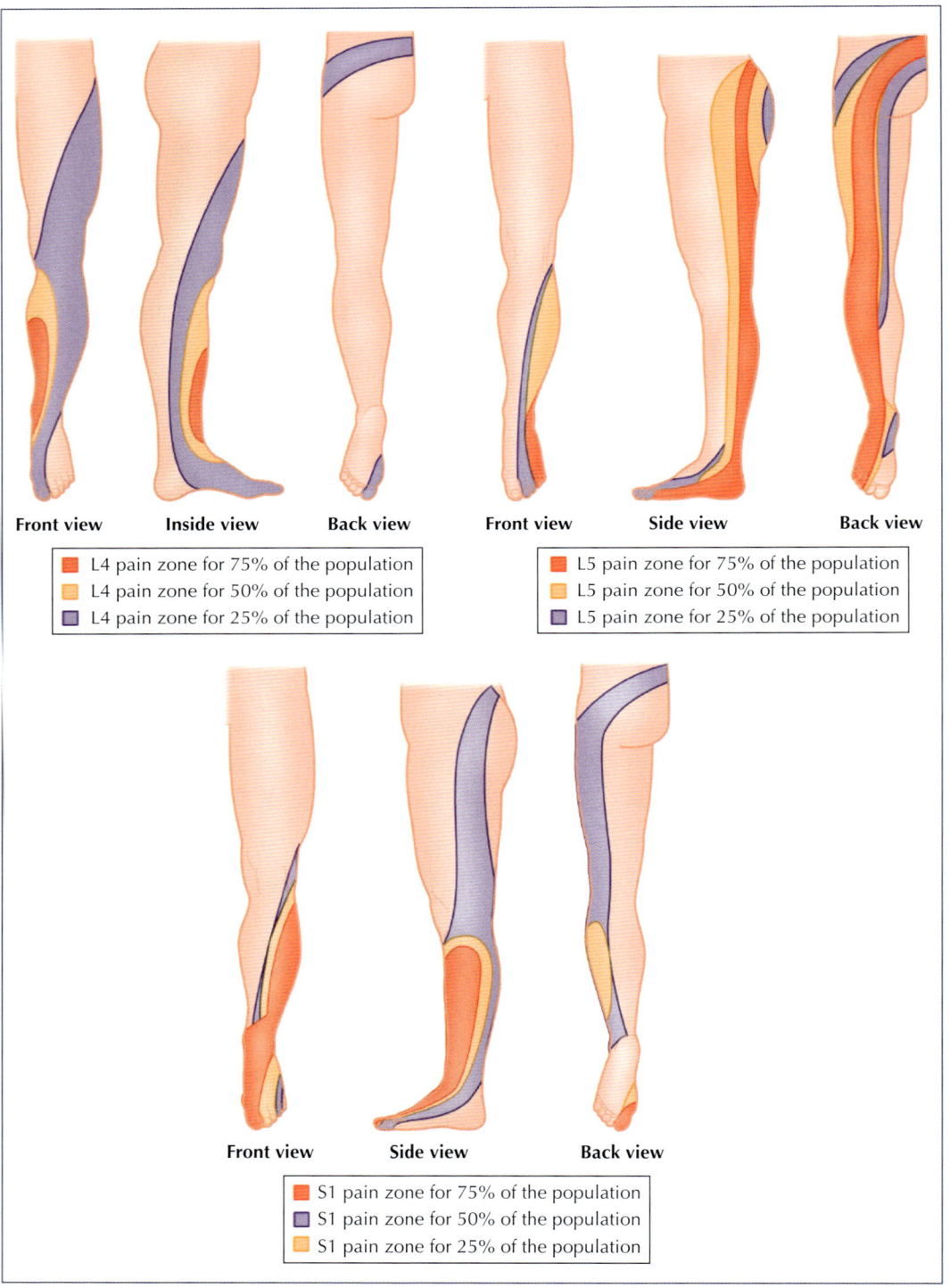

Figure 3.6. Dermatome pathways of pain for L4, L5, and S1 nerve roots.

the next space; therefore, the L4/5 disc will typically contact the *L5* nerve root rather than the L4 exiting nerve. The same applies in the case of the L5/S1 disc prolapse—this will typically contact the *S1* nerve root; although if the prolapse is severe enough it can contact the nerve roots of both L5 (exiting) and S1 (traversing).

In the cervical region, however, it is the actual nerve emerging through the intervertebral foramen that is contacted by the prolapse disc and *not* the one below; thus, a C4/5 prolapse (left or right) will contact *only* the exiting *C5* nerve root.

Central Disc Prolapse and Cauda Equina Syndrome

A large prolapsed disc within the cervical spine can contact the actual spinal cord and subsequently cause upper motor neuron symptoms. However, a central disc prolapse, located within the lumbar spine, can potentially contact the end component of the spinal cord, the *cauda equina*, so-called because it is formed of bundles of nerves and resembles the tail of a horse (figure 3.7).

This rare condition can cause a devastating neurological disorder called cauda equina syndrome (CES). If this is not diagnosed and treated in time, there can be serious consequences. Typically, the patient complains of urinary or rectal incontinence, with saddle anesthesia as well as bilateral leg pain and associated weakness. Patients might also mention lack of sensation

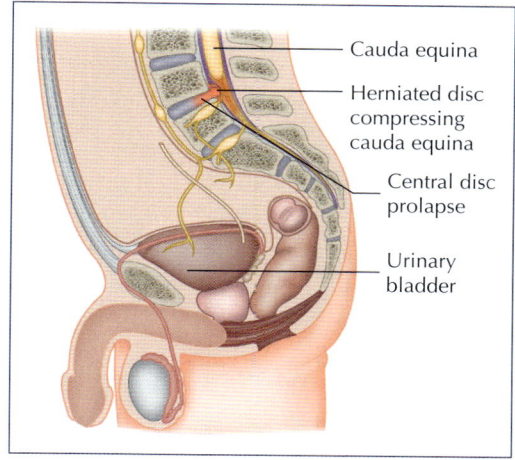

Figure 3.7. Central disc prolapse and cauda equina syndrome.

during sexual intercourse. Urgent surgery within 48 hours from the initial onset of symptoms is typically required to correct this serious medical condition.

Degenerative Disc Disease

Degenerative disc disease (DDD) tends to be linked to the aging process and is a syndrome in which a painful disc causes associated chronic lower back pain, which can radiate to the hip region (figure 3.8).

The condition is generally caused by some form of injury to the lower back and the associated structures, such as the intervertebral discs. A sustained injury can cause an inflammatory process and subsequent weakness of the outer shell of the disc (annulus fibrosus), which will then have a pronounced effect on the inner substance (nucleus pulposus). This reactive mechanism will create excessive movement, because the disc can no longer control the motion of

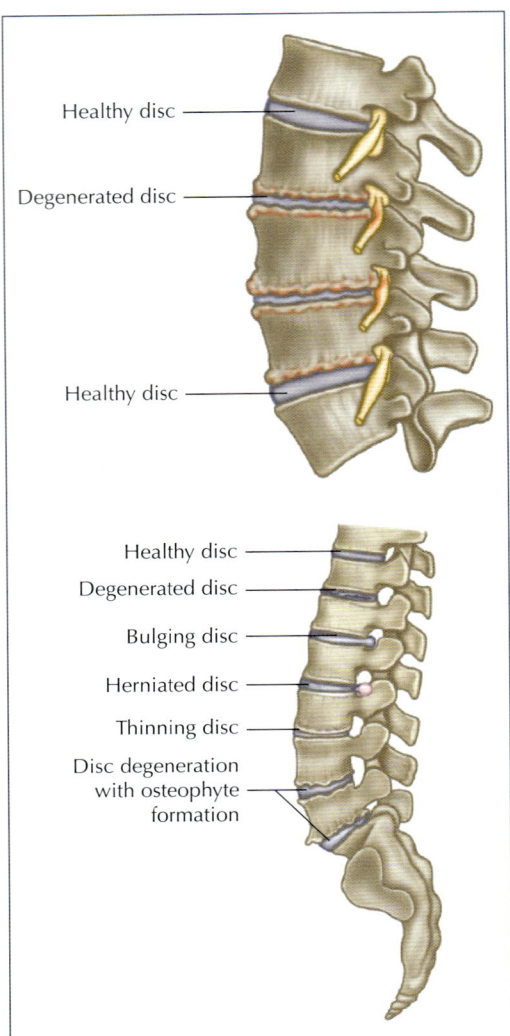

Healthy disc

Degenerated disc

Healthy disc

Healthy disc
Degenerated disc
Bulging disc
Herniated disc
Thinning disc
Disc degeneration
with osteophyte
formation

Figure 3.8. Degenerative disc disease (DDD).

the adjacent vertebral bodies, above and below. This excessive movement, combined with the natural inflammatory response, will produce chemicals that irritate the local area, which commonly produces symptoms of chronic lower back pain.

DDD has been shown to cause an increase in the number of clusters of chondrocytes

(cells that form the cartilaginous matrix, which consists mainly of collagen) in the annulus fibrosus (consisting of fibrocartilage). Over a prolonged period of time, the inner gelatinous nucleus pulposus can change to fibrocartilage, and it has been shown that the outer annulus fibrosus can become damaged in areas that allow some of the nucleus material to herniate through, causing the disc to shrink and eventually leading to the formation of bony spurs called *osteophytes.*

Unlike the muscles in the back, the discs of the lumbar spine do not have a natural blood supply and so cannot heal themselves. The painful symptoms of DDD can therefore become chronic, eventually leading to further problems, such as disc herniation, facet joint pain, nerve root compression, spondylolysis (defect of the pars interarticularis), and spinal stenosis (narrowing of the spinal canal).

Types of Pain

Shooting Pain

Another name for a shooting-type pain either in the arm or the leg is *radicular pain*. Sciatica is the most common type of radicular pain and tends to be sharp, bandlike, and electric in nature, and follows the nerve-root dermatome pattern. The mechanism of radicular pain is considered to originate from inflammation of the nerve root or compression of the dorsal root ganglion (DRG).

Radiculopathy Pain

Radiculopathy tends to coexist with radicular pain. Radiculopathy, however, is classified as either a neurological loss of sensation or a change in sensation; typically, these present as numbness and tingling and/or motor loss, where the patient will demonstrate loss of strength/weakness of the associated muscles and reduced reflexes.

Radiculopathy is generally caused by the compression of nerve roots. By far the most common cause of both types of radicular symptom are conditions mainly caused by spinal disc herniation. Pain can also result from hypertrophy of the spinal facet joints, osteophytes, and spinal stenosis.

Referred Pain

Referred pain is pain that is perceived in an area of the body distant from the site of its cause. For example, in a heart attack (myocardial infarction), the pain is often felt by patients not only in the central chest area (origin) but also at distant (referred) sites such as the jaw, back, arm, and hand.

Axial Pain

Typically, axial pain is thought of as "mechanical" in nature and tends to be local to the actual source. This type of pain can be dull and aching but may have a referred component to it as well.

For example, the lumbar facet joints can give local back pain, especially during particular movements such as exercises. However, the facets can also refer pain to the buttock and leg, so it is not always that easy to localize the source.

Another example of axial pain is if a patient has axial neck or axial lower back pain. In these cases, the pain is generally caused by a structural component within the neck or lower back and is also perceived by the patient in those areas.

Where is the Patient's Pain?

Let us take the cervical spine as an example of a potential location of your patient's presenting symptoms. It is important to try to ascertain the cause, because if the patient says that their pain is localized within the neck region, then it is probably going to be axial neck pain. If, on the other hand, the patient mentions that it is difficult to locate the pain, because it seems more widespread than just local to the neck—and is duller and achier in nature—then it is probably referred pain.

However, if the patient says that the pain is sharper, stabbing, and bandlike, then it is likely to be radicular pain.

To clarify—if radicular symptoms are suspected from the cervical spine at the level of the C5 nerve root, typically the patient will perceive altered sensations in the area of the lateral shoulder and lateral antecubital fossa. C6 nerve root radicular symptoms are most often associated with the first digit (thumb) and forearm, and those of the C7 nerve root with the third digit (middle finger). The C8 nerve root affects the fifth digit (little finger), and the T1 nerve root presents radicular symptoms in the region of the medial antecubital fossa.

My Own Case Study—Lumbar Spine

I have always been particularly stiff and inflexible, especially in my lower back and hips, and I can recall being this way as far back as my memory allows. I could never touch my toes, and when I joined the British Army at 16 years old, I remember failing the flexibility tests.

The problem started in 2008 and went on for more than three months. Being an osteopath who suffered from lumbar spine and leg pain was not a very good marketing strategy for business. I had decided to modify the fishpond in my garden, and after five hours of shifting huge quantities of earth and rock, my lower back felt very stiff. The next morning when I woke up, I felt like an old man, unable to move very well in bed because of the pain and stiffness in my lower back region. I eventually (very slowly) made my way to the medicine cabinet and took some anti-inflammatory medication as well as some painkillers. The pain slowly subsided and I was able to go through my daily routine.

A few days later, I started to feel some numbness in the lateral side of my left tibia, but also perceived a particularly sharp pain in my left quadriceps and tensor fasciae latae (TFL) muscle. This progressively worsened over a few days, to the point that I could not sleep on my back in a comfortable position, and walking to the shop was unbearable owing to the pain in my left anterior thigh.

I thought I had an L4/5-disc bulge that was pressing on my exiting L4 nerve. I also thought the bulge must be large enough to compress the L5 descending (traversing) nerve as well, mainly because of the dermatome distribution in my lateral tibia. What was strange with me, though, was that my anterior thigh pain on a dermatome map was located somewhere between the L2 and L3 nerves, and there was no medial tibia pain (L4). So, I was a bit confused, given that I also had excruciating pain in my left TFL, as well as groin pain on my left side. My overall conclusion was that my psoas must be involved, as the lumbar plexus penetrates the psoas muscle and could cause this muscle to produce a kind of protective spasm with a resultant referral pattern.

My deep tendon reflex of L4 was reduced to less than a 1+ (and still is, many years later). The muscle strength (myotome) of the left quadriceps muscles (knee extension) when tested was weaker, as was the strength of the left tibialis anterior muscle (ankle dorsiflexion). This confirmed to me that the problem was indeed a neurological one, and I thought it had manifested because of a disc bulge.

Strangely enough, I found that sitting was the most comfortable position for me. However, the pain resulted in 58 consecutive disturbed nights, trying to sleep on the floor with my legs on the sofa (psoas position), which was the only position that provided me with some pain relief, albeit for a few hours at a time, before I would sit again.

One week after an MRI self-referral, it was confirmed that I had an L4/5 bulging disc that was just in contact with the L4 nerve root. I consulted a neurosurgeon colleague, and almost immediately asked him to operate on me, which I thought was my only option. However, he said that he would prefer to wait, and that often the pain will subside; moreover, as my disc bulge was laterally placed, he would have to remove a facet joint to get to the bulge. The effect of this over time would be to make me less flexible, and to potentially cause ongoing back pain. His advice was to avoid bending for nine months and let things settle down on their own.

After the prescription of codeine, diclofenac, tramadol, and anything else I could try, I decided that medication was not the answer for me: none of the prescribed pills really seemed to help my symptoms.

So, what did I do? Well, having researched the most effective way of treating disc pain, I bought an inversion table. I used this table twice daily, and this helped to reduce my symptoms, on the basis that pain arises from a bulge that may be as little as 0.04 inches (1 mm) in the wrong direction. If the disc happens to be bulging away from the ligaments and nerves, there is either a reduction

in pain or no pain at all. However, a bulge 1 mm in the other direction results in considerable pain, and that is how it was with me: one day would be slightly better and another would be particularly painful.

Three months later, 22 pounds (10 kg) lighter and very depressed, I started to improve, albeit very slowly, but things were nevertheless moving in the right direction.

At least I could run again and had resumed training, although somewhat modified. Even today, I avoid lifting heavy objects and training with very heavy weights, and especially steer clear of movements such as deadlifts, and so on. I am acutely aware that if the disc moves just 1 mm in the wrong direction, I will feel it, but in particular it will remind me of the 58 nights lying on my back on the floor, with my legs over the sofa … not a good place to be!

Prognosis, Treatment, and Conclusion

As an osteopath, I have treated numerous patients with back pain, and I have referred a small number of them for an MRI scan, because I considered these particular patients to have suffered some form of disc condition. I have referred to the neurosurgeon for a second opinion approximately 10%–20% of the patients I see with a disc condition that is confirmed by the MRI. The neurosurgeon will then decide what the best options are for the patient; in reality, most patients

I refer to the surgeon will eventually have spinal surgery.

It is very difficult to say what is the best *conservative treatment* or even what is the best *management* of a disc bulge, because everybody will react slightly differently. My neurosurgeon friend's advice was to simply "not bend down for nine months and wait to see what nature will do." For me, as for others, that is very simple advice, and with the help of the inversion table, it actually helped reduce the presenting symptoms.

My Own Case Study—Cervical Spine

As part of an off-road motorbike group, I was following an elite rider who was riding pretty fast through some narrow forest trails. I was following at pace and didn't see him duck under a tree because I was focusing on the muddy terrain directly in front of me. In a split second I glanced upward and a tree branch caught my helmet visor, almost decapitating me as my cervical spine has never traveled that far into extension before. Somehow, I managed to stay upright on the bike; however, I almost passed out as I felt immediate pain to the base of my neck around the C7/T1 area with a sudden onset of strange tingling symptoms to my left arm and even to my left leg.

At the time, I seriously thought I had done some major damage, as I was frantically testing the power in my arms—groups of muscles supplied by a single spinal nerve root, known as *myotomes*—and I even

tested the dorsi- and plantar flexion of my ankles. I knew it was an L4/5 and S1 myotome, and remarkably they all seemed fine.

After a few minutes of panicking, I continued riding even though I didn't feel normal. That evening, I had some symptoms to my left anterior thigh as well as to the lateral side of my shin and some tingling to both hands (mainly around the little fingers, so a C8 dermatome). For the leg symptoms, I felt I might have *stretched* the spinal cord, especially where I had the L4/5 issue back in 2008, and I felt the impact had exacerbated that previous disc pathology.

The tingling type of symptoms in both hands fluctuated to C6, C7, and C8 dermatomes and stayed for many weeks, so I had an MRI scan as I wanted to ascertain the integrity of the spinal cord as well as to assess any further damage. The MRI mainly diagnosed two severe nerve root compressions caused by disc osteophyte complex—one at C6/7 affecting the C7 nerve root and mainly on the left, and also a bilateral nerve root compression at C7/8 affecting the C8 nerve root on both sides.

I had a consultation with the neurosurgeon, who did all the standard tests of reflexes, myotomes, and dermatomes. Each was relatively negative, so she said I wasn't a surgical case unless I develop weakness and pain, which I don't currently have. Her recommendation as gold standard would be an anterior cervical discectomy—essentially a removal of the disc—which in my case would be for two levels: C6/7 and C7/C8.

Her main advice was not to crash if I was to continue riding off-road, which is a natural hazard when you ride through wet and muddy terrain. So I bought a neck brace, and I wear it now for every ride, and this has helped to reduce the trauma to the neck because I have fallen many times since the accident.

In terms of conservative treatment, I have had some soft-tissue, mobilization, and manipulative techniques performed on me by various practitioners, and no doubt the treatment has helped. I have also bought a couple of cervical spine traction devices, which I use often, and these too relieve some of the ongoing symptoms.

Spinal Mobilization versus Manipulation and Contraindications

Joint manipulation has always been a part of medicine, with evidence of manual techniques being used in Thailand and Egypt as early as 2000 BC. During the 1800s, practitioners within the US and parts of Europe known as "bonesetters" developed what we know today as *joint manipulation techniques*.

Osteopathy and chiropractic originated in the early twentieth century, and the techniques used by these two professions have a similarity to those of the original bonesetters.

Osteopaths and chiropractors work on many conditions of the human body, and chiropractic philosophy maintained that the cause of the disease was a vertebral dysfunction that affected the exiting spinal nerve, and would focus their strategies and treatment protocols on purely spinal manipulation. Osteopaths can utilize and perform similar spinal manipulative techniques to the ones chiropractors use; however, in the US, for example, osteopaths have the same training as medical physicians with the added bonus of training in spinal manipulation, and are known as osteopathic physicians.

Many practitioners believe that any underlying vertebral dysfunction will have an effect on neural, vascular, and lymphatic connections, and they consider that correcting these dysfunctions through the use of spinal manipulative techniques will help restore homeostasis to the body.

When I studied osteopathy many years ago, it was mentioned to me many times by my tutors that "structure affects function" and "function affects structure." This means, quite simply, that if you have a *structural* abnormality within the vertebral column, potentially it might affect the *function* of anything that relates to that particular spinal segment—for example, the exiting spinal nerve.

Let's discuss the two common terms that physical therapists use often when they treat patients: *mobilization* and *manipulation*.

Mobilization and Manipulation

Definitions

Joint *mobilization* is defined as a slow, passive motion to encourage a separation of the articular surfaces of the joint planes.

Joint *manipulation* is defined as a quick thrusting motion of the articular joint capsule that subsequently moves the two surfaces in relation to one another and commonly causes an audible cavitation noise.

Chest of Drawer's Analogy

When I try to discuss the difference between the two techniques of mobilization and manipulation, I use an analogy that relates to the opening a chest of drawers.

Imagine one morning you go to get a pair of socks from the top drawer; as you pull the drawer back to expose the contents, it becomes stuck. At this point, you have two choices: a mobilization choice and a manipulative choice. It seems the natural option is to push the drawer back in, and then try to pull it out, and if it gets stuck for the second time then you will try again, and again, and so on until the drawer is *released*. Simply, a *push away* motion, then a *pull toward* motion … and then repeat …

This is a similar concept to a mobilization technique. If it is a gentle motion, then we can call it a *grade 1* mobilization; if it's not working particularly well and the drawer still feels a bit restricted, we can use more of an effort and call it a *grade 2*;

and so on, until a *grade 4* mobilization technique is achieved. However, if you wanted to continue and perform a *grade 5* technique, this is not strictly classified as a mobilization anymore but is now graded as a manipulation.

Osteopaths like myself don't generally tend to use grades per se, because they are mostly used within the realms of physiotherapy and physical therapy. What is known in physiotherapy and physical therapy terminology as a grade 5 manipulation, the osteopathic profession refers to as a *high velocity thrust* (HVT). Another term is *high velocity with low amplitude* (HVLA).

Let me return to the analogy of the chest of drawers and relate it now to a manipulative technique. At the end point where the drawer gets stuck, you will feel a *bind* or a point of resistance. If you want to perform a manipulation, then it will be executed at the *point of bind* (explained later), and instead of *pushing* the drawer back in you will now *pull* the drawer with a quick *thrusting* type of motion, with the distance of the pull being very small (the LA part of HVLA—low amplitude). Why? If you happen to pull the drawer too far, it will come out and fall to the floor. If you don't use a thrusting motion and rely on your strength to just pull the drawer, then the whole chest of drawers will start to move and tilt toward you, and the items on top of it will start to fall off.

I use this analogy a lot to explain the motion of a spinal manipulation. When you initiate a set-up to the specific level of the vertebra of your patient that you believe requires the manipulative technique, you would achieve this by specific positioning of the vertebra to the point of bind by potentially using something called *coupled motion* (see chapter 6 for further clarification). From this position of bind, the manipulative technique (HVT) is executed, and typically a cavitation is felt by the patient and subsequently heard by both parties.

This is where the ability of the practitioner comes in, because they need to be highly competent in what they are doing, as well as confident, to even try to perform these skilled maneuvers. It is not an easy skill to learn or even to be precise on your location for the set-up. However, like most skills, it is worth persisting, and with thousands of hours of practice it will eventually pay off.

Teaching Manipulative Techniques

I have probably performed spinal and joint manipulative techniques more than 150,000 times, and these manipulations have been focused to the area of the patient's vertebrae, pelvis, and even the peripheral joints, and for *each* person, the technique will be slightly different. This is difficult to explain to a group of students for the first time who want to learn everything in a very short space of time. I will mention to them that I personally have a tendency to modify the technique in a very subtle way for each and every patient—for someone watching it might look the same, but no two techniques I demonstrate and perform are ever *exactly* the same …

Before the pandemic, I would lecture to over 100 students a month and would

encounter all types and skill sets of physical therapists. Some would ask me if I would personally watch them demonstrate a spinal manipulation technique, because they had attended previous manipulative courses, and would I give my opinion on how I thought they performed the technique. I would wait a few moments before saying anything, as I watched exactly how the therapist was going through all the necessary procedures to set up the patient before they performed the actual manipulation. When the therapist was just about to manipulate, I would always ask, "What level of the spine are you planning to manipulate?" and "Why have you decided to manipulate this specific area?"

Once I had asked those two questions, I generally tended to get blank expressions, and eventually after repeating the questions I might get some explanation, but 90% of the time I got a response like "Mmm … not sure what exact level," or "I was shown just to set up like this and then just to go for it and hopefully it will get a noise from the joint," or "Got no idea, I'm just going for a crack" …

These responses are frustrating. Although the therapist has the best intentions for their patient, I believe that what they are doing is unsafe and can eventually cause damage to the underlying tissues. The therapist needs to understand *how* to assess the spinal column, at *what level* they are manipulating, and *why* they are doing it in the first place!

Mobilization and manipulative techniques for the spine, thorax, and pelvis are commonly performed for the treatment of pain and dysfunction, and the purpose of this textbook is to introduce qualified and experienced manual therapists' techniques to manipulate the pelvis and lumbar, thoracic, and cervical spine. The techniques that will be demonstrated throughout are very safe and effective if they are performed correctly.

Proficiency in their use requires training and practice on a continual basis. The term *manipulation* is often used to describe a range of physical therapy techniques. The techniques that will be demonstrated are a high velocity thrust (HVT) to achieve a joint cavitation that is accompanied by the cracking sound.

So, What Exactly is the Noise from the Cavitation/Manipulation?

I always get asked that question, and typically, before I answer, I click my thumb and say "That noise?" and then the person asking the question says, "Yes, that noise … that click – what is it?"

There are a few theories, but I believe that the noise of the cavitation from a spinal facet joint (*zygapophyseal joints* is the proper name for facet joints) is the release of a mixture of gases (oxygen, carbon dioxide, and nitrogen) that escapes through the synovial membrane lining the joint. The synovial fluid, which lubricates the joint, undergoes a rapid change in pressure, causing gas bubbles to form within the fluid and then collapse, or "pop." The noise typically happens when a force type of motion, like a thrust in HVLA, stretches the joint capsule, which causes the gases to quickly release,

producing the audible noise that you and the patient will hear.

This phenomenon can happen in various joints throughout the skeletal system, and is not specific to the spinal column.

Please note that the noise you hear is not an indicator of ligaments snapping or bones cracking together or even intervertebral discs going back in to position after they have slipped out of place. It is basically a normal procedure and a harmless occurrence, which as mentioned is associated with changes in joint pressure and gas bubble dynamics. A lot of patients experience instant relief of their symptoms after hearing the noise, although the therapeutic benefits of spinal manipulation on their spinal column extend way beyond just the audible sound you hear.

What Are the Benefits of Spinal Treatments?

Increasing Joint Range

Any type of joint mobilization or manipulative technique can promote pain-free movement, and can improve the range of motion of any articular surfaces that have become restricted, especially if the adhesion is within the joint capsule. When a joint has become immobilized, and this can happen for many reasons, a few changes occur, as the intracellular water content is reduced within the facet joint capsule owing to the lack of mobility. There is an increase in the cross-linking of localized fibers because of the lack of motion, which causes an increase in collagen tissue and fibro-fatty connective tissue proliferation, leading to the formation of scar tissue and subsequent adhesions. These changes to the joint perpetuate the joint restriction. Joint manipulation has been shown to reverse these changes by breaking adhesions within the joint capsule and breaking the intracapsular fibro-fatty adhesions.

Any form of inflammation will initiate the activation of the inflammatory mediators, and this over time can produce a hypertrophic thickening of the synovial membrane of the joint, resulting in fibrosis of the joint lining. Naturally, joint immobility will go hand in hand with inflammation. Specific joint treatments have been demonstrated to be effective at treating joint hypomobility due to inflammation.

Joint treatments of mobilization and manipulations will not only focus on the joint capsule, but will also have an effect on all of the surrounding tissues, including, muscles, tendons, ligaments, and the fascia.

Correcting Position

A word that is used often, especially within the chiropractic profession, to describe a vertebral positional fault is *subluxation*, meaning that the vertebra, for some reason, has been displaced and is now in a misaligned position. Within osteopathy we might call the vertebral position a *somatic* dysfunction, or simply a *positional* fault. However, to take it a stage further, I discuss in chapter 6 whether

the vertebral facet joint is fixed closed in a position of extension, combined with rotation and side bending, or if the facet joint is fixed in an open flexed position, combined with rotation and side bending (this will make more sense when you read that chapter). If either of these is the case, then the spinal techniques that will be demonstrated later will encourage the facet joints either to open (if fixed closed) or to close (if fixed open).

Spinal manipulation techniques (if chosen) are naturally more forceful, and one might even use the word *aggressive*, as you will need enough of a force to produce a change of position to the alignment of the two joint surfaces you are focusing the treatment on.

Promoting Adequate Nutrition

Maintaining the health of any synovial, freely movable joint within the skeletal framework relies generally on joint motion. Movements that occur through general activities will allow the synovial membrane to secrete synovial fluid into the joint cavity, and the fluid will circulate within the joint space. This lubricating fluid provides all the necessary nutrients to sustain and promote a healthy and functional joint, and will lubricate the articular joint surfaces. If a joint has become restricted for some reason (frozen shoulder, for example), then the nutrients available to the joint will be limited, because the lack of motion inhibits the secretion of synovial fluid. This condition is termed *adhesive capsulitis*, and can last for well over 12–18 months.

Pain Modulation

Pain modulation typically refers to the complex processes by which the body alters its perception of pain. This can happen at various levels within the nervous system, including the spinal cord, brainstem, and brain. There are multiple mechanisms involved in pain modulation, each playing a role in either enhancing or dampening pain signals.

Inflammatory mediators released at the site of injury (e.g., prostaglandins, bradykinin) can increase the sensitivity of nociceptors (pain receptors). The brain can send inhibitory signals down the spinal cord to suppress pain transmission. Neurotransmitters like serotonin and norepinephrine play key roles in this process. The brainstem releases natural pain-relieving chemicals like endorphins, enkephalins, and dynorphins, which bind to opioid receptors and inhibit pain transmission.

There are many factors that can influence pain modulation, and high levels of stress and anxiety can amplify pain perception by increasing the excitability of pain pathways. Hormones like adrenaline and cortisol modulate pain sensitivity, and these can increase pain during stressful periods. Medications like nonsteroidal anti-inflammatory drugs (NSAIDs) and opioids modulate pain by acting on various regions in the pain pathway, and local anesthetics provide pain relief as they assist in blocking pain signals at the site of injury.

One thing I often tell my students is that *swelling causes pressure, and pressure subsequently causes pain*, because it irritates the nociceptors (pain receptors) within the tissues. Naturally, if one can reduce the swelling—through whatever methods available—then the pain will eventually start to subside.

I personally believe that the mobilization and manipulation maneuvers I use—including soft-tissue techniques such as muscle energy techniques (METs)—will have a major effect on reducing the patient's painful symptoms. Heat can help relieve pain by increasing blood flow, reducing muscle tension, and improving flexibility. I discussed above how mobility promotes production of synovial fluid within the joint, and this will generate heat within the tissues. Soft-tissue massage techniques also stimulate a warming effect within the tissues by contracting and relaxing the muscles through METs—and again will have a major effect on reducing pain—as well as mobilization and manipulation. This overall reduction of pain will transmit to the soft tissues associated with the joint and subsequently cause the muscles to relax.

When I discuss general mobility exercises and the effect they have on joints, I compare the synovial fluid to engine oil: if the vehicle is cold, then most of the oil is located within the sump of the engine and is relatively thick. Once you start the vehicle, the oil starts to circulate around the engine to keep it lubricated and prevent it from breaking down.

The consistency of the oil changes too—it becomes warmer and less viscous through the motion of the moving parts of the engine.

Remember: *all* types of mobilization and manipulation techniques will have a direct effect on the two joint surfaces and help to promote and increase the secretion of the synovial fluid within the joint you are focusing your treatment on.

Grading Scale of Mobilizations

Below is a grading scale that can be used by physical therapists for the different grading of mobilizations (table 4.1).

Grades 1–4 will be classified as mobilization techniques, whereas a grade 5 will be classified as a manipulative technique.

Contraindications and Precautions

There are obvious risks with any type of manipulative spinal technique, especially HVT, but most published literature shows that injuries resulting from manipulative techniques are mostly from cervical spine manipulation, so you should be relatively safe when you treat the thoracic spine and ribs. However, there are some techniques discussed and demonstrated for the base of the cervical spine, known as the cervicothoracic (CT) junction, and one must be careful *not* to use the cervical spine as a *thrust lever* when performing these techniques.

Safety First

Before any treatment is carried out, we have to consider if there are any

Table 4.1. Grading of Mobilizations.

Grade	Action
1	Slow, small-amplitude oscillatory movement parallel to the concave joint surface in early range of movement
2	Large-amplitude, rhythmic oscillating mobilization in midrange of movement
3	Large-amplitude, rhythmic oscillating mobilization to point of limitation in range of movement
4	Small-amplitude, rhythmic oscillating mobilization at end of available range of motion
5 (thrust manipulation)*	Small amplitude, with a quick thrust at the end of the available end range of available motion

*"Thrust" is not intended to imply that specific chiropractic technique. Practices differ by region, and while "thrust" might be acceptable outside of the US, it has specific regulatory implications in the US.

contraindications present that might make treatment more likely to cause an injury or make the underlying problem worse.

We can classify contraindications as *absolute* (neurological, vascular, or bone), where you should *never* include any spinal manipulative techniques, and *relative*, where you might consider treatment would be beneficial to the patient, although you may, for example, avoid treating an area of the body where they have pathology; however, it would be valid to use some form of physical therapy treatment in other areas.

The distinction between absolute and relative is also influenced by factors such as the skill, experience, and training of the practitioner; the type of technique selected; the amount of leverage and force used; and the age, general health, and even the physique of the patient.

Absolute—Neurological

- Spinal cord compression or cauda equina syndrome: If an individual presents signs of spinal cord compression (such as muscle weakness or numbness) or cauda equina syndrome (a specific compression of the lower spinal cord nerve roots), spinal manipulation is contraindicated, and a medical referral is immediately required.
- Neurological symptoms
- Nerve root compression

Absolute—Vascular

- Aortic aneurysm
- Vertebrobasilar insufficiency
- Vertebral artery dissection: Spinal manipulation has rare but potential risks related to vertebral artery dissection—a spontaneous tear in the wall of the artery. Spinal manipulation is contraindicated in individuals with a history of vertebral artery dissection or those at higher risk.

Absolute—Bone

- Certain types of cancer: Spinal manipulation is contraindicated for patients with certain types of cancer, such as metastatic cancer of the spine. A healthcare professional should assess the individual's situation.
- Bone or joint infections: Active or suspected bone or joint infections in the spine require prompt medical treatment and should be managed by a healthcare professional.
- Tumors
- Metabolic bone disease
- Inflammatory joint diseases such as rheumatoid or psoriatic arthritis
- Severe osteoporosis: Individuals with severe osteoporosis may have weakened bones that can fracture or break more easily. Spinal manipulation could increase the risk of fractures.

Relative

- Reaction to previous treatment
- Disc herniation

- Pregnancy
- Facet joint pathology
- Spondylosis
- Spondylolysis
- Spondylolisthesis
- Ankylosing spondylitis
- Spinal stenosis
- Scheuermann kyphosis
- Scoliosis
- Early-stage osteoporosis
- Hypermobility or ligamentous laxity
- Arterial calcification
- Recent fractures or dislocations

It is important to remember that these lists are not exhaustive, and individual circumstances will influence the decision of whether to treat and when to refer to another professional.

General Considerations

- **Patient positioning:** Ensure that the patient is comfortable and positioned correctly before initiating any mobilization techniques. Proper positioning helps promote relaxation and prevents unnecessary strain on the body.
- **Communication:** Effective communication with the patient is vital throughout the procedure. Explain the technique, expected sensations, and any potential discomfort they might experience. Encourage them to provide feedback and inform you if anything feels unusual or painful.
- **Patient suitability:** Assess the patient's overall health, medical history, and any specific conditions or injuries they

may have. Certain conditions such as osteoporosis, arthritis, or spinal fractures may require modifications to the mobilization technique or be absolute contraindications.

- **Technique selection:** Select the appropriate technique based on the patient's needs and condition. Consider factors such as joint mobility, stability, and any existing pathologies. Use gentle and controlled movements during mobilization to minimize the risk of injury.
- **Gradual progression:** Start with low-force mobilization techniques and progress cautiously, considering the patient's response. Gradually increase the intensity and range of motion based on the patient's tolerance and comfort. Be mindful of any signs of adverse reactions, such as increased pain or neurological symptoms.
- **Rest periods:** Allow adequate rest periods between any type of spinal mobilization techniques to prevent overstimulation or excessive stress on the spine. This helps the body adapt and minimizes the risk of exacerbating any existing conditions.
- **Monitoring response:** Continuously monitor the patient's response to mobilization. Watch for signs of discomfort, adverse reactions, or changes in neurological status. If any concerns arise, modify or discontinue the technique accordingly, and seek appropriate medical advice.
- **Proper training:** Perform spinal mobilization techniques only if you have received proper training and have the necessary insurance and certification. It is essential to have

a thorough understanding of the functional anatomy, biomechanics, and indications/contraindications specific to any spinal mobilization and manipulative techniques prior to administering them to your patients.

Most of the techniques within this book are very safe to perform in your own clinic. If you are unsure of which technique (depending on your skill level and qualifications) is best applied to your patient, I would follow the soft-tissue muscle energy techniques (METs) approach initially, because generally these techniques will cause no harm but are very effective at correcting any malalignment presentations, especially when used properly.

However, there will come a time when you feel that a thrust technique (HVT) is needed, so you have a choice: either you can train in the appropriate field of manual therapy—for example, osteopathy or chiropractic—or it might be easier (in my opinion) to simply refer your patient to a suitably qualified practitioner who is skilled in the art of spinal manipulation.

Note: The techniques demonstrated in this book are mainly mobilizations using METs that are classified as soft-tissue techniques. However, since I am an osteopath and have trained in spinal manipulation, the word "thrust" or the words "high-velocity thrust" (or HVT) will be mentioned from time to time. These advanced techniques should be incorporated into the treatment plan only if one has the necessary training and qualifications to perform them.

Gait Cycle and its Relationship to the Vertebral Column

Whenever I assess patients who present with pelvic, lumbar spine, or hip pain, or a combination of all three, I would always include within my assessment the passive range of motion (PROM) of the associated joints that relate to the lower limb (including the hallux, or great toe, and ankle), working cephalic toward the knee, and then finally the hip joint—and this is prior to assessing the pelvis and lumbar spine. In my clinical experience, I typically find some dysfunctional motion or restriction somewhere within this initial assessment that I believe might be the missing piece of the puzzle as to why the patient is suffering this chronic pain.

For example, I always ask my patients if their previous therapist ever assessed their lower limb joints, including the hip, even though they have been diagnosed with piriformis syndrome or sacroiliac joint dysfunction, because they might consider these areas of the body irrelevant to what they are presenting with now. I find that most patients have not had any previous therapist assess either their hip or lower limb joints, only to discover on examination findings such hallux rigidus (restricted motion of the great toe into extension), hallux valgus, or even gout, a meniscal tear of the knee restricting full extension or full flexion of the knee joint, degenerative changes (osteoarthritis) of the hip joint, or even other pathologies of the hip like an acetabular labral tear or a cam lesion (part of a condition known as a femoral-acetabular impingement [FAI]). Any of the conditions mentioned here will cause a structural and functional compensation throughout the kinetic chain, and this, I believe, is very likely why the patient is presenting with chronic pelvic or back pain. These conditions will need to be addressed initially through physical therapy rather than merely treating where the symptoms are. Remember the famous quote by Doctor Ida Rolf that I adapt for my students: "Where the pain is, the problem is not."

I like to call practitioners "therapy detectives," looking for *clues* as to why the patient is presenting with their symptoms, and it is important to address

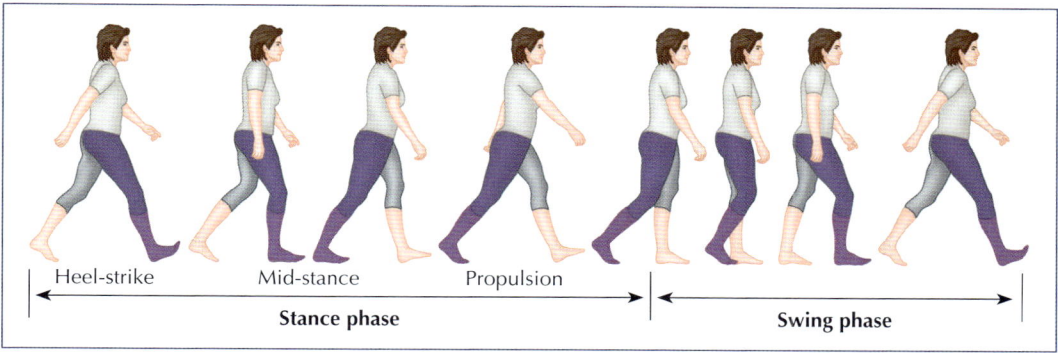

Heel-strike Mid-stance Propulsion

Stance phase **Swing phase**

Figure 5.1. Stance and swing phases of the gait cycle.

the cause and not treat just the symptoms. A hip pathology—such as a labral tear, as mentioned above—might be the reason why the patient is presenting with piriformis syndrome or sacroiliac joint dysfunction.

What I would like to do in this chapter is examine in detail what exactly takes place when we walk (you might want to go through some of the movements yourself as they are described) and the relationship of the gait cycle to the pelvic girdle and of course the vertebral column.

Gait Cycle

Definition: A *gait cycle* is a sequence of events in walking or running, beginning when one foot contacts the ground and ending when the same foot contacts the ground again.

The gait cycle is divided into two main phases: the *stance* phase and the *swing* phase. Each cycle begins at initial contact (also known as *heel-strike*)

of the leading leg in a stance phase, proceeds through a swing phase, and ends with the next contact of the ground with that same leg. The stance phase is subdivided into *heel-strike*, *mid-stance*, and *propulsion* phases.

Human gait is a very complicated, coordinated series of movements. An easier way of thinking about the gait cycle is to break it down into phases. The stance phase is the weight-bearing component of each cycle; it is initiated by heel-strike and ends with toe-off from the same foot. The swing phase is initiated with toe-off and ends with heel-strike. It has been estimated that the stance phase accounts for approximately 60% of a single gait cycle, and the swing phase for approximately 40% (figure 5.1).

Heel-Strike

If you think about the position of your body just before you contact the ground with your right leg during the contact phase of the stance phase, the right hip is in a position of flexion, the knee is

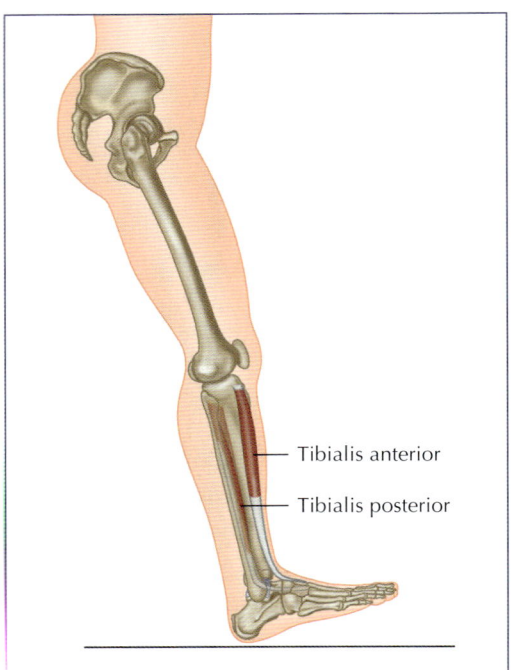

Figure 5.2. The position of the leg just before heel-strike.

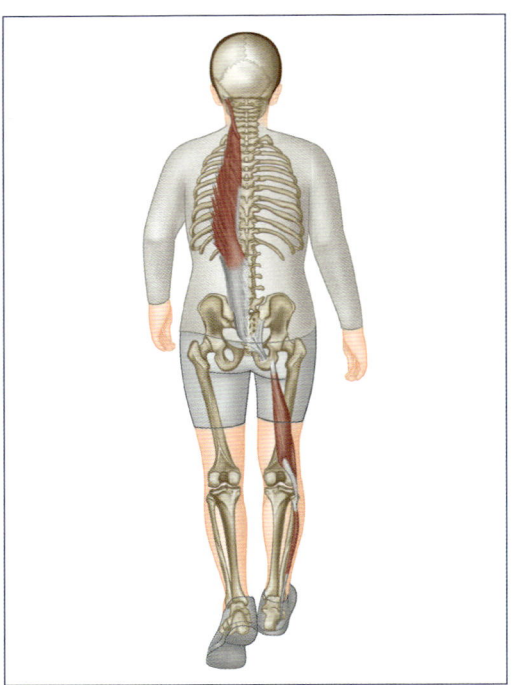

Figure 5.3. A person walking, with the posterior (deep) longitudinal sling muscles highlighted.

extended, the ankle is dorsiflexed, and the foot is in a position of supination (figure 5.2). The tibialis anterior muscle, with the help of the tibialis posterior, works to maintain the ankle/foot in a position of dorsiflexion and inversion (inversion is one part of the motion referred to as *supination*).

In normal gait, the foot strikes the ground at the beginning of the heel-strike in a supinated position of approximately 2 degrees. A normal foot will then move through 5–6 degrees of pronation at the subtalar joint (STJ) to a position of approximately 3–4 degrees of pronation, as this will allow the foot to function as a "mobile adaptor."

Myofascial Link

As a result of the ankle and foot being in a position of dorsiflexion and supination, the tibialis anterior (which is the main muscle responsible for this anatomical position, with an insertion on the medial cuneiform and first metatarsal on the foot) is now part of a link system that we will call a *myofascial sling*. This sling—the posterior longitudinal (PLS) or deep longitudinal sling (DLS), (figure 5.3)—starting from the initial origin of the tibialis anterior, continues as the insertion of the fibularis longus (onto the first metatarsal and medial cuneiform, as in the case of the tibialis anterior) to its muscular origin on the lateral side and head of the fibula. This bony landmark is also where the biceps femoris muscle inserts.

The sling now continues as the biceps femoris muscle toward its origin on the ischial tuberosity, where the muscle attaches to the tuberosity via the sacrotuberous ligament; often the biceps femoris directly attaches to this ligament rather than to the ischial tuberosity, and some authors have mentioned that potentially 30% or more of the biceps femoris attaches directly to the ILA of the sacrum. Vleeming et al. (1989a) found that in 50% of subjects, part of the sacrotuberous ligament was continuous with the tendon of the long head of the biceps femoris.

The sling continues its journey as the sacrotuberous ligament, which attaches to the inferior aspect of the sacrum at the ILA and fascially connects to the contralateral (opposite side) multifidi and to the erector spinae, which continue to the base of the occipital bone.

Even before you initiate the contact to the ground through heel-strike, dorsiflexion of the ankle (by the contraction of the tibialis anterior) initiates a coactivation of the biceps femoris and fibularis longus just prior to heel-strike. Studies have shown that the biceps femoris communicates with the fibularis longus at the fibular head, transmitting approximately 18% of the contraction force of the biceps femoris through the fascial system into the fibularis longus muscle. This co-contraction therefore serves to "wind up" the thoracolumbar fascia mechanism as a means of stabilizing the lower extremity; this results in the storage of the necessary kinetic energy that will subsequently be released during the propulsive phase of the gait cycle.

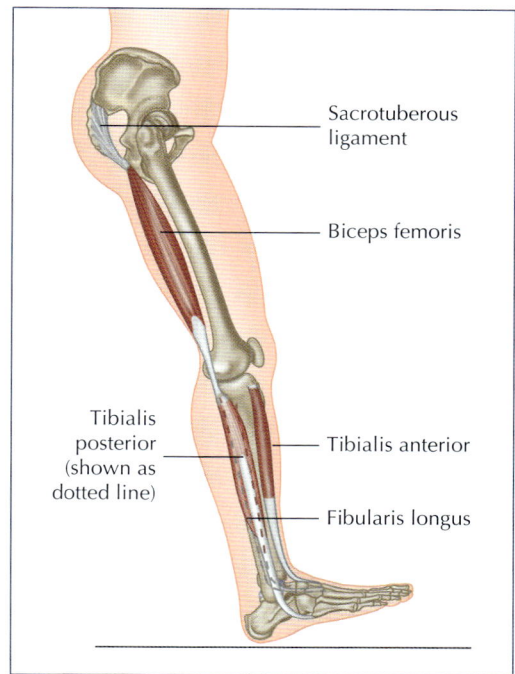

Figure 5.4 Position of the leg just before heel-strike, with the biceps femoris and sacrotuberous ligament tensioned.

The posterior (deep) longitudinal sling as described is being fascially tensioned; the increased tension is focused on the sacrotuberous ligament via the attachment of the biceps femoris (figure 5.4).

This connection will assist the *force closure* mechanism process of the SIJ (figure 5.5); in simple terms, this creates a self-locking and stable pelvis for the initiation of the weight-bearing gait cycle. You may also notice that the right ilium (figure 5.6(a–b)) undergoes posterior rotation during the swing phase, which will assist the force closure of the SIJ because of the increased tension in the sacrotuberous ligament.

You can also see from figure 5.6(b), that there is now tension developing within

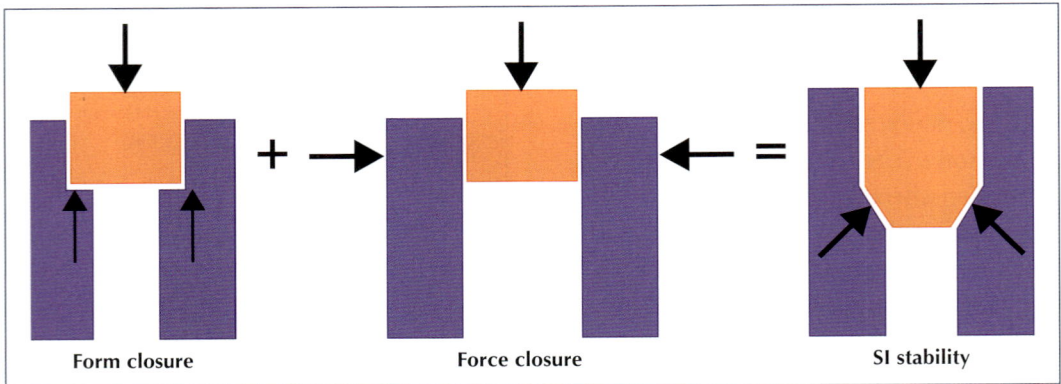

Figure 5.5. The relationship between form/force closure and sacroiliac stability.

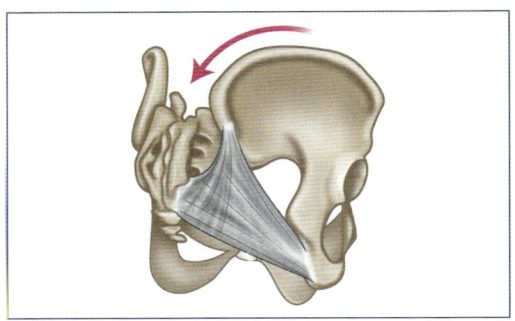

Figure 5.6. (a) Right ilium in posterior rotation—sacrotuberous ligament tensioned.

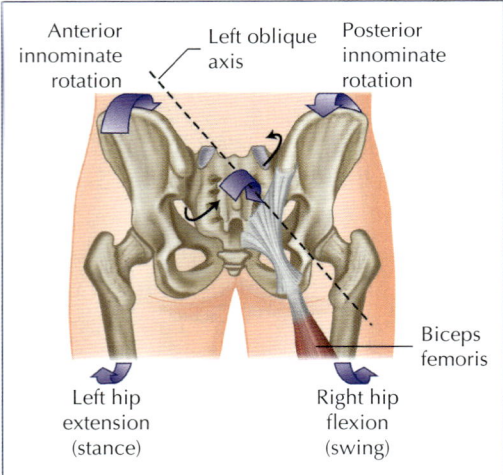

Figure 5.6. (b) Right ilium in posterior rotation—left ilium in anterior rotation and sacrum rotated on the L-on-L axis.

the right sacrotuberous ligament because of the contraction of the biceps femoris as well as the posterior rotation of the right innominate; at the same time, the left innominate is rotating anteriorly and the sacrum has rotated on the left oblique axis (L-on-L). This specific motion of the lumbopelvic hip complex occurs all at the same time as the right heel-strike.

For the next phase, you might want to stand and slowly go through the following movements so that you can get a sense of what happens with your body in the normal walking cycle. As explained above, just before the heel-strike phase your hip will be flexed, your knee extended, and your ankle dorsiflexed with the foot supinated. The tibialis anterior and tibialis posterior maintain this position of the ankle and foot, and as you contact the ground, these two muscles are responsible for controlling the rate of pronation through the STJ by contracting eccentrically.

As your right leg moves from heel-strike to toe-off (stance phase), your body weight begins to move over your right leg, causing your pelvis to shift laterally to the right.

As the movement continues toward heel-lift and toe-off, your right pelvic innominate bone begins to rotate anteriorly while your left innominate bone begins to rotate posteriorly.

As you proceed through the gait cycle, you now enter the mid-stance phase of gait. This is where the hamstrings should reduce their tension because of the natural anterior rotation of the pelvis and the slackening of the sacrotuberous ligament. Form closure at this point is gradually lost during the latter part of the stance phase, so that stability at this point is chiefly maintained through force closure. This is the point during the mid-stance phase where the Gmax on the right side should take the role of the continued movement of lower limb extension, as well as working in concert with the contralateral latissimus dorsi (left side). The active contraction of these two muscles increases the tension in the thoracolumbar fascia (posterior oblique sling), thus providing the necessary force closure stability to the right SIJ during the mid-stance phase of gait.

I would like to elaborate a little more on this process. Contraction of the Gmax occurs in the mid-stance phase; the Gmax simultaneously contracts with the contralateral latissimus dorsi—it is this muscle that will extend the arm through what is known as *counter-rotation*, to assist in propulsion. The thoracolumbar fascia, which is a sheet of connective tissue, is located between the Gmax and the contralateral latissimus dorsi; this fascial structure is forced to increase its tension because of the contractions of the Gmax and latissimus dorsi. This increased tension will assist in stabilizing the SIJ

of the stance leg through the force closure mechanism.

In figure 5.7 you can see that just before heel-strike, the Gmax will reach maximum stretch as the latissimus dorsi is being stretched by the forward swing of the opposite arm. Heel-strike signifies a transition to the propulsive phase of gait, at which time the Gmax contraction is superimposed on that of the hamstrings.

As explained in the previous paragraphs, activation of the Gmax occurs in concert with contraction of the contralateral latissimus dorsi, which is now extending the arm in unison with the propelling leg. The synergistic contraction of the Gmax and the contralateral latissimus dorsi creates a state of tension within the thoracolumbar fascia, which will be released in a surge

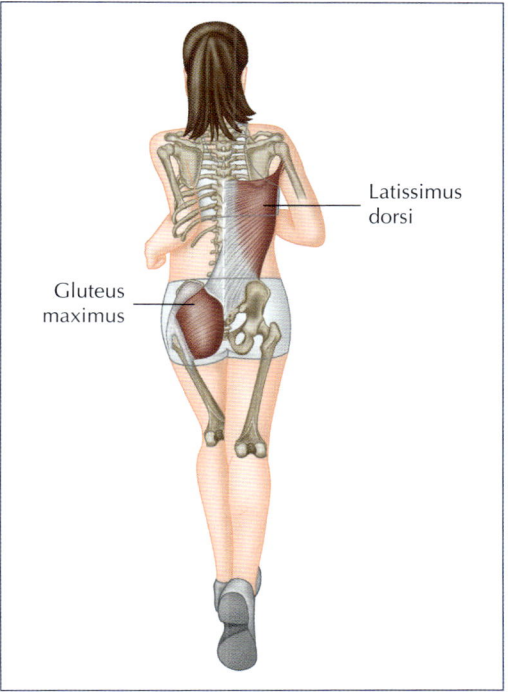

Figure 5.7. A person running, with the posterior oblique sling muscles highlighted.

of energy that will assist the muscles of locomotion. This stored energy within the thoracolumbar fascia helps to reduce the overall energy expenditure of the gait cycle. Janda (1992, 1996) mentions that poor Gmax strength and activation is postulated to decrease the efficiency of gait. The posterior oblique sling also contains a lower component (consisting of the continuations of the Gmax), which acts to increase the tension of the iliotibial tract (ITT); this helps to stabilize the knee during the stance phase of gait.

As we progress from the mid-stance phase to heel-lift, toe-off, and subsequent propulsion, the foot begins to re-supinate and passes through a neutral position when the propulsive phase begins; the foot continues in supination through toe-off. As a result of the foot supinating during the mid-stance propulsive period, the foot is converted from a "mobile adaptor" (which is what it is during the contact period) to a "rigid lever" as the mid-tarsal joint locks into a supinated position. With the foot functioning as a rigid lever (as a result of the locked mid-tarsal joint) during the time immediately preceding toe-off, the weight of the body is propelled more efficiently.

Pelvis, SIJ, and Lumbar Spine Motion

Next we will take a look at the pelvis and how it functions during the mid-stance phase of the walking cycle. As the right innominate bone starts to rotate anteriorly from an initial posteriorly rotated position, the tension of the right sacrotuberous ligament is reduced, and the sacrum will

be forced to move (passively) into a right torsion on the right oblique axis (R-on-R). In other words, the sacrum rotates to the right and side bends to the left, because the left sacral base moves into an anterior nutation position (this is also known as *Type I spinal mechanics*, as the rotation and side bending are coupled to opposite sides—see Chapter 6; the motion is illustrated in Figure 5.8(a).

We also need to mention and consider that, as the left side of the sacrum moves forward into nutation, the right side of the sacral base will move backward into counter-nutation *(R-on-R)*; this is mainly because of the slackening of the right sacrotuberous ligament and the continual anterior rotational movement of the right innominate bone during mid-stance.

Owing to the kinematics of the sacrum, the lumbar spine rotates left (opposite to the sacrum) and side bends to the right (Type I mechanics), as shown is

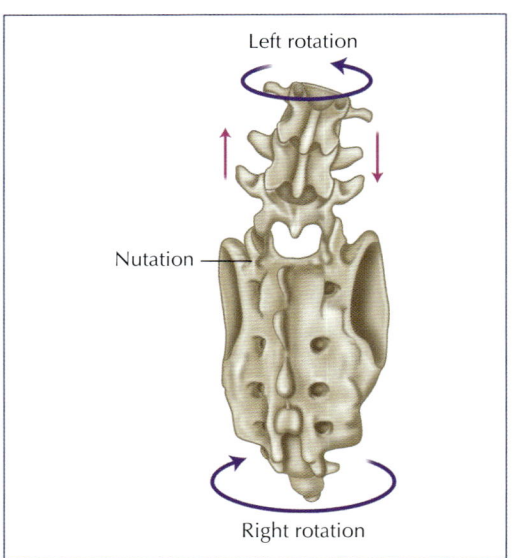

Figure 5.8. (a) Sacral rotation and lumbar counter-rotation.

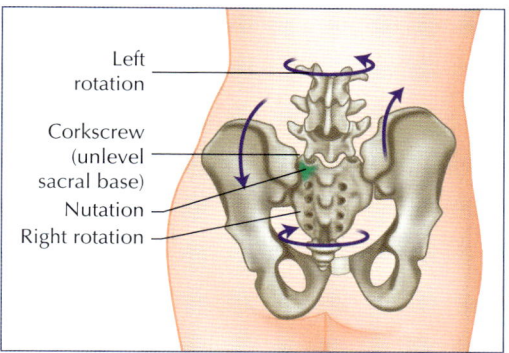

Figure 5.8. (b) Sacral rotation and lumbar counter-rotation superimposed on the pelvic girdle.

Figure 5.8(b). The thoracic spine rotates right (same as the sacrum) and side bends to the left, and the cervical spine rotates right and side bends to the right. The cervical spine coupling is opposite to that of the other vertebrae, since its specific spinal motion is classified as *Type II spinal mechanics* (Type II means that rotation and side bending are coupled to the same side—see Chapter 6 for more details).

The anterior oblique also works in conjunction with the stance leg adductors, ipsilateral internal oblique, and contralateral external oblique muscles (figure 5.9). These integrated muscle contractions help stabilize the body on top of the stance leg and assist in rotating the pelvis forward for optimum propulsion in preparation for the ensuing heel-strike.

The abdominal oblique muscles, as well as the adductor muscle group, serve to provide stability and mobility during the gait cycle.

When looking at the EMG recordings of the obliques during gait and

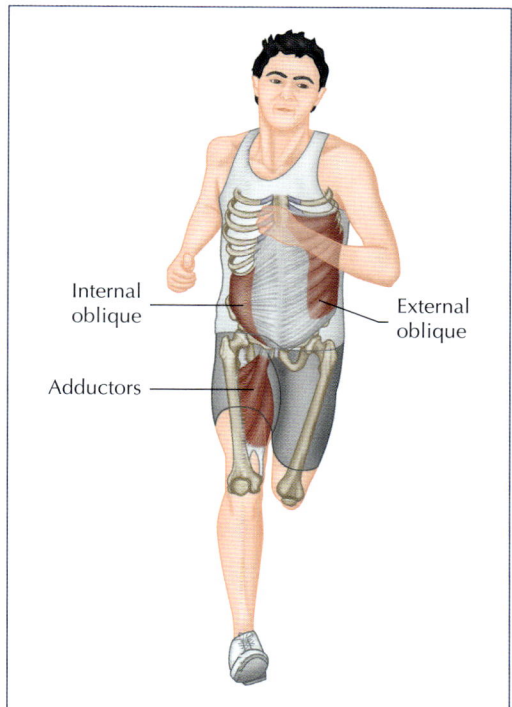

Figure 5.9. A person running, with anterior oblique sling muscles highlighted.

superimposing them on the cycle of adductor activity in gait, Basmajan and De Luca (1979) found that both sets of muscles (obliques and adductors) contribute to stability at the initiation of the stance phase of the gait cycle, as well as to the rotation of the pelvis and the action of pulling the leg through during the swing phase of gait. (This was also demonstrated by Inman et al. (1981).) As the speed of walking increases to running and sprinting speeds, the activation of the anterior oblique system becomes more prominent as well as a necessity.

The swing phase of gait utilizes the lateral sling system, as we have now entered the single-leg stance position (figure 5.10). This sling connects the Gmed and Gmin

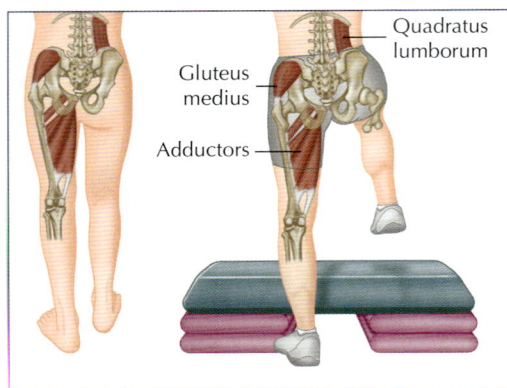

Figure 5.10. An example of the swing phase of gait, with lateral sling muscles highlighted on the single-stance leg.

of the stance leg, and the ipsilateral (same side) adductors, with the contralateral (opposite) QL. Contraction of the left Gmed and adductors stabilizes the pelvis, and activation of the contralateral QL will assist in elevation of the pelvis; this will allow enough lift of the pelvis to permit the leg to go through the swing phase of gait. The lateral sling plays a critical role, as it assists in stabilizing the spine and hip joints in the frontal plane and is a necessary contributor to the overall stability of the pelvis and trunk.

Not only does the lateral sling system provide stability that protects the working spinal and hip joints, but it is also a necessary contributor to the overall stability of the pelvis and trunk. Should the trunk become unstable, the diminished stability will compromise one's ability to generate the forces necessary for moving the swing leg quickly, as required in many work and sports environments. Attempts to move the swing leg, or to generate force with the stance leg during gait and other functional activities, can easily disrupt the

SIJs and symphysis pubis and cause kinetic dysfunction in joints throughout the entire kinetic chain (Chek 1999).

Maitland (2001) mentions that proper body movement while walking is influenced by the ability of the sacrum to cope with left torsion on the left oblique axis (L-on-L) and right torsion on the right oblique axis (R-on-R). Since most walking is accomplished with the vertebral column relatively upright and vertical, for the purpose of this discussion we will assume that your spine and sacrum are in neutral while you walk.

The way our axial skeletal system alternately undulates in side bending and rotation as we walk is very interesting and extremely important to our overall well-being. It is a movement that is reminiscent of the undulating action of a snake as it slithers through the grass. The big difference between a snake and a human, of course, is that our snakelike spine has ended up being given two legs on which to walk.

Summary of the Sacrum and the Gait Cycle

To summarize the gait cycle and the specific motion of the sacral spine, the sacrum is capable of left rotation on the left oblique axis (L-on-L), from which it then returns to a neutral position. From this neutral position the sacrum then rotates to the right on the right oblique axis (R-on-R) and again returns to neutral. The movement of the sacrum is *anterior* in its nature as it undergoes the earlier-described motion of nutation. The forward nutational movement during walking is anterior on one side, followed by a return to the neutral position; anterior nutation then occurs on the opposite side, before the sacrum again returns to neutral. This process is continually repeated. According to various studies, the motion of posterior nutation (counter-nutation) does not appear to extend past the neutral position during the normal walking/gait cycle.

You might not see the relevance of discussing the gait cycle and its relationship to the kinetic chain of the spinal column; however, I consider the human ability to perform the gait cycle on a day-to-day basis to be of significant relevance, as our role as healthcare practitioners is to provide treatment, advice, and even guidance to our patients,

to address their various health concerns, alleviate symptoms, manage medical conditions, and promote recovery. The ultimate goal of treating patients is to help them feel better, recover from illnesses or injuries, and maintain or improve their overall quality of life.

Recall my first paragraph in this chapter, where I discussed the importance of screening for PROM of the lower limb, and especially to include the hip joint. This is prior to assessing and treating the area of the patient's presenting pain, because the missing piece of the puzzle might be located within the intricacies of the gait cycle. If you don't look at the patient's movement patterns, you will be treating only their symptoms, meaning that in theory, the patient—in terms of what they are presenting with—might not actually improve … ever!

Biomechanics of the Vertebral Column

This chapter, in my opinion, is one of the most important because it focuses on the biomechanics of the spinal column, an important and invaluable topic if you want to understand the motion of the spine fully. If you are a practitioner assessing and treating patients that present with any type of spinal pain or pathology with or without symptoms, a good understanding of the specific biomechanics is essential.

Spinal Mechanics: Fact or Fiction?

A medical doctor by the name of Robert Lovett was the first person (I believe) to confirm coupled spinal motions, other than the standard primary motion of flexion and extension (Lovett 1903). He believed that side bending and rotation of the spine are parts of one compound movement and cannot be dissociated: he found that a flexible rod bent in one plane could not bend in another plane without twisting. In all his experiments Lovett proved that if the spine was in a position of lordosis, it rotated in the

opposite direction to that of the side bending motion; moreover, if the spine was in a position of kyphosis, it rotated in the *same* direction as that of the side bending motion.

He considered that only three spinal movements were possible within the vertebral column: (1) flexion; (2) extension; and (3) side bending with rotation. He also concluded that side bending, or lateral flexion, must accompany spinal rotation (i.e. the motions are coupled).

Lovett proposed that coupled motion occurs in a second plane of motion within a joint system, and is part and parcel of the primary motion. Two or more motions are considered "coupled" when it is not possible to produce one motion without inducing the second; spinal coupling occurs because of the morphological shape of the facet joint surfaces and the connecting ligaments and spinal curvatures.

In the early 1900s the osteopath Harrison M. Fryette contributed some pioneering work on the mechanics of spinal motion. He spent many years of his life researching this topic and eventually presented a paper in 1918 on the principles of spinal motion, which was sent to the American Osteopathic Association (Fryette 1918).

Regarding the motion of the spine, Stoddard (1962) states the following in his manual on osteopathic technique:

"Rotation of the spine is always accompanied by some degree of lateral flexion. Likewise, lateral flexion of the spine is accompanied by some degree of vertebral rotation."

How All This Came About

Fryette utilized and established correlations with a lot of the earlier work conducted by Lovett in 1903. The research methodology consisted of cadaveric study and in vivo research via the application of gummed paper stickers. These bits of sticky paper were attached to the spinous processes of the vertebrae of a small number of individuals; the results were then obtained by observing the relative spinal motion of these gummed paper stickers.

Research into spinal mechanics has progressed considerably over the last 50–100 years, from the simple observatory techniques of Fryette employing sticky paper to the use of advanced technology such as computer simulation, computerized tomography (CT scan), magnetic resonance imaging (MRI scan), and cineradiology (viewing an organ in motion with a special movie camera). We can even detect motion of

the spine and pelvis by implanting gallium balls and Steinman pins.

If we were able to look into the future, it would be very interesting to see what actually changes in terms of research and technology. It goes without saying, especially as time passes, that the more we are able to visualize and research living spinal motion, the more complex and unpredictable the precise combination of individual spinal joint motion becomes for each particular area and segment of the vertebral column.

I have read numerous articles and many books by various authors over the last few years while researching the subject of spinal motion, before eventually deciding to write this particular book on spinal manipulation and mobilization techniques. However, rather than having what we call definitive "laws of spinal motion" or "principles of spinal motion," there are substantial individual and regional variations, and, as yet, no true accurate model for predicting the behavior of the vertebral column as regards specific motion.

Koushik physio (2011) says in his website blog:

"The work of Fryette must be applauded for its longevity and insight, and celebrated as part of our osteopathic heritage and history, but the "laws" can no longer be viewed as such, nor do they serve as a viable explanation of physiological motion behavior. With all this uncertainty why do some of us still persist in promoting a model for physiological motion based on work conducted over 100 years ago?"

Gracovetsky's "Spinal Engine Theory"

Serge Gracovetsky (1988) elaborated on a particular idea of spinal motion, which he discussed in his book *The Spinal Engine*. He considered the spine to be the "primary engine" in the role of locomotion and proposed that the legs were not responsible for gait, but were merely "instruments of expression" and extensions of the spinal engine. He argued that the spine was not a rigid lever during the gait cycle and that its ability to produce axial compression and torsion was a fundamental driving force during locomotion.

In his discussions, Gracovetsky says that during heel-strike, kinetic energy is not displaced into the earth as in the pedestrian model, but efficiently transmitted up through the myofascial system, causing the spine to resonate in the gravitational field. He did not view the spine as a compressive loading system, whereby the intervertebral discs act as shock absorbers; he regarded the outer anulus fibrosus disc fibers and their accompanying facet joints as dynamic antigravity torsional springs that store and unload tensional forces to lift and propel the body in space. He also considered that the natural process of interlocking of the facet joints and intervertebral discs transmitted virtually all of the available counter-rotational pelvic torque that is needed to aid the inner and outer core muscles for locomotion.

A quote from Gracovetsky:

"The spine is an engine driving the pelvis. Human anatomy is a consequence of function. The knee cannot be tested in isolation, as it is part of the overall function and purpose of the musculoskeletal system. The leg transfers the heel-strike energy to the spine. It is a mechanical filter. The knee is a critical part of that filter and improper energy transfer will affect spinal motion. Functional assessment of the spine ought to be part of the assessment of knee surgery."

Let's think back to the earlier concept of Lovett: it is this lumbar lateral flexion/rotation coupling that serves as the Gracovetsky spinal engine "drivetrain." For example, left lateral lumbar flexion will drive right rotation of the lumbar spine, and subsequently the SIJ and pelvis.

What I would like to do now is to briefly mention the gait cycle (figure 6.1), and

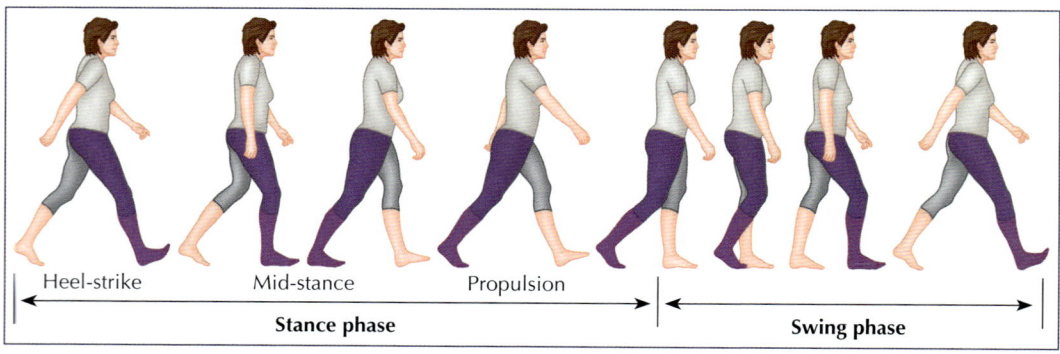

Heel-strike   Mid-stance   Propulsion

Stance phase   **Swing phase**

Figure 6.1. The gait cycle.

the interaction of spinal motion, and look at this concept in a slightly different way. Some authors have considered that the biceps femoris muscle of the hamstring group, along with its connection to the posterior (deep) longitudinal sling (figure 6.2), effectively starts the spinal engine. The biceps femoris has been likened to the *pull cord* of the spinal engine in view of its action of inducing a "force closure" mechanism in the SIJ. This closure of the SIJ will naturally lead to a subsequent transmission of force up into the osteo-articular-ligamentous tissues of the lumbosacral spine; this force will eventually continue into the muscles of the lumbar erector spinae.

EMG studies have demonstrated that the biceps femoris muscle is particularly active at the end of the swing phase of gait, through the early loading of the stance phase. During the transition from swing to stance, the heel contact phase of the gait cycle effectively closes the kinetic chain, and the biceps femoris can now perform its work in a manner that is commonly called a *closed kinetic chain*. Within the closed chain, the biceps femoris acts on its more proximal attachment within the chain, namely the pelvis. The biceps femoris attaches directly to the ischial tuberosity and also to the sacrotuberous ligament, sacrum, iliac crests, and up through the multifidi and lumbar erector spinae (figure 6.2).

At heel contact, the ipsilateral (same side) hip and contralateral (opposite side) shoulder are in a position of flexion, which effectively preloads the posterior oblique sling (figure 6.3(a)),

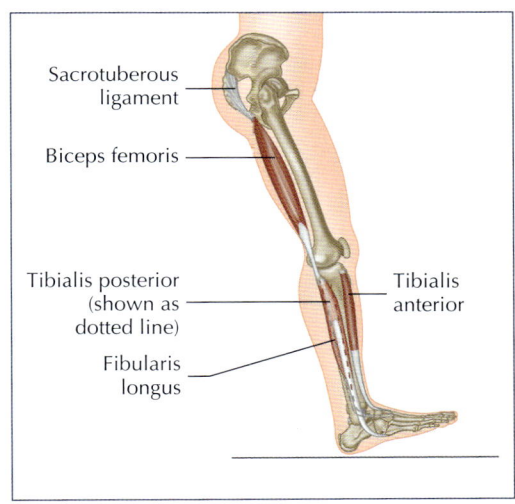

Figure 6.2. Posterior (deep) longitudinal sling.

specifically the ipsilateral Gmax and contralateral latissimus dorsi. This allows extra-spinal propulsion in a "sling-like" manner, with the superficial lamina of the thoracolumbar fascia serving as an intermediary between these kinetically linked muscles (figure 6.3(b)).

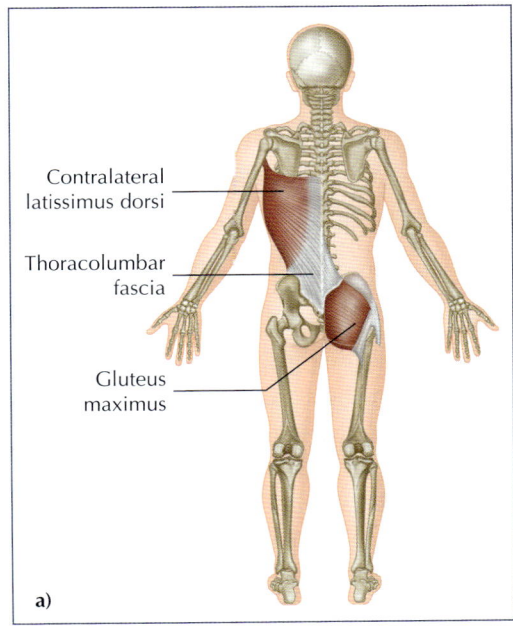

Figure 6.3. (a) Posterior oblique sling.

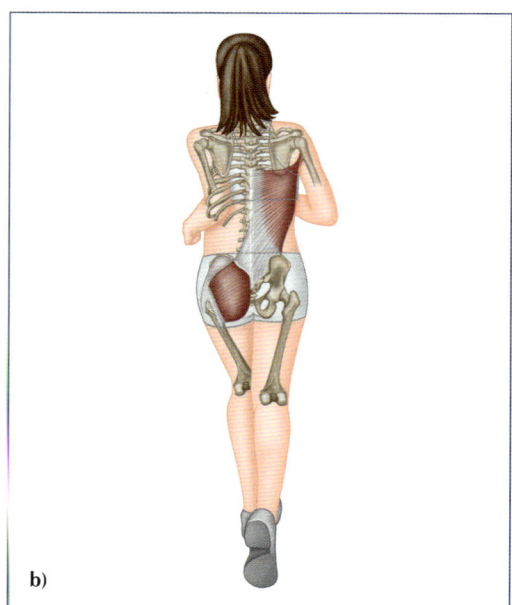

b)

Figure 6.3. (b) Posterior oblique sling utilized whilst running.

The force transmitted through the osteo-articular-ligamentous structures induces "form closure" of the spinal facet joints and rotation in the lumbar spine; coupled with a lateral flexion moment, the spinal engine *initiates and selects the gears* to drive the pelvis into a forward rotation. The induced lumbar rotation effectively stores elastic energy in the spinal ligaments and the anulus fibrosus of the intervertebral discs, and it is this return of energy that drives gait.

To return the energy, the spine must be stabilized from above: this is accomplished via contralateral arm swing and trunk rotation produced by the contralateral Gmax and latissimus dorsi involvement. The coupling patterns of the spine have evolved to facilitate the return of this force. The counter-rotation is considered to be recruited directly from the spine and not from the legs.

Spinal Mechanics Explained

Every patient, especially from a spinal mechanics point of view, should be assessed on the basis that they are unique, especially since some people present with vertebral anomalies, which may cause abnormal physiological movement. The following information relating to spinal physiological movement is based on empirical experience rather than on scientific theory; however, it is dependable and useful in helping the budding therapist to understand what they should expect to palpate in most people.

By developing good hand–eye coordination and tactile tissue tension sense, it is certainly possible to detect spinal lesions or, in modern terms, *somatic spinal dysfunctions*. These dysfunctions can be palpated as abnormal vertebral positioning; they function either statically or dynamically, while surrounding abnormal soft tissue texture is a common feature. Once the somatic spinal dysfunctions have been identified and appropriately treated, the offending vertebral segment(s) can be re-evaluated to determine whether the treatment approach has been successful. This whole process can be demonstrated clinically, provided that the underpinning knowledge of basic spinal physiological movement has been studied and put into practice by the practitioner.

Fryette's Laws (1918) consist of two laws (originally known as *principles*) pertaining to spinal positioning.

These laws only relate to the thoracic and lumbar vertebrae, and the motion available is only considered to be governed by the patterns of force generated by the intervertebral discs, ligaments, and associated musculature. On the other hand, cervical spine motion, which is not classified as a motion that follows Fryette mechanics, is mainly determined by the orientation of the facet joints. We can, however, describe the cervical spine motion as Fryette-*like* mechanics because of the similarity.

Law 1: Neutral Mechanics—Type I

Neutral mechanics relates to standing or sitting in a relaxed upright position, with normal neutral spinal curves. But what is neutral? *Neutral* in the world of spinal mechanics is not defined as a single point, but rather as a range in which the weight of the trunk is borne on the vertebral bodies and intervertebral discs, and the facet joints are in an idle state.

Fryette wrote: "Neutral is defined to mean the position of any area of the spine in which the facets are idling, in the position between the beginning of flexion and the beginning of extension."

This basically means that in neutral, the facet joints are neither in a state of extension (closed) nor in a state of flexion (open)—they are simply idling or resting between these two positions.

According to Fryette, when the spine is in a *neutral* position, side bending to one side will be accompanied by horizontal rotation to the *opposite* side: this is referred to as

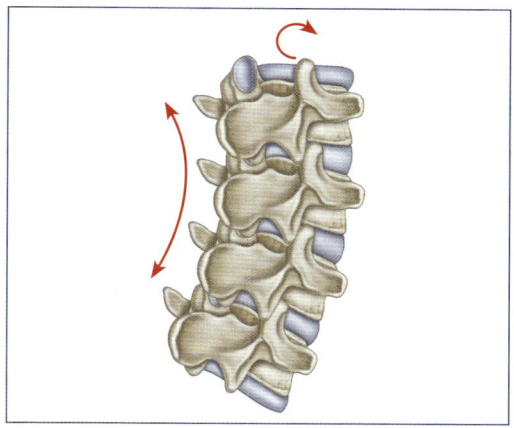

Figure 6.4. Type I spinal mechanics—side bending left, rotation right.

Type I spinal mechanics (figure 6.4). This first law is observed in what is known as a *Type I spinal dysfunction*, where more than one vertebra is out of alignment and cannot be returned to neutral by flexion or extension of the vertebrae. The group of vertebrae in question demonstrates a coupled relationship: when side bending forces are induced in a group of typical vertebrae to one side, the entire group will rotate to the *opposite* side, in other words obeying Type I or Law 1 spinal mechanics. This spinal motion will produce a convexity similar to a spinal curvature known as a *scoliosis*.

Type I (neutral) dysfunctions generally occur in groups of vertebrae, for example T1–7, and are typically seen in spinal conditions such as scoliosis. The vertebrae of a Type I dysfunction tend to compensate for a single Type II dysfunction, and are usually at the beginning or the end of the group dysfunction, although the dysfunction can sometimes be located at the apex of the curvature.

Another way of looking at Type I spinal mechanics is as follows. In the neutral position for the thoracic and lumbar spines, side bending will create a concavity to the same side as the side bend and a convexity to the side of the rotation (opposite side). For example, side bending to the left will create a concave curve on the left side of the body and a convex curve on the right side.

Neutral spinal mechanics is a naturally occurring motion of the spine that is required to promote Gracovetsky's spinal engine, due to the side bending and rotation to the opposite side. Any spinal dysfunction present will reduce the overall efficiency of the 'engine' (spinal).

Law 2: Non-Neutral Mechanics— Type II

Fryette states that when the spine is in a position of flexion or extension, by either standing or sitting while in a forward- or backward-bent position (also known as *non-neutral*), side bending to one side will be accompanied by rotation to the *same* side: this is referred to as *Type II mechanics* (figure 6.5).

This second law is observed in Type II spinal dysfunctions, where only one vertebral segment is restricted in motion, and becomes much worse in a position of flexion or extension. As mentioned above, there will be a coupled spinal motion, with side bending and rotation in the *same* direction when this dysfunction is present.

Let's look at this from another angle. Put simply, if the thoracic or lumbar spine is sufficiently forward or backward bent,

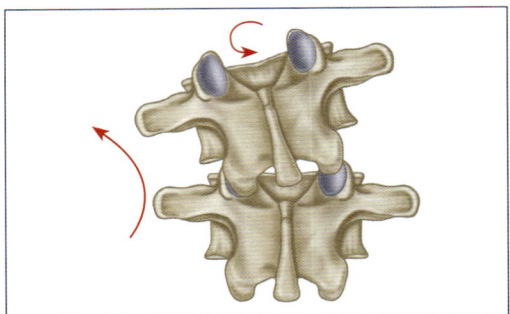

Figure 6.5. Type II spinal mechanics—side bending left, rotation left.

the coupled motions of side bending and rotation of a single vertebral unit will occur in the same direction (i.e. to the same side).

Type II (non-neutral) spinal dysfunctions are generally thought to occur in a single vertebral segment. However, two Type II dysfunctions can appear next to each other at the same time, but the occurrence of more than two is rare.

Viewing Perspective

When assessing for spinal movement, the spine is usually viewed from behind. Typically, a spinal dysfunction exists when we try to place the patient's spine in a neutral position, but this position of symmetry cannot be achieved; the likely reason being a dysfunction of either a group of vertebrae or a single spinal segment.

It is possible to detect an abnormal or restricted ROM of the spine when patients perform flexion, extension, side bending, and rotation in the cardinal planes.

The following sections detail the specific spinal mechanic motion for the whole of the vertebral column.

1. Lumbar Spine

Neutral Mechanics: Type I

When side bending to one side, the vertebral bodies rotate to the *opposite* side.

Non-Neutral Mechanics: Type II

When side bending to one side, the vertebral bodies rotate to the *same* side.

L5 is one exception to the rule. In neutral mechanics, during side bending to one side L5 may rotate to either the opposite side or the same side (obeying non-neutral mechanics, even though the spine is in a relatively neutral position) whenever there is some asymmetry/dysfunction of the sacral base or if there are facet joint anomalies present.

2. Thoracic Spine

Neutral Mechanics: Type I

When side bending to one side, the vertebral bodies rotate to the *opposite* side.

Non-Neutral Mechanics: Type II

When side bending to one side, the vertebral bodies rotate to the *same* side.

3. Cervical Spine

Spinal motion in the cervical spine is mainly determined by the orientation of the facet joints and does not come within the realm of Fryette's laws; however, we can say these mechanics are Fryette-*like*, because the motion is similar.

Atlanto-Occipital Joint (AOJ)

The AOJ always follows Type I (like) mechanics: in side bending to one side, the occiput rotates to the *opposite* side, independent of whether the occiput is in a neutral or a non-neutral position (flexion or extension).

Atlanto-Axial Joint (AAJ)

The AAJ (C1/C2) is mainly considered to only rotate. There has been some discussion suggesting that, in either neutral or non-neutral mechanics, during side bending movements the atlas (C1) is capable of rotating to either side. Dysfunctions typically found at this level are thought to consist mainly of a rotational component.

The level of C2–C6 is believed to only follow Type II (like) mechanics, in that side bending and the rotation are always coupled to the *same* side, regardless of whether the cervical spine is in a neutral position or a non-neutral position (flexion or extension).

C2–C6: Neutral Mechanics

When side bending to one side, the vertebral bodies rotate to the *same* side, i.e. Type II-*like* mechanics.

C2–C6: Non-Neutral Mechanics

When side bending to one side, the vertebral bodies rotate to the *same* side, i.e. Type II-*like* mechanics.

C7 has facet joints that are orientated in a similar way to the thoracic spine, so this spinal level will follow the classic law of Fryette.

Spinal mechanics

Spinal Mechanics: Definitions

The specific position of a vertebra can be referenced in two different ways:

1. The position of the vertebra, relative to the vertebra below.
2. The direction of the motion restriction of the vertebra, relative to the vertebra below.

In other words, the same vertebral segment can be described from two different points of view.

For example, let's say T4 is fixed in an extended, side-bent right, and rotated-right position. This simply means that the T4 is fixed in a position of extension, side bend, and rotation, all to the right side, on top of the vertebra immediately below, i.e. T5. This is because the right T4 inferior facet is fixed in a *closed* position on the superior facet on T5. The motion restriction has to be in forward flexion as well as in left side bending and left rotation

(opposite to the fixed position). This type of dysfunction obeys Type II mechanics, as already explained earlier; however, taking it a stage further, we would now classify the spinal dysfunction as a *T4 extension, rotation, side bend right*, or *T4 ERS(R)*, which will be discussed shortly.

In terms of diagnosing somatic spinal dysfunction, the positional diagnosis is determined and named according to the direction of the vertebra that has the easiest motion. Let's take a look at what I mean by that in more detail.

Spinal dysfunction is typically described as either *extended* or *flexed*, with a rotation and a side bending component to the same side, or possibly to the opposite side, as you will read later.

Before we define the terminology for spinal dysfunctions, we first need to confirm the presence of a spinal dysfunction by ascertaining the specific position and motion of the vertebra being tested. We can establish this by asking our patient to adopt three different positions of the vertebral column: neutral, extension, and flexion. The vertebral position through palpation simply becomes either symmetrical (level) or asymmetrical (not level) in these three positions, depending on the type of spinal dysfunction/ facet restriction present at the time.

If there are no facet restrictions present, when you forward bend your spine, the left and right facet joints (top vertebra in relation to the bottom vertebra) will slide forward in a superior and anterior direction to open; conversely, when you backward bend your spine, the left and right facet joints will slide backward in an inferior and posterior direction to close. However, if the facet joints are for some reason restricted in either a flexion or an extension position, the restricted joint will now act as a pivot point, especially when performing the spinal motion of forward and backward bending.

To illustrate this, ask your patient to adopt a neutral position (normally a sitting position, for the thoracic spine) and lightly place your left and right thumbs on the T4/5 transverse process (TP). Lightly palpate for a few seconds and compare the left and right TPs to see if there is any asymmetry; if so, you have now identified the presence of a spinal dysfunction—in a very simple way, you have located a facet restriction. For instance, if the left thumb, while in contact with the left TP, appeared to palpate *shallow* (i.e. the TP feels closer to the surface of the skin), whereas the right thumb (on the right TP) palpated *deep* (i.e. the thumb traveled further to reach the right TP), this would be indicative of T4 (superior) having rotated to the left side on T5 (inferior) below (see figure 6.6(c)).

What this does not tell you, however, is whether the *left* facet joint is fixed in a *closed* position or whether the *right* facet joint is fixed in an *open* position. That is why it is necessary to palpate the TPs in the position of spinal extension (backward bending) and spinal flexion (forward bending) in order to confirm or discount the presence of a fixed closed facet joint or a fixed open facet joint.

Let's try to look at this concept in a relatively simple way (I hope) by using T4/5 as an example. As already discussed, we should now know that when the patient

is in a neutral position, T4 has rotated to the left side, because the left TP palpated as shallow (more prominent) and the right TP palpated as deep (less prominent). From the neutral position, we now ask our patient to forward bend, while the thumbs are still in contact with the TPs; you notice the left and right TPs in the forward-bent position become more asymmetrical (the TP on one side becomes more prominent, and the TP on the other less prominent).

Imagine for a moment that you consider the left thumb to feel more prominent (think of it as a bump) and now the right thumb feels even deeper (less prominent); this must mean that the left facet joint is fixed in a *closed* position on the *left* side, see figure 6.6(g). Why? When the patient forward bends, the right facet joint is free to glide anteriorly as normal, but the left facet joint is now fixed posteriorly; because the left facet cannot open normally during forward bending, the left facet joint that is fixed in a closed position becomes a pivot point. Because of this pivot, one could say that the right facet basically has to open even more during forward bending, but ends up rotating around the left fixed facet joint that cannot open; this is why the left and right thumbs appear even more asymmetric. In this case the left thumb has become more prominent (the bump increases because the left TP is fixed posteriorly) in the forward-bent position.

When you ask the patient to adopt a position of extension, the thumbs will now palpate level (symmetric), because the left facet joint is already fixed posteriorly in a closed position, and the right facet joint simply continues its natural motion of closing. The left and right thumb positions on the TPs therefore become symmetric (level) in extension (the bump on the left TP disappears), see figure 6.6(e).

Consider now another type of dysfunction—the case where the right facet joint is fixed in an open position. When we palpate the T4/5 TP in neutral, we will still notice the left thumb is shallow (bump) and the right thumb is deeper, indicating a left rotation, see figure 6.10(c). However, when the patient forward bends their spine, the thumbs now become symmetric (i.e. the thumbs are now level and the bump disappears), see figure 6.10(g). By contrast, when the patient backward bends their spine, you notice that the thumbs become asymmetric (i.e. symmetry is lost in extension—the bump felt by the left thumb on the TP increases), see figure 6.10(e). This time the left thumb actually appears more prominent (bump present), and the right thumb appears to travel deeper in the backward-bent position. Why? In a forward-bent position, both of the facet joints are able to open as normal, hence the thumbs becoming level in this position; however, in a backward-bent position of extension, because the *right* facet is fixed in an *open* position (even though it has rotated to the left side), the facet joint cannot close on the right side, but the fixed pivot point created by the right open facets keeps the right TP fixed anteriorly. Since the backward bending motion causes the left side to move more posteriorly, the left TP appears to move further into left rotation. The thumbs therefore appear asymmetric and now, in the backward-bent position, the left thumb on the left TP becomes more prominent (bump appears) than the right thumb.

Note: The above dysfunction relates to the right facet joint fixed in an open position. This is called an FRS(L) as you will read shortly.

One way of remembering these two processes, as it will help you with your own patients, is to understand the following two rules:

Rule 1: In forward bending, if the prominent TP becomes even more prominent (bump appears), then that side is fixed closed.

Rule 2: In backward bending, if the prominent TP becomes more prominent (bump appears), then the opposite side is fixed open.

Maitland (2001) offers another explanation, which might help you better understand what I am trying to say. First, you determine rotation in a neutral position. Then, keeping your thumbs on the TPs of the rotated vertebra, forward and backward bend your client, and feel and watch what happens under your thumbs. Look for the position where the bump (the posterior or prominent vertebra TP of the rotated vertebra) disappears. Maitland says that the position where the bump disappears (or vertebral de-rotation appears to occur) is the position in which the facets are restricted:

"If the bump disappears in forward bending, the facets are fixed in the forward-bent position, which means the facets are fixed open (flexion fixed)."

"If the bump disappears in back bending, the facets are fixed in the back bent position, which means the facets are fixed closed (extension fixed).”

We will now look at some of the typical terminology that practitioners use in their clinics, along with a few common examples of spinal dysfunctional patterns that patients might present with in your own clinic. Hopefully, once you have read all the information in this chapter, and practiced all the necessary spinal positions in order to confirm or discount the presence of either a fixed facet or an open facet, we can look at some form of treatment strategy, especially for the thoracic spine and ribs, which will be discussed in later lessons.

Extension, Rotation, Side Bending Left—ERS(L)

> **Definition:** An *extension, rotation, side bending (ERS) dysfunction* involves a facet joint (inferior and superior component) which is fixed in a closed position. It is classified as a *non-neutral (Type II) spinal mechanics dysfunction.*

This is a situation in which the *left* facet joint is fixed in a *closed* position.

ERS(L) refers to the orientation of an uppermost vertebra that is fixed in an extended, side-bent, and rotated position to the left side (figure 6.6(a)).

Consider this example: T4 is assumed to be fixed in a closed position on the left side on T5. We will now test the levels of T4/5 in the three positions of neutral, flexion, and extension.

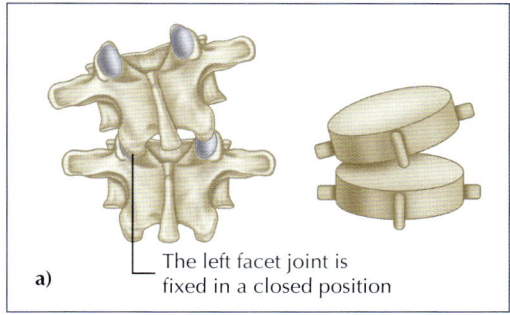

a) ⎣ The left facet joint is fixed in a closed position

Figure 6.6. (a) Extension, rotation, side bending left—ERS(L).

Neutral Position

With the patient in a neutral position, place your thumbs approximately 1” (2.5 cm) lateral to the T4 and T5 spinous processes, so that the thumbs are in gentle contact with the left and right TPs. If there is an ERS(L) present, you will notice that the left thumb appears to be more prominent (shallow) and the right thumb appears to be deeper in the neutral position (figure 6.6(b–c)), indicating that the vertebra has rotated to the left side.

Extension Position

As the patient backward bends, observe the relative levels of your thumbs. You will notice that the left and right thumbs are level (figure 6.6(d–e)).

Flexion Position

Next, look at the relative positions of your thumbs as the patient forward bends. This time you will notice that the left thumb appears to become more prominent (bump appears) and that the right thumb appears

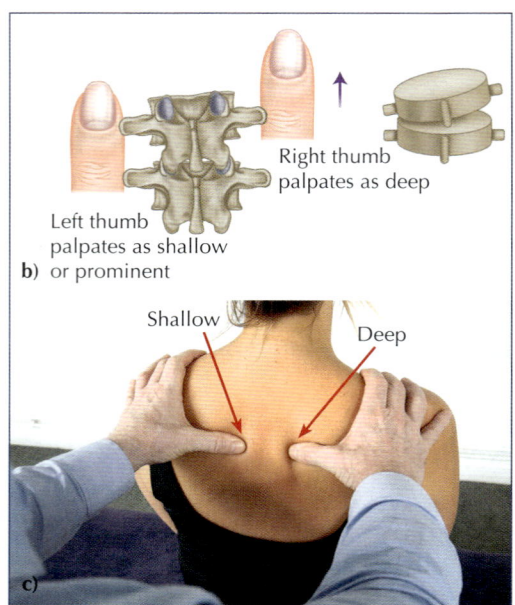

Figure 6.6. (b) Neutral position—the left thumb appears shallow and the right thumb appears deeper, indicating a left rotation of the vertebra. (c) Thoracic spine T4/5.

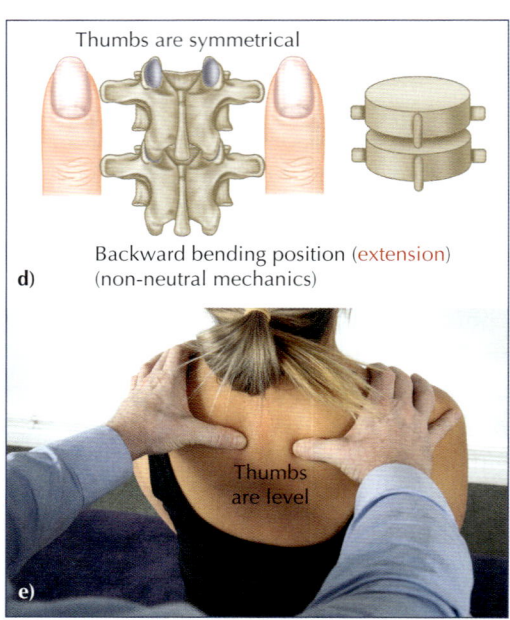

Figure 6.6. (d) Extension position—the left and right thumbs now appear to become level. (e) Thoracic spine T4/5.

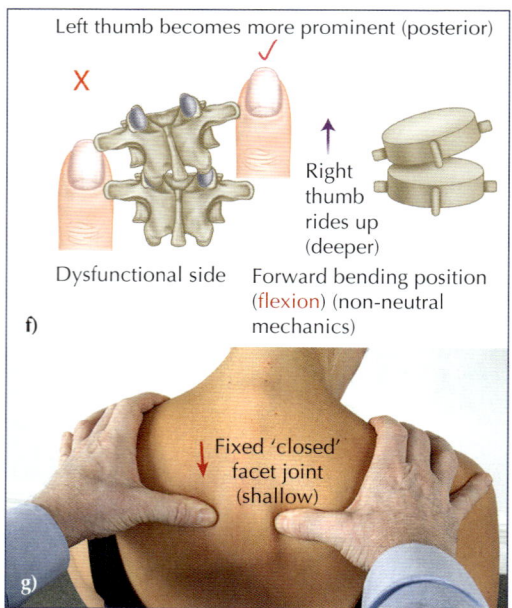

Figure 6.6. (f) Flexion position—the left thumb appears more prominent and the right thumb appears deep, indicating a fixed closed vertebra on the left side. (g) Thoracic spine T4/5.

to travel deeper (figure 6.6(f–g)). This asymmetric positioning of the thumbs indicates a fixed closed facet joint on the left side. Figure 6.7 recaps the thumb position for neutral, extension, and flexion.

Extension, Rotation, Side Bending Right—ERS(R)

This is a situation in which the *right* facet joint is fixed in a *closed* position.

ERS(R) refers to the orientation of an uppermost vertebra that is fixed in an extended, side-bent, and rotated position to the right side (see figure 6.8(a)).

Consider this example: T4 is assumed to be fixed in a closed position on the right side on T5. We will now test the levels of

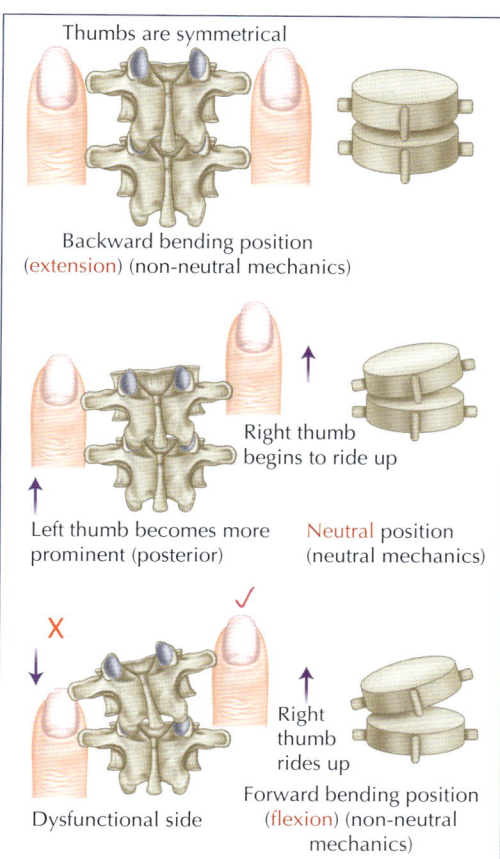

Figure 6.7. Thumb positions in neutral, extension, and flexion for ERS(L).

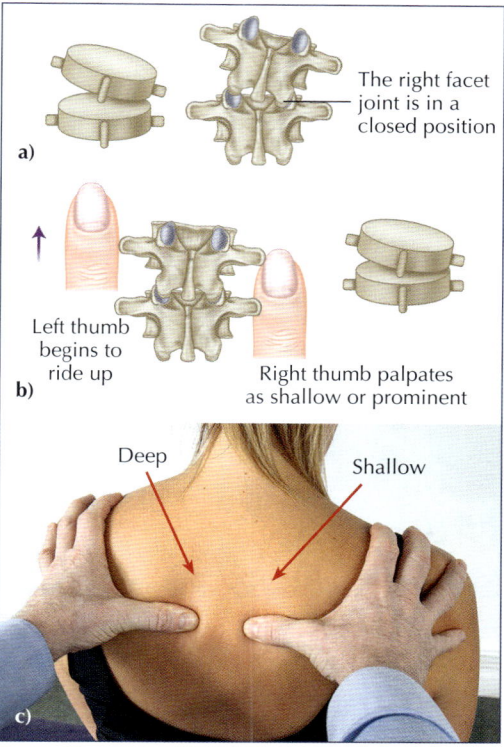

Figure 6.8. (a) Extension, rotation, side bending right—ERS(R). (b) Neutral position—the right thumb appears more prominent and the left thumb appears deeper, indicating a right rotation of the vertebra. (c) Thoracic spine T4/5.

T4/5 and L5/S1 in the three positions of neutral, flexion, and extension.

Neutral Position

With the patient in a neutral position, place your thumbs approximately 1" (2.5 cm) lateral to the T4 and T5 spinous processes, so that the thumbs are in gentle contact with the left and right TPs. If there is an ERS(R) present, you will notice that the right thumb appears to be shallow and the left thumb appears to be deeper in the neutral position (figure 6.8(b–c)), indicating a right rotation of the vertebra.

Extension Position

As the patient backward bends, observe the relative levels of your thumbs. You will notice that the left and right thumbs are level (see figure 6.8(d–e)).

Flexion Position

Next look at the relative level of your thumbs as the patient forward bends. You will notice that the right thumb appears to become more prominent (bump appears) and the left thumb appears to travel deeper (see figure 6.8(f–g)). This asymmetric

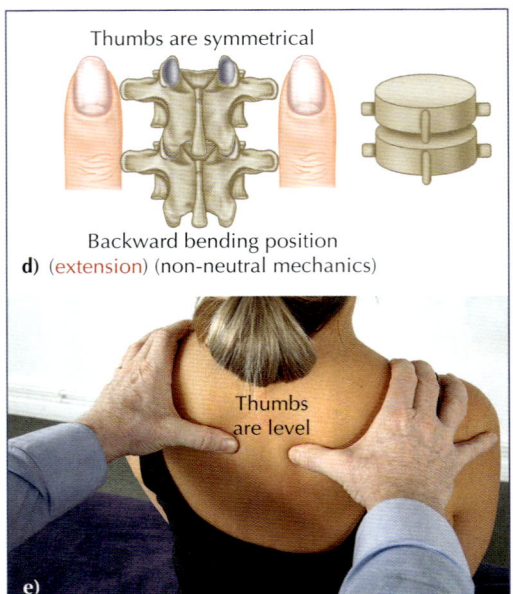

Figure 6.8. (d) Extension position—the left and right thumbs now appear to become level. (e) Thoracic spine T4/5.

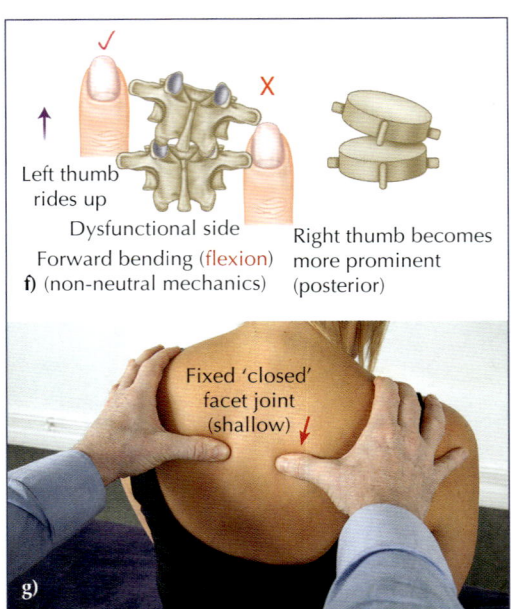

Figure 6.8. (f) Flexion position—the right thumb appears more prominent and the left thumb appears deeper, indicating a fixed closed vertebra on the right side. (g) Thoracic spine T4/5.

positioning of the thumbs indicates a fixed closed facet joint on the right side. Figure 6.9 recaps the thumb position for neutral, extension, and flexion.

Flexion, Rotation, Side Bending Left—FRS(L)

> **Definition:** A *flexion, rotation, side bending (FRS) dysfunction* involves a facet joint which is fixed in an open position. It is classified as a *non-neutral (Type II) spinal mechanics dysfunction.*

This is a situation in which the *right* facet joint is fixed in an open position.

Note that, although the dysfunction is to the *right* facet, *FRS(L)* refers to the orientation of an uppermost vertebra that is fixed in a flexed, side-bent, and rotated position to the *left* side. It is the *right* facet, however, that is dysfunctional, because it is fixed in an open position (see figure 6.10(a)).

We will now test the levels of T4/5 in the three positions of neutral, flexion, and extension.

Neutral Position

With the patient in a neutral position, place your thumbs approximately 1" (2.5 cm) lateral to the T4 and T5 spinous processes, so that the thumbs are in gentle contact with the left and

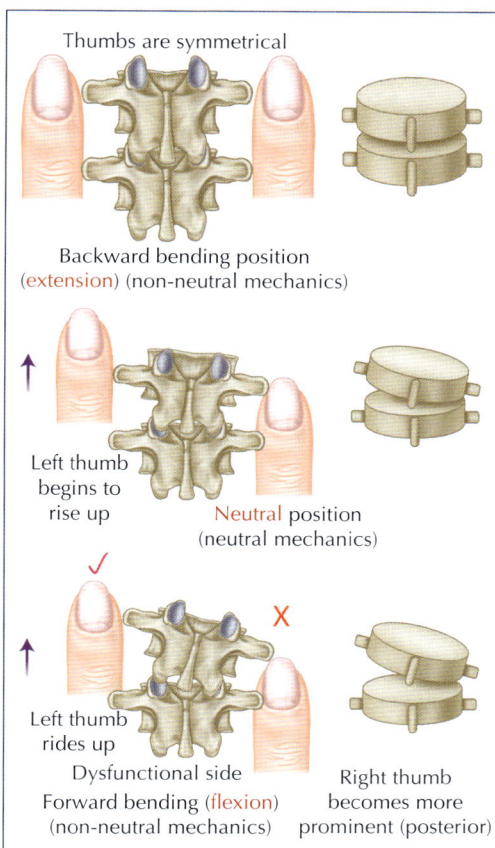

Thumbs are symmetrical

Backward bending position
(extension) (non-neutral mechanics)

Left thumb
begins to
rise up
Neutral position
(neutral mechanics)
✓
✗
Left thumb
rides up
Dysfunctional side
Forward bending (flexion)
(non-neutral mechanics)
Right thumb
becomes more
prominent (posterior)

Figure 6.9. Thumb positions in neutral, extension, and flexion for ERS(R).

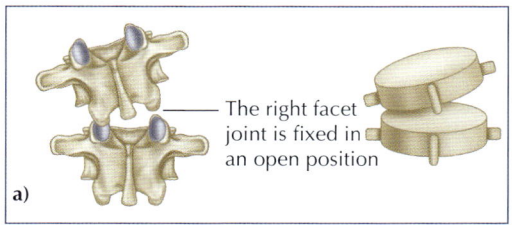

The right facet
joint is fixed in
an open position

a)

Figure 6.10. (a) Flexion, rotation, side bending left—FRS(L).

right TPs. If there is an FRS(L) present, you will notice that the left thumb appears to be more prominent and the right thumb appears to be deeper in the neutral position (figure 6.10(b–c)), indicating that the vertebra has rotated to the left side.

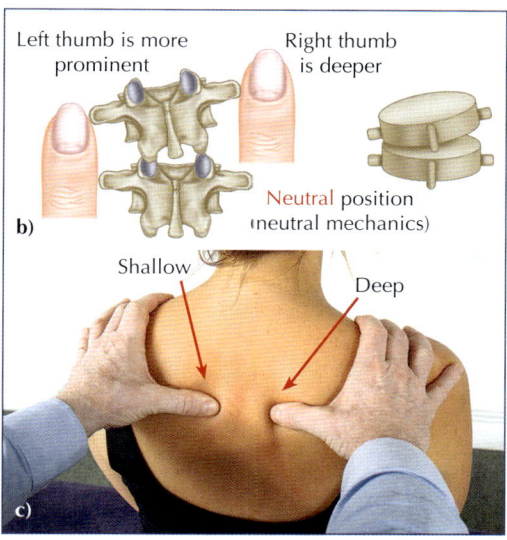

Left thumb is more
prominent
Right thumb
is deeper

Neutral position
(neutral mechanics)

b)

Shallow

Deep

c)

Figure 6.10. (b) Neutral position—the left thumb appears shallow and the right thumb appears deeper, indicating a left rotation of the vertebra. (c) Thoracic spine T4/5.

Extension Position

As the patient backward bends, observe the relative position of your thumbs. You will notice that the left thumb appears to become more prominent (bump appears) and the right thumb appears to travel deeper (Figure 6.10(d–e)). This asymmetric positioning of the thumbs indicates a fixed open facet joint on the right side (side opposite to rotation).

Flexion Position

Next look at the relative position of your thumbs as the patient forward bends. You will notice that the left and right thumbs are now level (Figure 6.10(f–g)). Figure 6.11 recaps the thumb position for neutral, extension, and flexion.

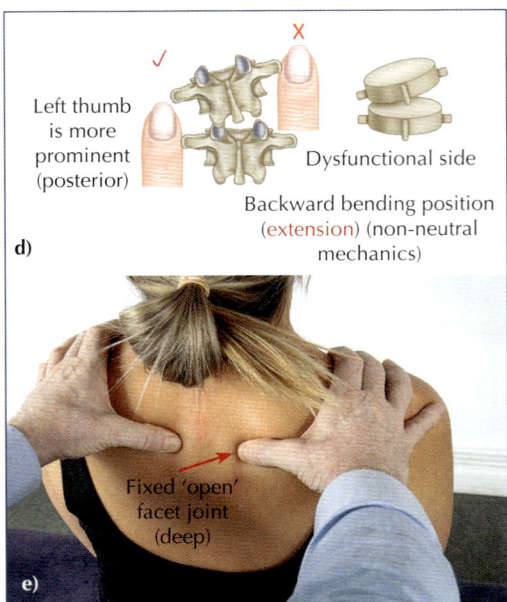

Figure 6.10. (d) Extension position—the left thumb appears more prominent and the right thumb appears deeper, indicating a fixed open facet joint on the right side. (e) Thoracic spine T4/5.

Flexion, Rotation, Side Bending Right—FRS(R)

This is a situation in which the *left* facet joint is fixed in an open position.

Note that, although the dysfunction is to the *left* facet, *FRS(R)* refers to the orientation of an uppermost vertebra that is fixed in a flexed, side-bent, and rotated position to the *right* side. It is the *left* facet, however, that is dysfunctional, because it is fixed in an open position (Figure 6.12(a)).

We will now test the levels of T4/5 and L5/S1 in the three positions of neutral, flexion, and extension.

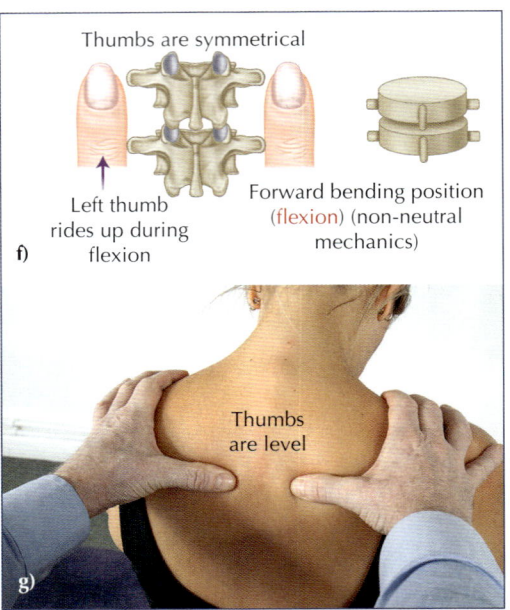

Figure 6.10. (f) Flexion position—the left and right thumbs now appear to become level. (g) Thoracic spine T4/5.

Neutral Position

With the patient in a neutral position, place your thumbs approximately 1" (2.5 cm) lateral to the T4 and T5 spinous processes, so that the thumbs are in gentle contact with the left and right TPs (repeat the same process when you are ready to do L5/S1). If there is an FRS(R) present, you will notice that the left thumb appears to be deep and the right thumb appears to be shallow in the neutral position (Figure 6.12(b–c)), indicating that the vertebra has rotated to the right side.

Extension Position

As the patient backward bends, observe the relative position of your thumbs. You

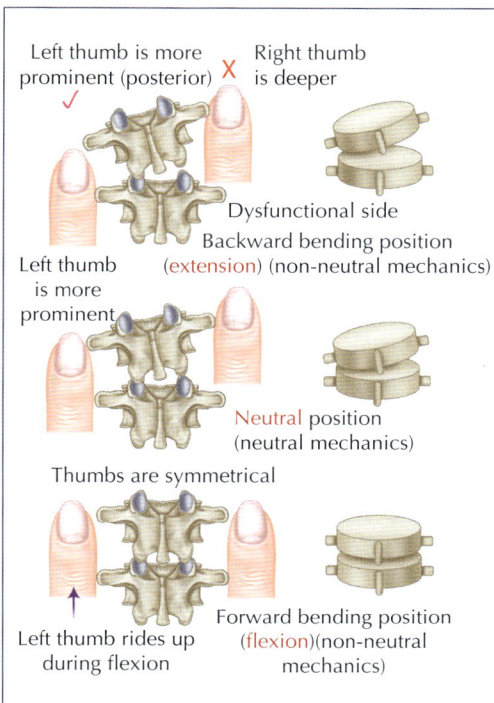

Left thumb is more prominent (posterior) ✓ X Right thumb is deeper

Dysfunctional side
Backward bending position (extension) (non-neutral mechanics)

Left thumb is more prominent

Neutral position (neutral mechanics)

Thumbs are symmetrical

Left thumb rides up during flexion

Forward bending position (flexion)(non-neutral mechanics)

Figure 6.11. Thumb positions in neutral, extension, and flexion for FRS(L).

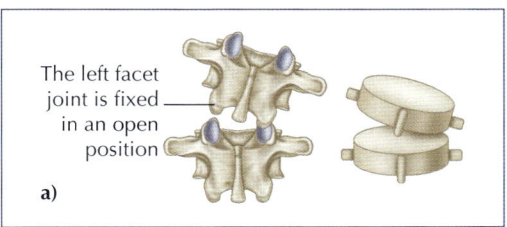

The left facet joint is fixed in an open position

a)

Figure 6.12. (a) Flexion, rotation, side bending right—FRS(R).

will notice that the right thumb appears to become more prominent (bump appears) and the left thumb appears to travel deeper (Figure 6.12(d–e)). This asymmetric positioning of the thumbs indicates a fixed open facet joint on the left side (side opposite to rotation).

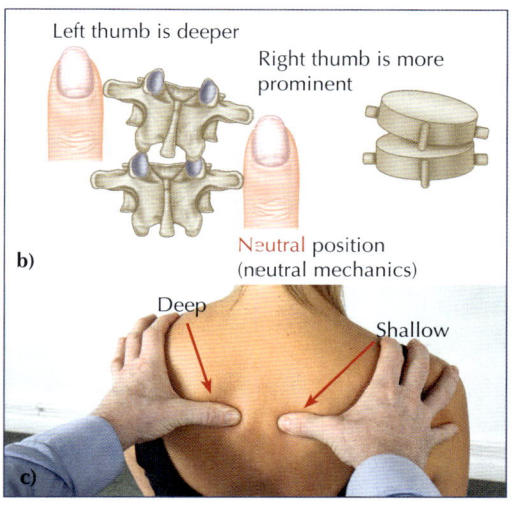

Left thumb is deeper

Right thumb is more prominent

Neutral position (neutral mechanics)

Deep   Shallow

b)

c)

Figure 6.12. (b) Neutral position—the right thumb appears shallow and the left thumb appears deeper, indicating a right rotation of the vertebra. (c) Thoracic spine T4/5.

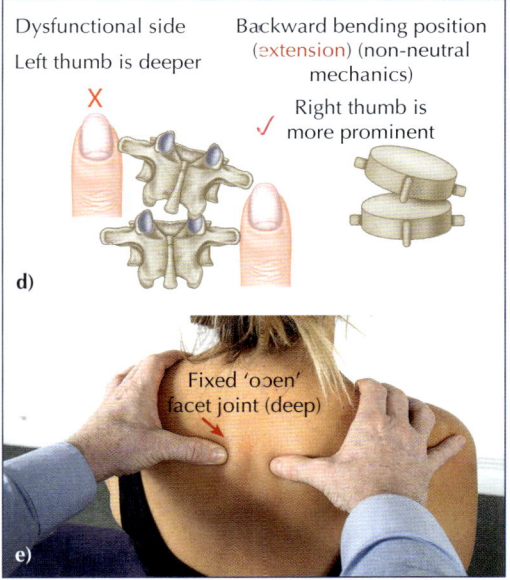

Dysfunctional side
Left thumb is deeper

Backward bending position (extension) (non-neutral mechanics)

X ✓ Right thumb is more prominent

d)

Fixed 'open' facet joint (deep)

e)

Figure 6.12. (d) Extension position—the right thumb appears more prominent and the left thumb appears deeper, indicating a fixed open facet joint on the left side. (e) Thoracic spine T4/5.

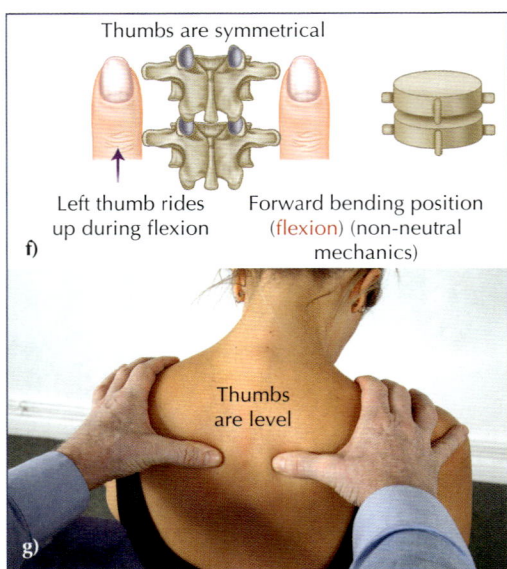

Thumbs are symmetrical

Left thumb rides up during flexion

Forward bending position (flexion) (non-neutral mechanics)

f)

Thumbs are level

g)

Figure 6.12. (f) Flexion position—the left and right thumbs now appear to become level. (g) Thoracic spine T4/5.

Flexion Position

Next look at the relative position of your thumbs as the patient forward bends. You will notice that the left and right thumbs are now level (Figure 6.12(f–g)). Figure 6.13 recaps the thumb position for neutral, extension, and flexion.

Remember the following because this will help you when assessing your patient's thoracic spine:

> "If the bump disappears in forward bending, the facets are fixed in the forward-bent position, which means the facets are fixed open (flexion fixed)."

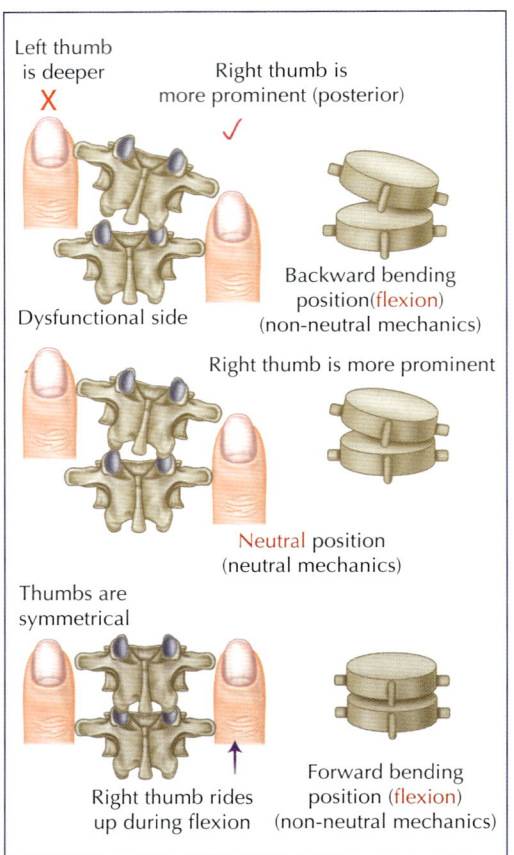

Left thumb is deeper ✗

Right thumb is more prominent (posterior) ✓

Dysfunctional side

Backward bending position(flexion) (non-neutral mechanics)

Right thumb is more prominent

Neutral position (neutral mechanics)

Thumbs are symmetrical

Right thumb rides up during flexion

Forward bending position (flexion) (non-neutral mechanics)

Figure 6.13. Thumb positions in neutral, extension, and flexion for FRS(R).

> "If the bump disappears in backward bending, the facets are fixed in the back bent position, which means the facets are fixed closed (extension fixed)."

Spinal motion assessment

PART II

PRACTICE

Techniques for the Cervical Spine

I believe the cervical spine (CSp) has a direct relationship to all the unique components that make up the spinal column. There are at this moment probably thousands of people throughout the world who think their presenting shoulder or upper limb pain is coming from the shoulder joint or its associated structures. For the majority, however, the underlying causative factor is likely the cervical spine—not only of their presenting shoulder pain but also for other symptoms they might have radiating to the arm, hand, and even to the lower limb.

I see the relationship of the cervical spine to the rest of the spinal column like a marriage or a conjoined partnership: simply speaking, if one breaks down or becomes dysfunctional (or maybe pathological, as this is a medical relationship), the other will not be able to cope and might have to compensate in one way or another.

I always teach the following concepts: if one has a problem at the thoracic spinal level, or even lower down the kinetic chain like the lumbar spine, pelvis, or the lower limb, then eventually this becomes a problem with the cervical spine, and vice versa. In other words, a problem with the cervical spine eventually becomes a problem with the rest of the spinal complex, and even through compensatory mechanisms with the lower limb. Remember that we have 24 movable parts in the spinal column, and because of this, I believe it fits perfectly to one of my sayings: where the pain is (symptoms), the problem (cause) might not be.

As an example during class, I asked the attendees whether anyone had shoulder pain, since that was going to be the next topic we covered. Within a microsecond, a gentleman shot his hand up, waving his arm vigorously in the air to me from the back of the class, saying, "Yes, I have a *big* problem with my shoulder" (while keeping his arm in the air!). I responded that I doubted the pain was in the arm that was currently still in the air, especially given the speed he lifted it. No, said the man, it *was* the arm that was in the air that had the pain. There lies the problem. To him, it was a *big* problem with his shoulder. However, I would classify it as a *little* problem, especially after the assessment and treatment, because the pain he felt in his shoulder was in fact referred and radiating from his cervical spine.

Case Study

A personal trainer friend who runs a cross-fit gymnasium referred one of his clients to me because she had difficulty performing one of the exercises in the routine. The exercise was to simply lie on a bench and then to extend the elbows using two dumbbells (figure 7.1). You can see that the left arm cannot extend as far as the right one because of weakness. This exercise is designed to strengthen the triceps muscle group.

However, what I found interesting was the patient did not mention that she had any form of pain or even restriction in the neck, shoulder, or arms; she simply had a weakness in performing that particular

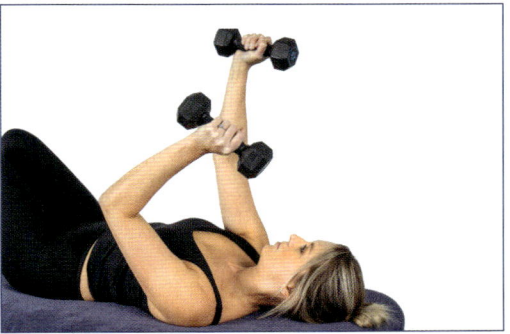

Figure 7.1. Elbow extension exercise using the triceps—left side limited due to weakness.

maneuver. The personal trainer took a video of her performing the motion so that I could have a better understanding of the underlying problem.

I remember once watching a Canadian chiropractor called Mike who traveled to the UK for some seminars and while there, visited Oxford University to treat a few of the rowers, previous Olympians from Canada whom Mike knew well. Initially, he would test the power (myotomes) of the upper and lower limbs, and when he found a specific neurological weakness, he would then proceed to adjust/manipulate that specific level of the spine. After the treatment he would then retest the power of the motion, and hopefully the power would be seen to test as normal, graded as a 5 on a scale ranging from 0 to 5.

I have been trying to use similar concepts ever since, so when I tested this patient, I tried to focus initially on the power of elbow extension. I found the left side of her arm was very weak compared with the right side.

If you have a good understanding of myotomes, then you will consider that the C7 myotome might be the level that was the underlying problem (she also had weakness of wrist flexion and finger extension, but only to her left side). The C7 nerve root passes between the level of C6 and C7, so it could also have been disc pathology. However, because there was no altered sensation or pain, I thought she had a rotated vertebra (*subluxation* in chiropractic terms) that was tensioning the exiting C7 nerve and thereby giving her weakness on extending the left elbow.

An analogy I sometimes use is of a dimmer switch: if one turns the switch in one direction the light becomes dimmer—there is less power going down the wire to the light bulb; if we turn it the other way, the bulb gets brighter. If the nerve (like the wire) is being turned or compressed for some reason (vertebral rotation, for example) then the signal it carries along the C7 nerve pathway (like the power to the bulb) is reduced, and the movement or power of elbow extension will test or show weakness (the bulb becomes dimmer).

My treatment consisted mainly of a specific cervical spinal mobilization and then a manipulation technique to the left side of C6/7, and an audible cavitation was heard. I then retested her power of left elbow extension, and was very happy to report to the patient that the power had returned to normal. The personal trainer messaged me a few days later to say training had recommenced, and there was no weakness present.

The reason I discussed this case study is to illustrate an alternative way of assessing the upper limb, through myotome testing of the neurological system. I know many therapists who consider pain in the shoulder complex, arm, and hands must come only from the cervical spine. That means all the treatments they perform are biased toward the cervical spine and the exiting nerve pathways, rather than treating the painful areas their patients are presenting with.

Anatomy of the Cervical Spine

The human cervical spine has seven vertebrae (C1–C7) and eight cervical nerves (C1–C8). The upper cervical complex is composed of the atypical segments of the atlanto-occipital (C0–C1) joint and the atlanto-axial joint (C1–C2) between the *atlas* (C1) and the *axis* (C2). The lower, typical segments of the cervical spine continue through C3–C7.

In functional terms, the vertebral column of the cervical spine should also include the occipital condyles, which transfer the weight of the head to the uppermost cervical vertebra (C1). This atypical vertebral structure is a highly specialized vertebra aptly named after the Titan Atlas in classical mythology, whose role it was to support the whole of the world on his shoulders. The second cervical vertebra, the axis, is also a specialized structure, since its function is mainly to assist in rotation of the head.

Atlanto-Axial Joint

The atlanto-axial joint (AAJ) has four articulations. The first two are formed from the left and right inferior concave facets of the atlas, which articulate with the superior convex facets of the axis, and these are known as the *lateral atlanto-axial joints* and are classified as gliding or plane joints (figure 7.2).

The main articulation, however, is called the *median atlanto-axial joint* and is classified as a synovial pivot joint, and this relates to the odontoid process (also called

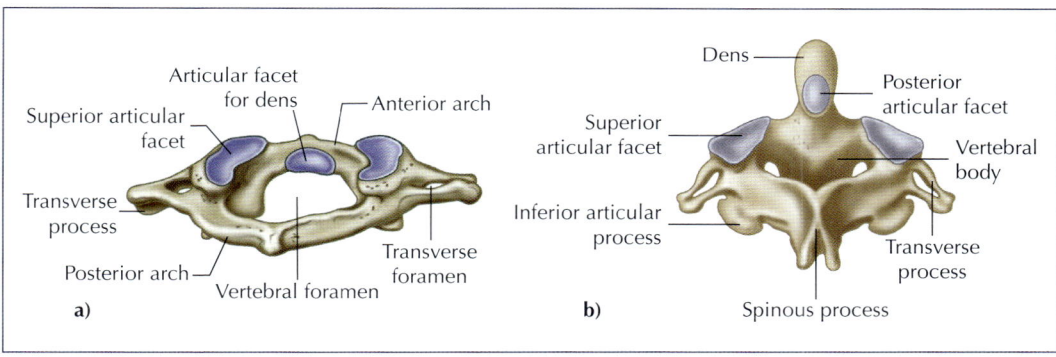

Figure 7.2. Anatomy of (a) the atlas (C1); (b) the axis (C2), posterosuperior view.

the dens), as the anterior surface of the odontoid process articulates with a small facet on the posterior region of the anterior arch of the atlas. On the posterior facet of the odontoid process is another articulation (the fourth articulation), directly connected with the anterior surface of the transverse ligament of the atlas.

The primary motion of the median atlanto-axial joint is rotation, and it allows the atlas, combined with the head, to rotate on an axis around the odontoid process. This movement allows us to look left and right and to shake our head from side to side, as when saying the word "no"; whereas the atlanto-occipital joint (discussed later) allowing us to nod, as when saying the word "yes."

C3–C7 Cervical Vertebrae

The lower cervical spine, comprising the remaining five cervical vertebrae (C3–C7), has structural features that are more typical of other spinal levels (figure 7.3). The facet joints between the levels of C3 and C7 are located posterolaterally, whereby the two articulating pairs of facet joints, which comprise the superior

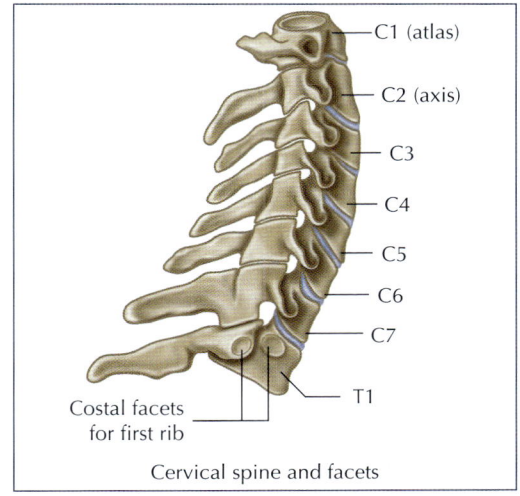

Figure 7.3. Anatomy of the cervical spine and the intervertebral discs.

and inferior components (on both sides), form the articular pillars, which are easily palpable. The superior facets face backward and upward, and this allows rotation and side bending to be coupled to the same direction (type 2 coupled movement). There is no obvious neutral position for the cervical spine, as there is with the thoracic and lumbar (according to Fryette), because there is a natural lordosis; therefore, when the cervical spine is placed into extension, the primary motion is side bending, owing to the orientation of the facet joints in

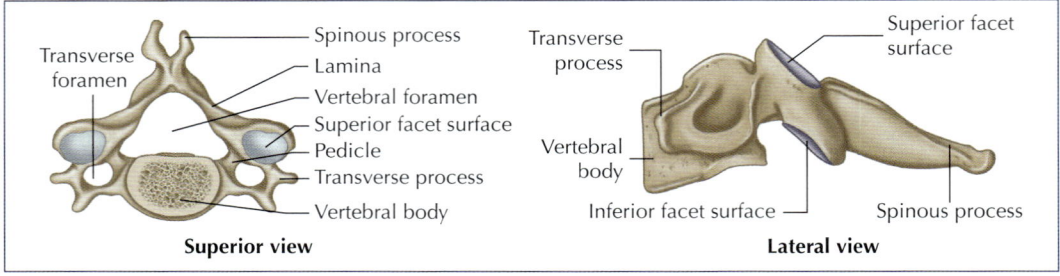

Figure 7.4. A typical cervical vertebra (C3).

the frontal plane. In cervical flexion, rotation is the primary motion because of the orientation of the facet joints being more horizontal.

General Components of a Typical Cervical Vertebra (figure 7.4)

- Vertebral body
- Spinous process
- Transverse process
- Facet joint
- Intervertebral foramen
- Spinal canal
- Lamina
- Pedicle
- Intervertebral disc: nucleus pulposus and annulus fibrosus (see figure 3.1b)

Vertebral Artery

This anatomical structure is very important because it supplies blood to the upper part of the spinal cord, brainstem, cerebellum, and part of the brain. The vertebral artery originates from the subclavian artery; it enters between the transverse processes of C6/C7 and immediately turns cephalad through the transverse foramina of C6, continues vertically, and exits through the transverse

process of the atlas (C1), where it acutely turns in a posterior direction over the posterior arch of the atlas before entering the foramen magnum, where it joins the opposite vertebral artery to become the basilar artery.

The reason for mentioning this artery is that during cervical spine rotation (without pathology) it can narrow as much as 80%–90% on the side contralateral (opposite) to the side of rotation. This narrowing may be exacerbated during extension of the cervical spine. The vertebral artery is at risk due to the acute angle change at C6/7 and especially at the atlanto-occipital region before the artery enters the foramen magnum.

It is recommended that prior to any type of manual therapy for the cervical spine, the practitioner uses provocative diagnostic tests that can ascertain the integrity of the vertebral artery. One such test is DeKleyn's test (see page 107).

Neurological Anatomy of the Cervical Spine

There are eight cervical nerves that exit the cervical spine. C1–C4 will exit through the

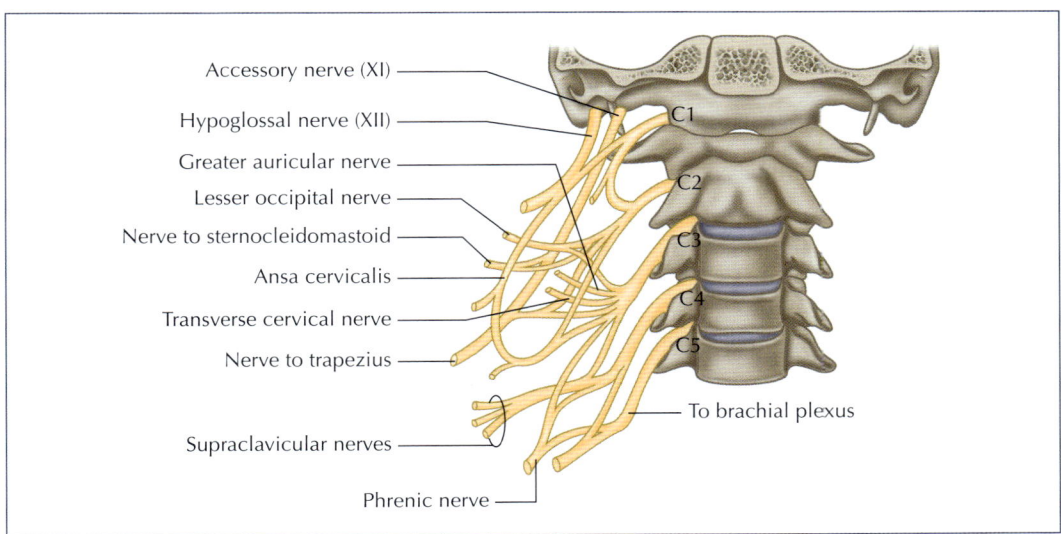

Figure 7.5. Anatomy of the cervical plexus and the levels of the exiting nerve roots.

cervical plexus (figure 7.5) and C5–T1 will exit through the brachial plexus. However, there are only seven cervical vertebrae.

The first (C1) through the seventh (C7) cervical nerves exit above the level of the cervical vertebra with the corresponding number (e.g., C1 nerve exits above the level of C1 vertebra), while the eighth cervical nerve exits below the seventh cervical vertebra and above the first thoracic vertebra (C8 nerve exits between the levels of C7 and T1). The first thoracic nerve (T1 nerve root) then exits below the first thoracic vertebra (the T1 nerve root exits between the levels of T1 and T2).

If you have disc pathology between C5 and C6, then the exiting nerve root of C6 could be contacted by the disc pathology. However, if you have disc pathology in the lumbar spine between the levels of L4 and L5, it will be the L4 exiting nerve root that is affected because the nerve exits at the level below in the lumbar

(and thoracic) spine, rather than the level above as in the cervical spine.

Brachial Plexus

The brachial plexus is composed of nerves emanating from the four lower cervical vertebrae and the first thoracic vertebra (nerves C5–T1). The brachial plexus passes through the space that is formed between scalenus anterior and scalenus medius, known as the *interscalene triangle* (figure 7.6). The nerve roots of C5 and C6 join to form the upper trunk. The nerve roots of C8 and T1 join to form the lower trunk. C7 does not join with any other nerve root; it alone makes up the middle trunk.

As the trunks pass beneath the clavicle, they divide to form cords. The upper and lower trunks contribute to the middle trunk to form the posterior cord. The middle trunk, in turn, sends a contribution with C5 and C6 to form the

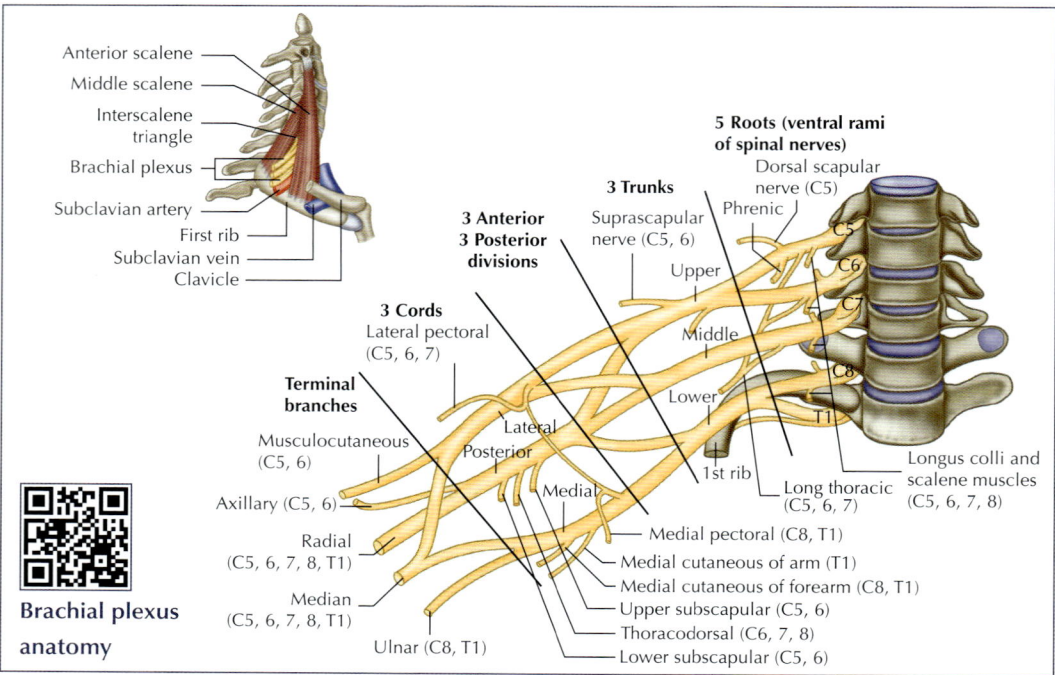

Figure 7.6. Anatomy of the brachial plexus.

lateral cord. The remainder of C8 and T1 form the medial cord.

Branches now continue, emanating from the cords: The lateral cord sends one branch to become the musculocutaneous nerve. The other branch of the lateral cord joins with a branch from the medial cord to form the median nerve. The second branch of the medial cord becomes the ulnar nerve, and the posterior cord becomes the axillary and radial nerves.

Cervical Intervertebral Discs

As explained in chapter 3, between adjacent vertebrae there is a structure known as an intervertebral disc. A disc is made up of three components: a tough outer shell, the annulus fibrosus;

an inner gel-like substance in the center, the nucleus pulposus; and an attachment to the vertebral bodies, the vertebral end plate. As we age, the center of the disc starts to lose water content, a process that will make the disc less elastic and less effective as a cushion or shock absorber.

The ratio of disc height to vertebral body height in the cervical spine is approximately 2:5, meaning cervical discs are the thickest of all the 23 intervertebral discs in the spinal column relative to their vertebrae. The cervical discs are wedge shaped, which assists in maintaining the cervical lordosis. The cervical discs are slightly thicker anteriorly than posteriorly.

Cervical nerve roots exit the spinal canal through small passageways between the vertebrae and the discs known as intervertebral foramina. Pain and other symptoms can develop when a damaged disc pushes into the spinal canal or nerve roots—a condition commonly referred to as a herniated disc.

In a severe disc herniation the bulging tissue may press against one or more of the spinal nerves, which can cause local and referred pain, numbness, or weakness to the cervical spine as well as to the upper limb, arm, and hand (see figure 3.4).

Approximately 85%–95% of cervical spine disc herniations occur at the cervical segments C4–C5, C5–C6, or C6–C7; the nerve compression caused by contact with the disc contents may result in perceived pain along the C5, C6, or C7 nerve root pathway (figure 7.7).

Cervical Spine Facet Joints

Located within the cervical spine are the facet joints (figure 7.8). These structures can be responsible for provoking a lot of pain, especially to the region of the shoulder, and in some instances it can radiate into the arm and hand.

The facet joints lie posteriorly and laterally to the vertebral body, and their role is to assist the spine in performing movements such as flexion, extension, side bending, and rotation. Depending on their location and orientation, these joints will allow certain types of motion but restrict others: for example, rotation is freely permitted in

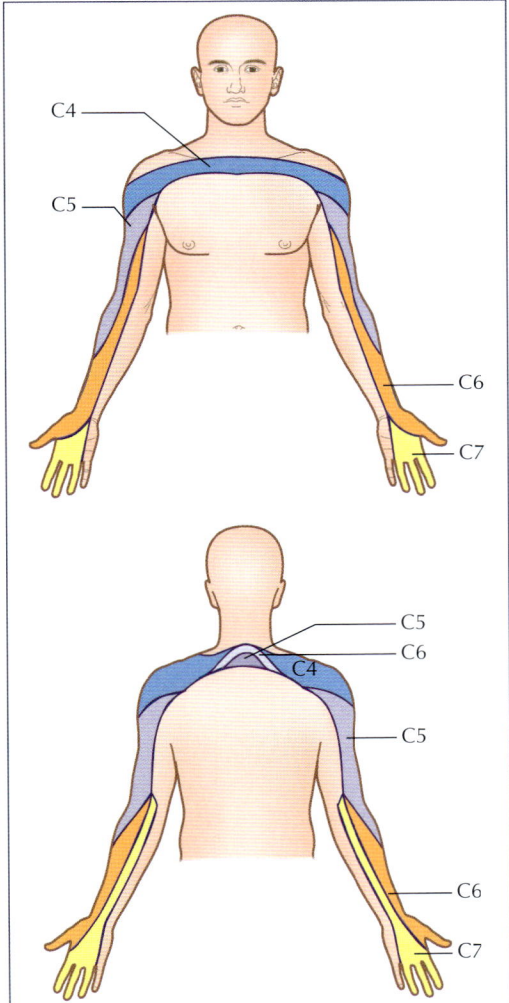

Figure 7.7. C4, C5, C6, and C7 dermatome pain pattern.

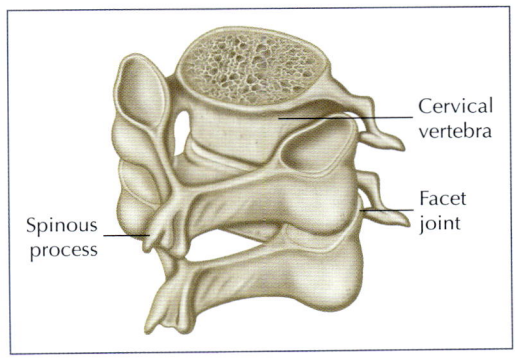

Figure 7.8. Cervical spine facet joint.

the cervical spine, but there is less range in lateral flexion.

Each individual vertebra has two facet joints on each side: the superior articular facet faces upward and articulates with the inferior facet of the vertebra above, and the inferior articular facet articulates with the superior facet of the vertebra below. The C4 inferior facet, for example, articulates with the C5 superior facet. The facet joint works similarly to a hinge.

Like all synovial joints in the body, each facet joint is surrounded by a capsule of connective tissue and produces synovial fluid to nourish and lubricate the joint. The articular surfaces of the joint are coated with cartilage, which helps the joint to move (articulate) smoothly. The facet joint is highly innervated with pain receptors, making it susceptible to producing neck, shoulder, and arm pain.

Many of my patients have had cervical facet joint injections (guided through ultrasound) in spinal pain clinics before they have come to me to see if these structures are responsible for their shoulder pain. If the injection reduced the symptoms for the patient, the doctor confirms a facet joint as the possible causative factor.

However, in my opinion, if the patient has experienced ongoing neck and shoulder pain, it is probably the result of many small musculoskeletal manifestations that have caused long-term dysfunctional changes over the preceding years, and

these small inconsequential changes have slowly become a larger problem.

Here is an analogy that might fit the description for these and other patients. Everyone has a reservoir of compensation; for some people it is the size of a large lake that will never run dry because it contains so much water—for these people, their body will always be able to compensate, no matter what the problem. You will know friends and athletes like this who can participate in every sport, do everyday tasks, and never complain of pain. However, for most patients, the lake is a lot smaller, contains less water, and is slowly starting to dry up because of a continuous hot spell. For these people, their body struggles to compensate, and this could be the reason for their presenting symptoms. For example, a friend of yours has been a runner for 20 years, running three times a week, and mentions to you that, suddenly, in the last two months, their knee, or hip, or foot (or any other body part) has become painful. Why? Quite possibly, because their reservoir of compensation is starting to dry up.

It is considered that most shoulder and arm pain is directly or indirectly related to the cervical spine, and so I would like to discuss briefly some very common musculoskeletal structures that can be responsible for the pain perceived in the upper limb. Most of these pathologies are contraindications for spinal manipulative techniques, although spinal mobilizations would probably still be recommended.

Facet Joint Syndrome/Disease

Facet joints tend to slide over each other, so are in constant motion with the spine, and like all types of weight-bearing joint, they can simply wear out and start to degenerate over time.

When facet joints become irritated (the cartilage can even tear), this will cause the bone underneath the facet joint to start producing osteophytes, leading to facet joint hypertrophy—the precursor of facet joint syndrome/disease (figure 7.9)—this eventually leads to spondylosis, in its purest form, osteoarthritis (OA) of the spine. This type of disease process is very common in older patients presenting with chronic neck and shoulder pain.

Unfortunately, sooner for some than others, age typically comes with some natural degenerative changes, and certain areas of the human body, such as the hip and knee, are particularly likely to suffer. That is also true for the lower three components of the cervical spine (C4/5, C5/6, and C6/7). In the spine, we call this spondylosis (*spondyl* means "of the spine" and *osis* means "abnormal or diseased condition"). Spondylosis generally affects the vertebral bodies as well as the facet joints.

The intervertebral (neural) foramina where the nerves exit can eventually narrow owing to the underlying pathology and cause painful symptoms.

Case Study

A 72-year-old female came to the clinic with generalized aching to both shoulders, especially in the morning upon waking. This ache would settle down after about 20 minutes, and she found that having a hot bath or shower would reduce some of her symptoms. Her active range of cervical rotation was limited, especially to the left, and she kept saying that her neck "just feels stiff all the time."

When I performed passive rotation to her cervical spine in a supine position, her motion was still very restricted and uncomfortable. Surprisingly, the deep tendon reflexes (DTRs) and specific myotome power testing for the cervical spine all tested normal. Her trapezius muscles felt exquisitely tender and very rigid on palpation; however, she felt a good massage would be of benefit.

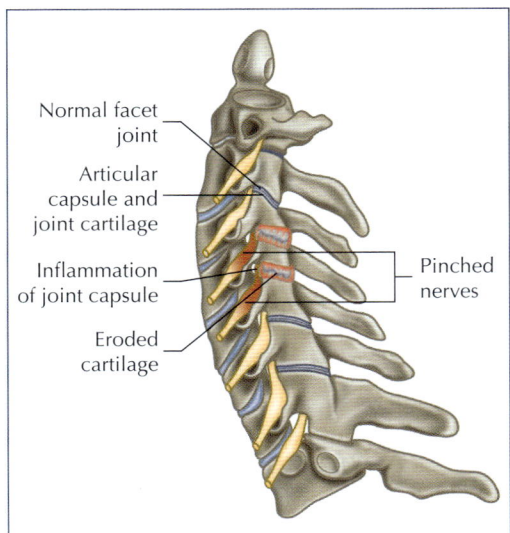

Normal facet joint

Articular capsule and joint cartilage

Inflammation of joint capsule

Eroded cartilage

Pinched nerves

Figure 7.9. Facet joint syndrome and cervical spondylosis.

I mentioned to her that I considered she had degenerative changes, and a week later, an MRI scan proved that she had multilevel disc dehydration and degeneration to the vertebral bodies and facet joints with osteophytic changes (bony spurs), especially to the lower three bodies of the cervical spine.

With regard to treatment strategy, the patient asked me if I was going to manipulate her neck (using an HVT), and I said that under the circumstances, and especially since there are bony spurs and multilevel degenerative changes present, these techniques were not appropriate and potentially very dangerous.

I told the patient that I would never be able to *fix* her neck because of what was shown on the scan; however, I recommended some soft-tissue techniques, gentle mobilizations, and METs to correct some of the shortened muscular tissues, as well as some postural reeducation exercises.

Some of the techniques I performed are covered later in this chapter.

Motion of the Cervical Spine

The cervical spine is capable of motion through all three axes/planes of movement, allowing flexion/extension in the sagittal plane, side bending in the frontal plane, and rotation in the transverse plane. Circumduction is also possible as a gross movement, through the summation of the other movements, although this is not recommended. The extent of these movements that is possible varies through the cervical spine owing to the shape of the facet joints, which assist in guiding the movements for the different spinal cervical segments and provide different emphasis of motion at different levels.

Motion of the Atlanto-Axial Joint

The AAJ is a pivot joint, and around 50% of the rotation (left or right) of the cervical spine is from the atlas, C1, rotating on the axis, C2 (figure 7.10), with this motion occurring 500–600 times daily. If we consider a normal range of motion for cervical rotation is approximately 80°, then 40° of that movement will occur between the levels of C1 and C2.

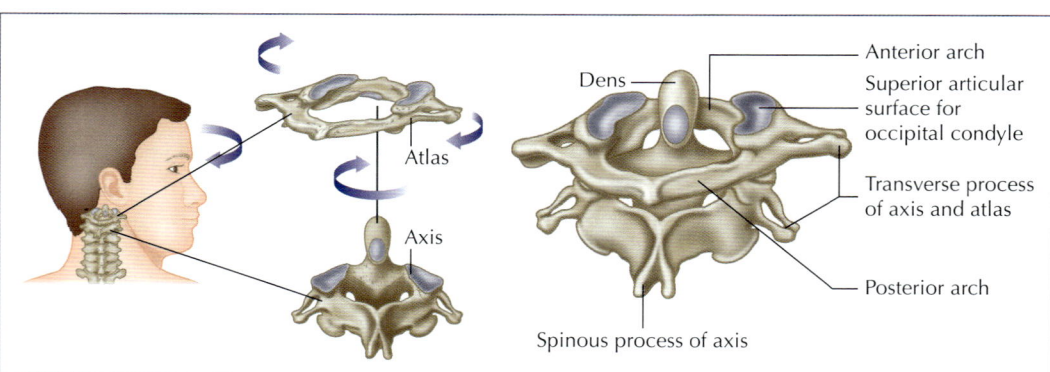

Figure 7.10. C1 motion on C2.

Assessment of the Cervical Spine

You will need to ascertain whether you consider the cervical spine to be involved in the symptoms for the patient's presenting shoulder pain.

Initially ask the patient to perform simple movements of rotation, flexion, extension, and side bending to see if these exacerbate the shoulder symptoms. If they perform one of these motions and feel an increase in symptoms in the cervical spine or shoulder region, it's reasonable to say that it requires further investigation and subsequent treatment.

Active Range of Motion (AROM)

Ask the patient to sit on a couch and to rotate their neck to the right and then to the left as far as they are comfortably able. Note if they feel any symptoms, restriction, or pain anywhere, focusing on their shoulder, arm, and hand (figure 7.11).

Then ask the patient to slowly flex their neck by bringing the chin toward their chest and then to extend their neck by slowly looking up toward the ceiling, once again mentioning if they feel any symptoms (figure 7.12).

Next, ask the patient to side bend (laterally flex) their neck by bringing the right ear down toward their right shoulder and to repeat on the other side, again noting if they feel any symptoms (figure 7.13).

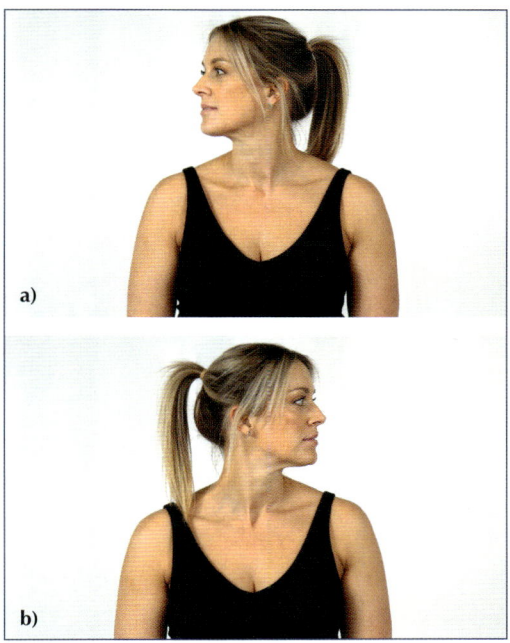

Figure 7.11. Patient rotates their neck to the right (a), and then to the left (b).

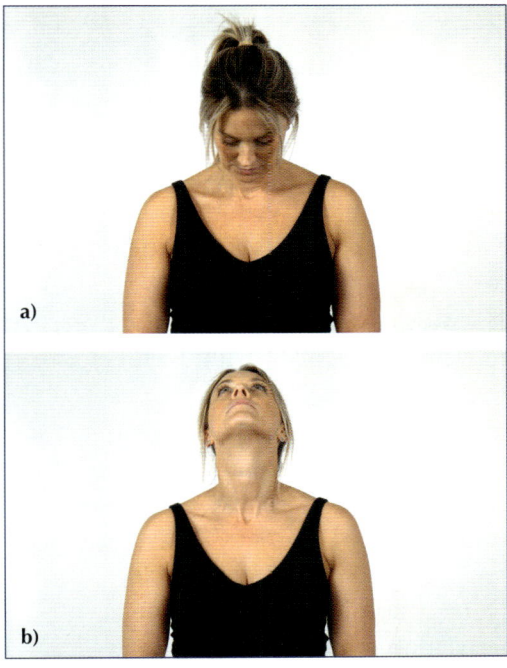

Figure 7.12. Patient flexes (a) and extends (b) their neck.

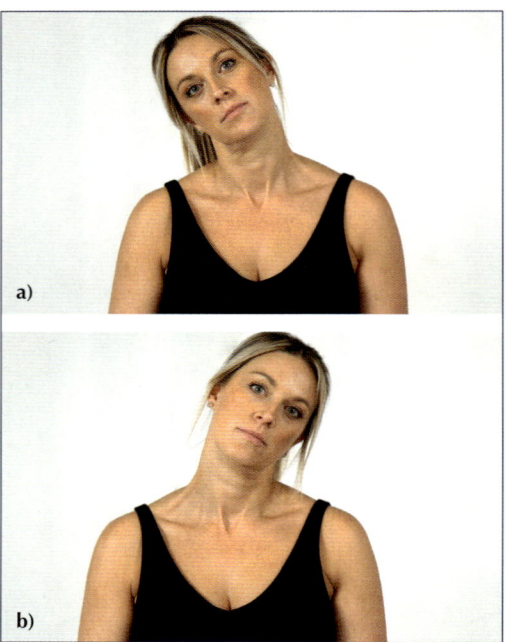

Figure 7.13. Patient side bends their neck to the right (a) and to the left (b).

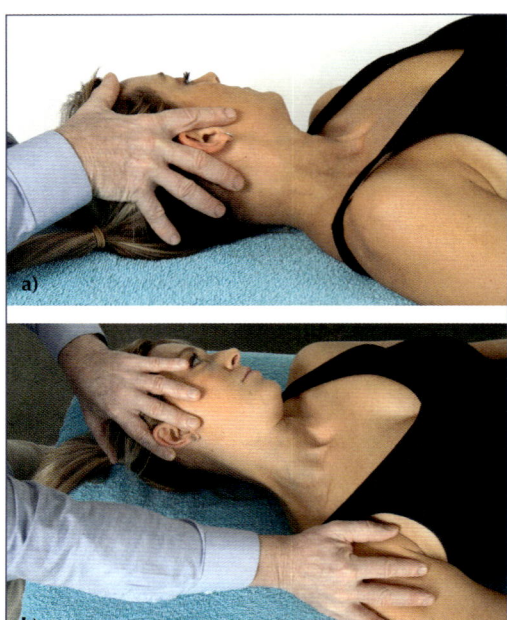

Figure 7.14. PROM for the cervical spine: (a) rotation; (b) lateral flexion.

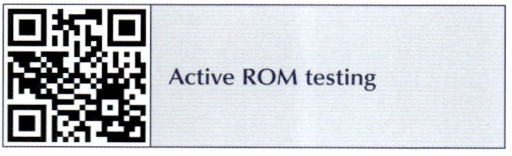

Active ROM testing

Passive Range of Motion (PROM)

It is possible to perform all the above movements passively with the therapist in the sitting position; however, the movements are typically done with the patient in the supine position. Figure 7.14 shows a couple of examples of passive rotation and passive lateral flexion.

Note: If the patient has any pain or restriction on the active movements but is pain-free when these movements are performed passively, this generally indicates the soft tissues of the muscles and tendons are involved in the pathology.

If, on the other hand, active and passive movements both cause increased symptoms to the patient, then one can assume that the cervical spinal joints are involved and will need further investigation.

Let me give you a couple of examples.

A 20-year-old patient has strained one of their neck muscles, so that when they rotate their neck to the left or right, they are aware of the pain. However, if I passively rotate their neck, the movement is almost pain-free.

A 65-year-old patient has confirmed degenerative cervical spondylosis (OA). When they rotate their neck to the left or right, it is very stiff, restrictive, and painful at certain ranges. If I passively rotate this patient's neck to the right and to the left,

I also feel the restrictive motion because of the underlying degenerative changes to the joints, and the patient is more than likely aware of some discomfort during the passive motions.

 Passive ROM testing

Passive Motion Testing of the Cervical Spine at C3–C7 (Translation Test)

Passive motion testing of the cervical spine, which can identify *facet restriction*, is known as the *translation test.* Osteopaths, in particular, have devised this specific motion test so that they can accurately identify which level of the cervical spine will require treatment.

The test is very simple and rather elegant: You start with your patient in a supine position and the cervical spine in neutral. Using your fingertips, you gently glide each vertebra from right to left and repeat from left to right along the horizontal plane. Simply speaking, if you find a vertebra is capable of gliding in one direction but not the other, you have discovered a facet restriction.

Next, you gently forward bend (flex) and backward bend (extend) your patient's head and repeat the process of gliding from one side to the other. What you feel will indicate any underlying restrictive tissue and the specific facet joint involved.

For example, when you hold your patient's neck in the forward bending position while you translate the vertebra, you are testing to see if the facet joints will open. If there are no facet restrictions, the facets will open and you will be able to translate the vertebra from left to right and right to left.

However, if you find that you can translate from left to right but not from right to left in forward bending, then you have discovered *fixed closed* facets that will not permit translation movements. Likewise, when you place your patient's neck in a backward bending position of extension and repeat the process of translation, you are testing whether the facets can close. If you find you can translate from left to right, however, and feel resistance from right to left, you have discovered *fixed open* facets that will not allow the necessary translation motion.

The absence of translation motion indicates the location of the facet restriction. In flexion, the facet restriction is on the opposite side to the motion restriction, and in extension the facet restriction is the same side as the motion restriction. This may sound odd but makes sense once you understand the logic of the test and the type 2 coupled movement biomechanics of C3 to C7 mentioned in chapter 6.

Before you concern yourself with the logic of the test and how to determine which side the facet restriction is, you must first learn the difference between a *facet restriction* and a *motion restriction*.

A facet restriction is the simple cause of a motion restriction. If you cannot translate a cervical vertebra in one direction, this is because of a facet restriction. Therefore, you will find facet restrictions in the cervical spine by feeling for motion restrictions and not by how the vertebra appears to de-rotate, as you would with the lumbar spine.

Remember this distinction. Your reference point is from motion restriction and NOT from rotation.

To understand what translation is and how it works, ask your patient to lie on the couch in a supine position with their head and neck in a neutral position, resting on the couch. There is no need to flex or extend the patient's neck, but rather try to develop a feel for the translation motion.

Let's start by translating C3 on the underlying level of C4. To do this, place the tips of your index and middle fingers on either side of the articular pillar of C3, or you can use the transverse process (TP). However, these landmarks can be exquisitely tender to palpate, so be careful. Use your palms and thenar eminences to stabilize and hold the upper part of the cervical spine and the head (figure 7.15).

Using the whole of your hands to stabilize the head and neck, perform the translation motion from left to right and then right to left along the horizontal plane. Be very careful to ensure you introduce motion back and forth along the horizontal plane with no side bending of your client's neck. The neck and C3 will automatically side bend as a result of moving sideways, so if you inadvertently side bend your client's neck to start with, you will get a false reading.

Using the sensitivity in your fingertips, try to feel if you have easier movement in

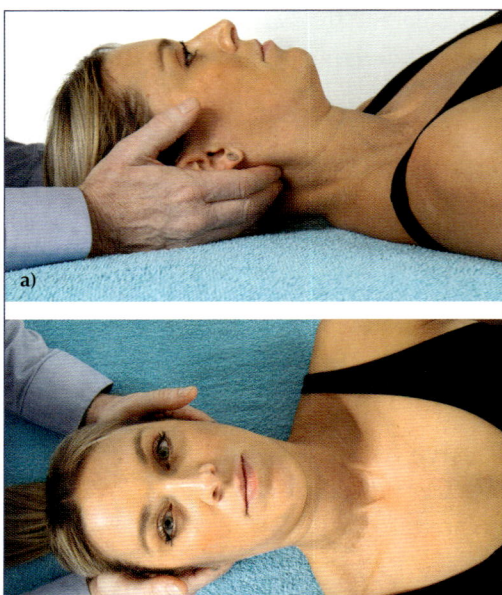

Figure 7.15. (a) Therapist cradling the cervical spine in a neutral position. (b) Overhead view of the hand placement of the therapist's hands.

one direction, either left to right or right to left. If it feels equal, try C4 and repeat the process until you can clearly feel a restriction of a vertebra. It takes time to develop a feel for this, and you may even find that some vertebrae don't translate (move sideways) at all. Ignore these and try to find one that is clearly easier to translate in one direction than in the other.

When you feel comfortable and can confidently translate C3 to C7 without inadvertently introducing side bending into your motion, you can try the next stage of translation: forward bending (flexion) of the cervical spine.

Prop your elbows on the table and carefully cradle and stabilize your patient's head and cervical vertebra at C3

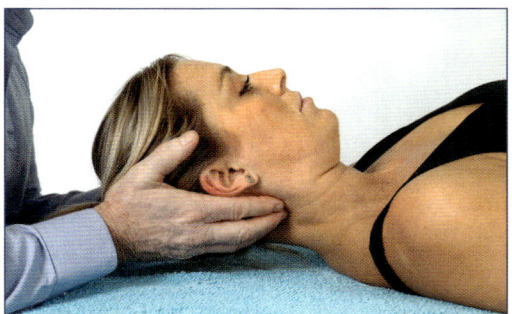

Figure 7.16. Therapist cradling the cervical spine in a flexed position.

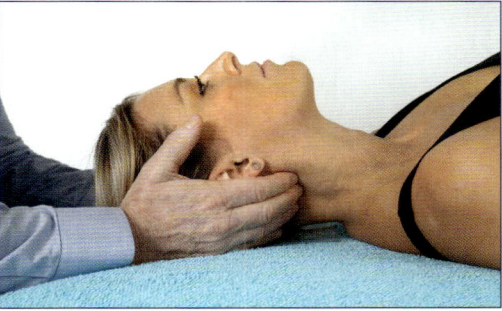

Figure 7.17. Therapist cradling the cervical spine in a backward bending (extension) position.

with your palms and thenar eminences the same as before, but this time carefully lifting the head off the table (figure 7.16). Having your arms propped up on your elbows will help take the effort out of supporting your client's head and holding it still. Many people struggle to relax and relinquish control of their head, and the more stable the platform, the more they will relax. You may prefer to use a face cradle as a head support to help you.

In a flexed position, stabilize the head and C1–C2 with your palms and thenar eminences and translate from left to right and right to left as before. Let's assume you have found a motion restriction from *left to right* and the translation from right to left tested normal. In flexion, this means the motion restriction is located on the *right* (opposite side). At this stage, we are not concerned with which side has a fixed facet, just with being able to feel it.

Now let's try translating in the backward (extended) position. To achieve an easy extension of the neck, simply slide the lateral edge of your forefinger under

the neck and gently push in an anterior direction while you simultaneously and gently push your client's head in an inferior position (figure 7.17).

Again, translate across the horizontal plane, feeling for a restriction in one direction. If the motion test shows a vertebra to translate from right to left but not *left to right*, then the motion restriction is located on the *left* (same side).

Practice translation from C3 to C7 in both flexion and extension until you are confident that you can locate each individual vertebra and feel if it has a free or restricted motion.

As you practice on a few different patients, you will be amazed at the vast differences between people. Some necks will be very flexible, with soft and supple tissues, and yet still show facet restrictions. Other necks will feel very tight and inflexible but be equal in motion testing with no facet restrictions. Experience will teach you that we are all different and what is restriction in one individual is a normal range in another.

Now you have some familiarity with translation, let's look a little more closely at motion testing and the information you can glean from it.

As we know, translation automatically introduces some side bending and rotation to the same side. Since side bending and rotation are always coupled to the same side in the neck (except for C1), if you know which way the vertebra cannot side bend, you also know which way it cannot rotate. Regardless of whether you translate your client's head in flexion or extension, if C3 can translate from right to left but not from left to right, you know that the vertebra is *right side bent* and *right rotated*, with fixed facets somewhere that are preventing left side bending and left rotation.

Suppose in forward bending you can translate C3 from right to left but it feels restricted from left to right. The discovery of a motion restriction on the right means that C3 is right side bent and right rotated on C4, and that C3 cannot left side bend and left rotate. Since you are testing in forward flexion, you also know that you have discovered fixed closed facets. So, since C3 has fixed closed facets and is right side bent and right rotated, you know the fixed closed facets must be on the *right side*. The terminology for this dysfunction is ERS(r), which means C3 is fixed closed on C4 in extension, rotation, and side bending (ERS) to the right side, indicating something has interfered with the right facet joint opening. This means the *motion restriction* is flexion, left rotation, and left side bending.

Let us suppose that you test another client's neck, but this time you have tested in extension and have found a motion restriction on the left. C3 translates easily from right to left but not from left to right. This tells you that C3 is right side bent and right rotated on C4, and the facets must be fixed open on the *left side*, known as an FRS(r), meaning the vertebra has flexed, rotated, and side bent to the right, but it is the *left* facet that is fixed in an open position. This means the *motion restriction* is extension, left rotation, and left side bending.

Two simple rules immediately emerge from this exercise:

- When you translate in flexion and meet a motion restriction, the facets are fixed closed on the *opposite side* to the motion restriction.
- When you translate in extension (backward bending) and meet a restriction, the facets are fixed open on the *same side* as the motion restriction.

This is quite different from, and shouldn't be confused with, testing for the thoracic and lumbar spine. Remember you are deducing where the cervical facet restriction is, having first determined the motion restriction.

In the cervical spine, you deduce that the fixed closed facets are on the same side as the rotation and the fixed open facets are on the same side as the motion restriction. With cervical translation, the reference point is the side to which the facet fixation is either the opposite or the same side, and this is reversed in relation to the forward and back bending test for the thoracic and lumbar spines.

If there are no fixed closed facets, when you forward bend (flex) your patient's cervical spine, *all* the facets will open, and when you translate from side to side you will not meet any motion restriction. Therefore, if you translate in forward flexion and meet a motion restriction, this simply tells you the facet joints are stuck closed because you can only translate in this flexed position with the facets open.

If there are no fixed open facets, when you backward bend (extend) your patient's cervical spine, *all* the facets will close, and when you translate from side to side you will not meet any motion restriction. Therefore, if you translate in extension and meet a motion restriction, this simply tells you the facet joints are stuck open as you can only translate in this extended position with the facets closed.

Summary

If translation reveals a motion restriction in backward bending (extension) of the cervical spine, the facets are fixed or stuck open on the same side as the motion restriction. If translation reveals a motion restriction in forward bending (flexion), the facets are fixed closed on the opposite side to the motion restriction.

I use two abbreviations to help me to remember this procedure:

FOC: Flexion, opposite, and closed

For example: When you translate from left to right with the patient in a flexed

position and you feel a restriction, it will be a FOC—so the opposite side (right) is fixed closed.

ESO: Extension, same, and open

For example: When you translate from left to right with the patient in an extended position and you feel a restriction, it will be an ESO—so the same side (left) is fixed open.

Motion testing cervical spine using translation test

Special Tests

There are numerous tests that we can incorporate, and we should already have a good idea if the cervical spine is involved with the patient's presenting upper limb symptoms. Below are some examples I use in clinic.

In terms of cervical spine and special tests, I would consider one of the best ways of assessing the cervical spine is using the C5–C7 reflexes, as well as individual power testing of the specific spinal myotomes and sensory testing through the dermatomes. These specific testing procedures should have already been included with the physical therapist's initial training, and I would expect them to be conducted on every patient who presents with any type of cervical, shoulder, or arm pain.

However, there are also some extra specific tests we can include to help with the overall diagnosis, and these are included here.

Spurling's Compression Test

This test for cervical nerve root pain was first described in 1944 by Roy Spurling and William Scoville, two US neurosurgeons, and a few variations of the procedure were described in 2012 by Anekstein et al. They suggested that a maneuver consisting of extension and lateral bending, which reproduced the patient's complaints in a tolerable fashion, be conducted first, followed by addition of axial compression in the case of an inconclusive effect. The test has also been called the foraminal compression test, the neck compression test, and the quadrant test, and it is considered to be highly specific as a provocation test for spinal assessment.

This test is performed with the patient in a sitting position, and the therapist guides their head into extension and lateral flexion (figure 7.18). If there are no symptoms reproduced, then the therapist gently applies a downward pressure to

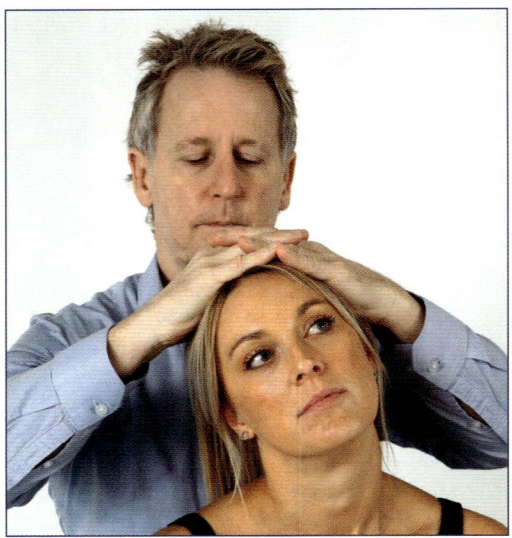

Figure 7.19. The therapist applies a downward pressure on top of the patient's head.

the top of the patient's head (figure 7.19). A positive sign is when the patient complains of pain that radiates into their shoulder or arm (dermatome).

Spurling's test

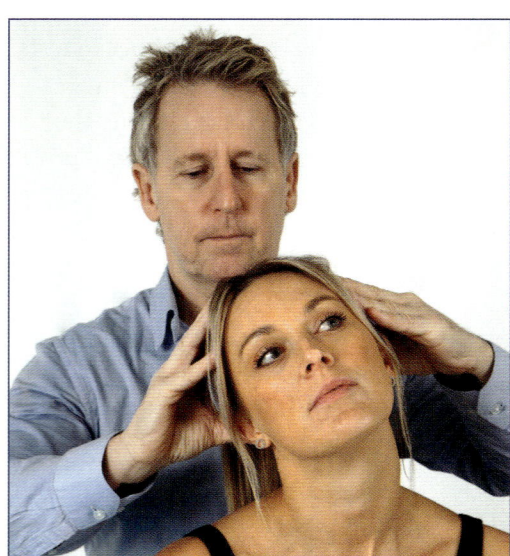

Figure 7.18. The patient extends and side bends their neck to the right.

Valsalva Maneuver

This test is named after Antonio Maria Valsalva, a physician specializing in the human ear. The Valsalva maneuver is used in diving to equalize pressure within the middle ear for descent.

With regard to the cervical spine and nerves, the Valsalva maneuver can increase spinal pressure, and the neural pain from any space-occupying lesion such as a disc prolapse can be exacerbated by increasing pressure (figure 7.20).

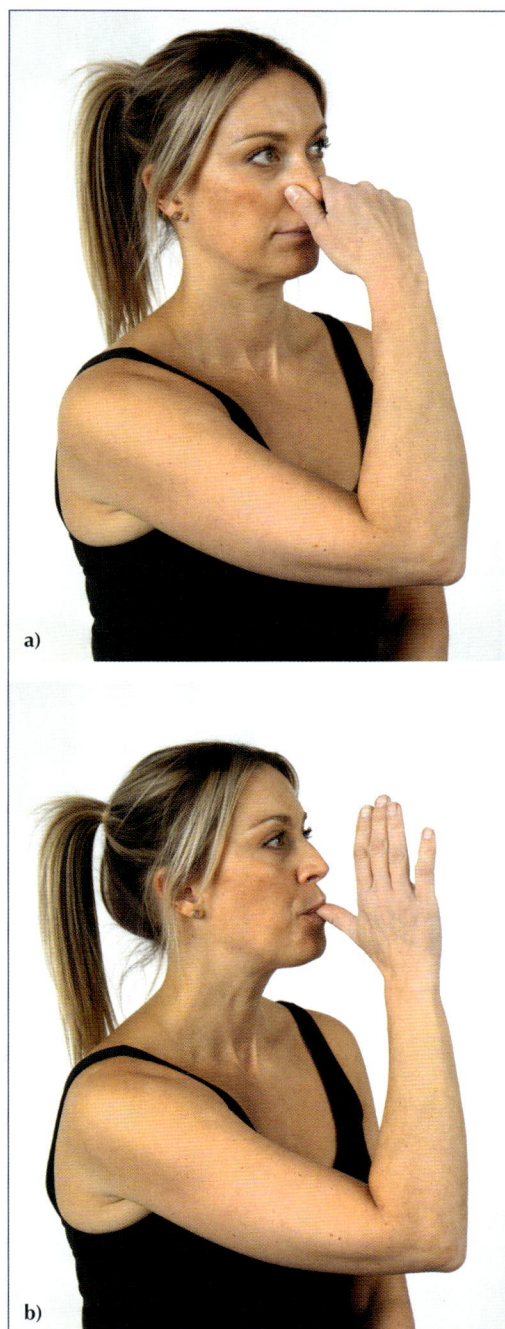

a)

b)

Figure 7.20. Valsalva maneuver: (a) the typical maneuver, trying to equalize the pressure within the ears by blowing out through the pinched nostrils; (b) an alternative method, either sucking the thumb or blowing out on the thumb.

DeKleyn's Test

As explained earlier, this provocation test is designed to ascertain the integrity of the vertebral artery. The practitioner must err on the side of caution when performing this test. It is also known as the vertebral basilar insufficiency (VBI) test.

With the patient supine, the practitioner controls the patient's head and slowly extends their head and neck over the end of a couch (figure 7.21). Next, the practitioner introduces rotation to the right (figure 7.22) and to the left (figure 7.23) and holds the head in each extended and rotated position for at

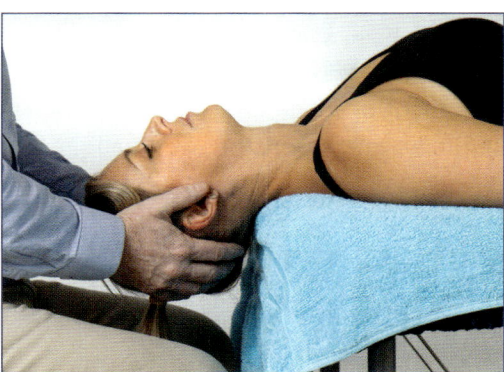

Figure 7.21. Practitioner controls the patient's head and neck into extension.

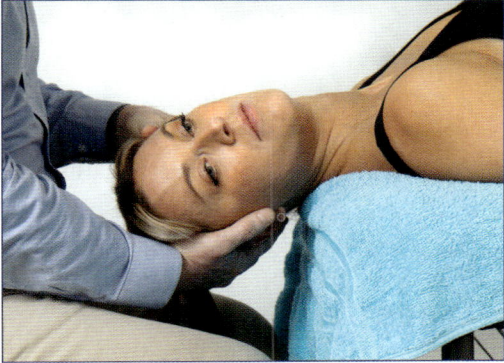

Figure 7.22. Practitioner rotates the patient's cervical spine to the right.

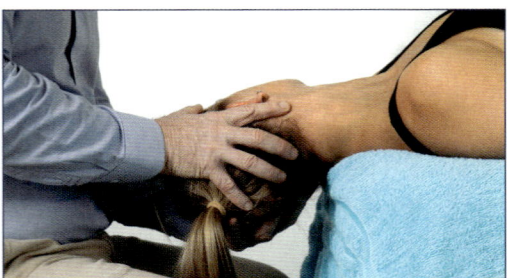

Figure 7.23. Practitioner rotates the patient's cervical spine to the left.

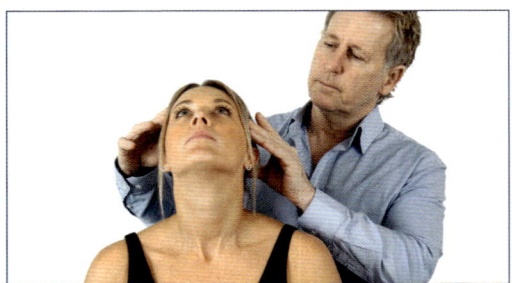

Figure 7.24. Patient is asked to look toward the ceiling.

least 30 seconds, while observing for any type of eye flickering, called *nystagmus*, due to a decrease in the blood flow of the opposite vertebral artery, and/or any symptoms such as nausea, dizziness, vertigo, and so on.

If any signs or symptoms are positive during this provocative evaluation test, the practitioner should stop immediately and recommend further investigations for potential vascular compromise.

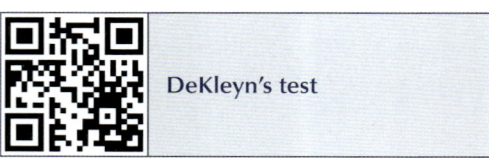

DeKleyn's test

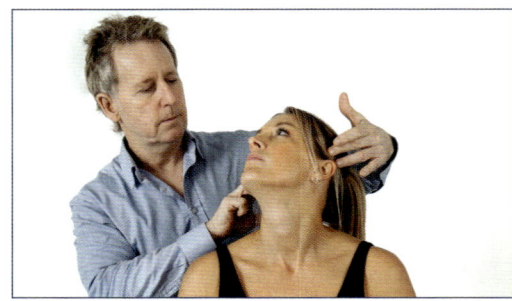

Figure 7.25. Patient rotates their cervical spine to the right.

Alternative Tests for VBI

These are another couple of recommended tests for VBI, which is more favored by some authors because the motion is controlled actively by the patient rather than passively by the practitioner as in DeKleyn's test.

The patient sits on a couch and the practitioner asks them to look toward the ceiling (figure 7.24) and from this position to look to the right (figure 7.25)

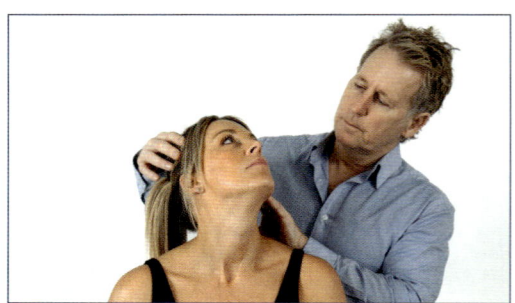

Figure 7.26. Patient rotates their cervical spine to the left.

and to the left (figure 7.26). The practitioner looks for any symptoms detailed in the previous test.

There is another procedure similar to the one above named Hautant's test, the difference being that the patient is asked to flex their shoulder to 90° with arms supinated and to extend the cervical spine (figure 7.27).

If there are no signs or symptoms with the cervical spine in extension, the patient is asked to rotate their cervical spine to the right (figure 7.28) and if a lowering of the opposite arm is seen it is classified as a positive test. If this test is negative the patient is asked to rotate the cervical spine to the left (figure 7.29), and if one observes

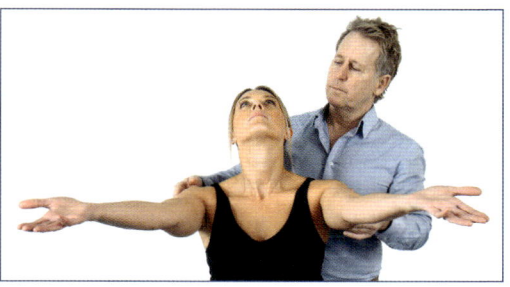

Figure 7.27. Patient is asked to flex shoulders to 90° with supination of the forearm and to look toward the ceiling.

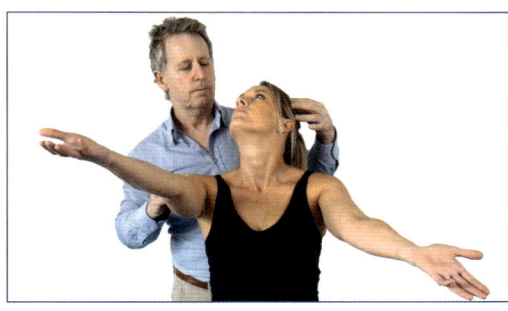

Figure 7.28. Patient rotates their cervical spine to the right and the left arm is seen to drop.

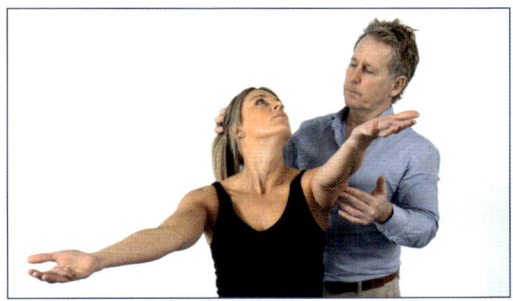

Figure 7.29. Patient rotates their cervical spine to the left and the right arm is seen to drop.

a lowering of the opposite arm, the test is classified as positive.

Please note: The test is positive if the patient reports dizziness or vertigo or the practitioner observes a lowering of the patient's arm. If the test is positive, naturally the test is stopped immediately as this potentially signifies a compromised vertebral arterial supply to the brainstem and vertebrobasilar system.

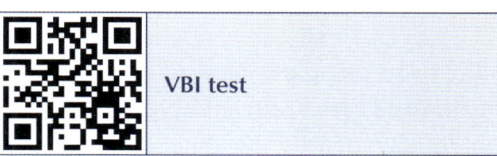

VBI test

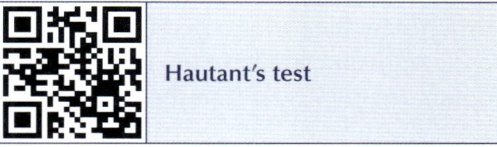

Hautant's test

Assessment of the AAJ

When you passively rotate the cervical spine in a neutral position, how would you know you are focusing the assessment purely on the AAJ? In reality, you are ascertaining only passive range of motion for the whole of the cervical spine, because this is simply a general passive range of motion testing and not specific for the AAJ.

One technique I use works exceptionally well because I feel I can ascertain motion of the AAJ. From here, the therapist can treat the AAJ as well as any restriction that occurs.

With the patient supine, initially you gain a general view of the passive range available by gently rotating the head to the left and to the right, as this will identify any possible restriction within the cervical spine.

Next, you take the cervical spine into approximately 30°–40° of flexion. This motion will pretension the ligamentum nuchae, and tensioning this ligament will restrict the lower cervical spine from rotating, allowing the AAJ to rotate relatively freely.

When you rotate the cervical spine in flexion and feel a restriction, you can now potentially identify the issue as being located within the AAJ. For example, if you rotate the patient's cervical spine to the right and you have full range of motion (figure 7.30a), and then rotate

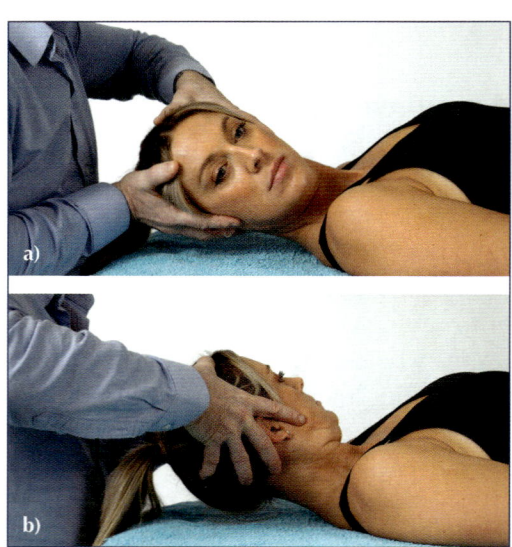

Figure 7.30. (a) Therapist places the cervical spine into flexion and rotates the cervical spine to the right, indicating a normal range of motion for the AAJ; (b) Therapist places the cervical spine into flexion and rotates the cervical spine to the left, indicating a right restriction of the AAJ.

the patient's cervical spine to the left side and you feel a restriction, I would consider the restricted side is on the right, therefore the dysfunction is located on the opposite side to the side you are rotating to (figure 7.30b).

Assessment of the AAJ

Treatment of the Cervical Spine

The following treatment techniques demonstrated for the cervical spine (plus the rest of the spinal column and pelvis) will be a mixture of METs, mobilizations, and manipulations. We will start with METs that are classified as soft-tissue techniques, although I will show you how to use them to specifically mobilize the spinal column. I will also explain and demonstrate HVT techniques. For further reading on METs, read *Muscle Energy Techniques* by Gibbons (2022).

The techniques demonstrated for the cervical spine are generally mobilizations; however, these techniques can be adapted and modified so that a gentle thrust can be incorporated, as demonstrated shortly.

General Treatment Techniques

The first treatment protocol I suggest for the cervical spine is through the simple use of an MET, because naturally this technique is the safest option and can be very effective.

There are two main effects of METs, and these are explained by two distinct physiological processes:

- Post-isometric relaxation (PIR)
- Reciprocal inhibition (RI)

PIR results from neurological feedback through the spinal cord to the muscle itself when an isometric contraction is sustained, causing a reduction in tone of the muscle that has been contracted. This reduction in tone lasts for approximately 20–25 seconds, so you now have a perfect window of opportunity to improve the ROM, because during this relaxation period the tissues can be more easily moved to a new resting length.

When RI is employed, the reduction in tone relies on the physiological inhibitory effect of antagonists (opposite muscles) on the contraction of a muscle. When the motor neurons of the contracting agonist muscle receive excitatory impulses from the afferent pathway, the motor neurons of the opposing antagonist muscle receive inhibitory impulses at the same time, preventing contraction. It follows that contraction or extended stretch of the agonist muscle must elicit relaxation or inhibit the antagonist; however, a fast stretch of the agonist will facilitate a contraction of the same muscle (agonist) via the activation through the muscle spindles sensing the sudden change of length.

Note: When utilizing the MET, the resistance is usually 10%–20% effort applied from the patient, because typically they have some discomfort present, and you don't want to exacerbate their condition. The muscular contraction

is approximately 10 seconds, and the technique is generally performed three times, with the final position being maintained for approximately 25–30 seconds, so that the neurological system can maintain this new position.

Side Bending MET

This PIR technique will predominantly encourage lengthening of the muscles involved with cervical spine side bending and shoulder girdle elevation—the upper trapezius and levator scapulae muscles. This MET will encourage lengthening of the muscles but will also promote the cervical facet joints opening and closing; therefore, it can be classified as an articular technique as well as a soft-tissue technique.

Place the patient's left cervical spine into a right-side bending position until a point of bind is felt. From this position, ask the patient to take a breath in, and on the out breath ask them to either side bend the cervical spine to the left or elevate the left shoulder against a resistance for approximately 10 seconds. Alternatively, you can request the patient to perform both actions at the same time against your resistance (figure 7.31).

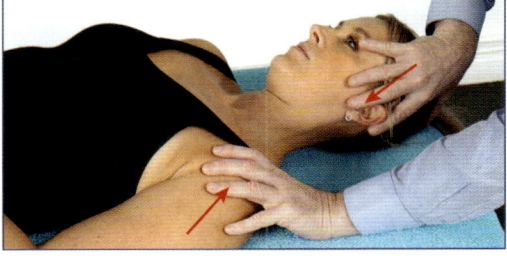

Figure 7.31. The patient is asked to side bend the cervical spine to the left, or elevate the left shoulder, or sometimes both.

Another way of communicating the technique is to ask the patient to bring their ear to their shoulder, or the shoulder to the ear, against a resistance, holding for 10 seconds. After the 10-second contraction, ask the patient to relax, take a breath in, and on the relaxation phase, the cervical spine is taken further into a right-side bend (figure 7.32). If the cervical side bending causes any discomfort, the shoulder can be taken into further depression, because this will also have the effect of lengthening the upper trapezius.

For an RI method, take complete control of the patient's cervical spine and shoulder as described above. From this position, ask the patient to reach slowly toward their lower left leg with their left hand, until a point of bind is felt (figure 7.33).

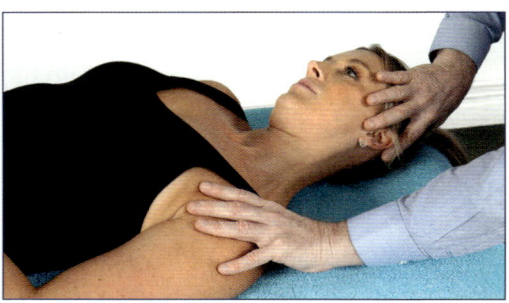

Figure 7.32. The therapist guides the cervical spine into right-side bending to lengthen the upper trapezius.

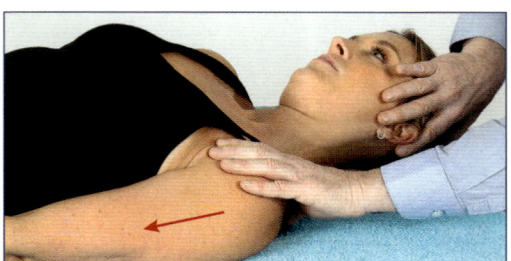

Figure 7.33. The patient is asked to depress the shoulder girdle, activating the lower trapezius; this will relax the upper trapezius through RI.

This approach will activate the lower trapezius, as the patient is causing a depression of the left shoulder girdle. This will induce an inhibition of the left upper trapezius, allowing a safe way of lengthening because it will override the activation of the muscle spindles.

Rotation MET

This PIR technique will predominantly encourage lengthening of the muscles involved with cervical spine rotation, including the SCM and scalene muscles.

With the patient in supine, gently rotate the patient's cervical spine into right rotation until a point of bind is felt. From this position, ask the patient to take a breath in, and on the out breath to rotate the cervical spine to the left against a resistance for 10 seconds (figure 7.34).

After the 10-second contraction, ask the patient to relax, take a breath in, and on the relaxation phase, you take the cervical spine further into right rotation (figure 7.35).

If an RI method would be preferable because the PIR method might cause some

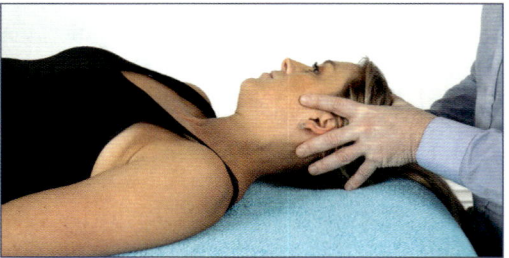

Figure 7.34. From a position of bind, the patient is asked to rotate to the left.

discomfort to the patient, from the position of bind, instead of asking the patient to rotate to the left against a resistance, ask them to rotate to the right (figure 7.36). This approach will activate the right rotators of the cervical spine and as above will induce an inhibition of the left cervical spine rotators, allowing a safe way of lengthening, as it will override the activation of the muscle spindles. After the 10 second contraction of the cervical spine to the right, the therapist encourages further right rotation.

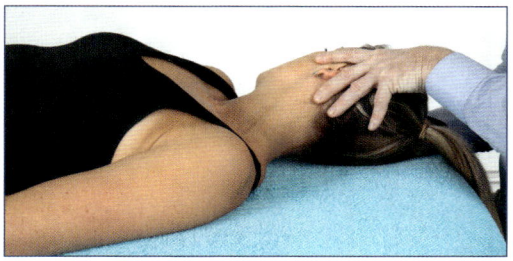

Figure 7.35. After the contraction the therapist passively encourages further right rotation.

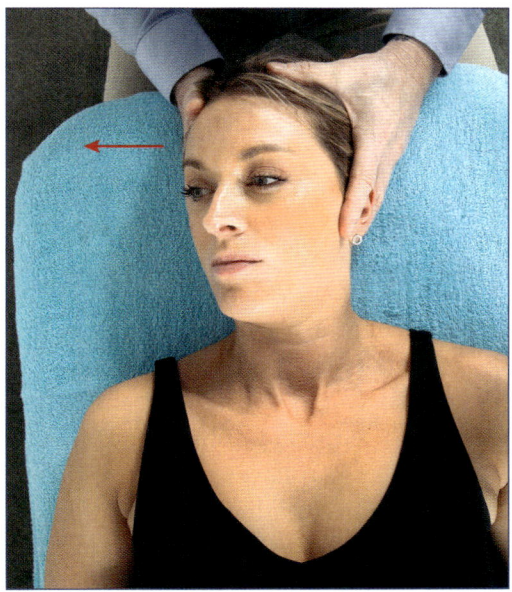

Figure 7.36. From the position of bind, the patient is asked to rotate the cervical spine to the right (RI).

MET treatment of cervical spine

Treatment of AAJ (C1/C2)

Diagnosis: Atlas Rotated Right

Motion restriction: The atlas is restricted to left rotation on the axis.

- With the patient supine, cradle their head with both hands and gently apply the second metacarpophalangeal (MCP) joint of your right hand and contact the posterior arch of the atlas, while your left hand is controlling the patient's head.
- Initially guide the cervical spine into approximately 30°–40° of flexion. This will reduce the mobility of the typical cervical vertebra because of the tensioning of the nuchal ligament.
- Slowly rotate the patient's neck to the left until you feel the restriction barrier.
- Next, fine-tune the position with a motion of right-side bending, flexion/extension, until there is a feeling of bind.
- From this position, ask the patient to look to the right (right rotation) for approximately 20% effort and for 10 seconds (figure 7.37).
- After the contraction and on the relaxation phase, increase further the left rotation of the AAJ (figure 7.38).
- This is typically repeated three times, and the last time, the position is held for approximately 25 seconds.

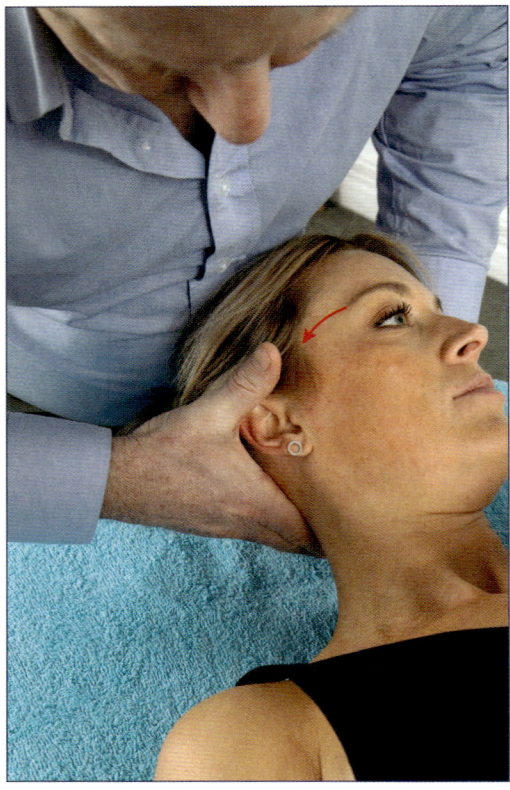

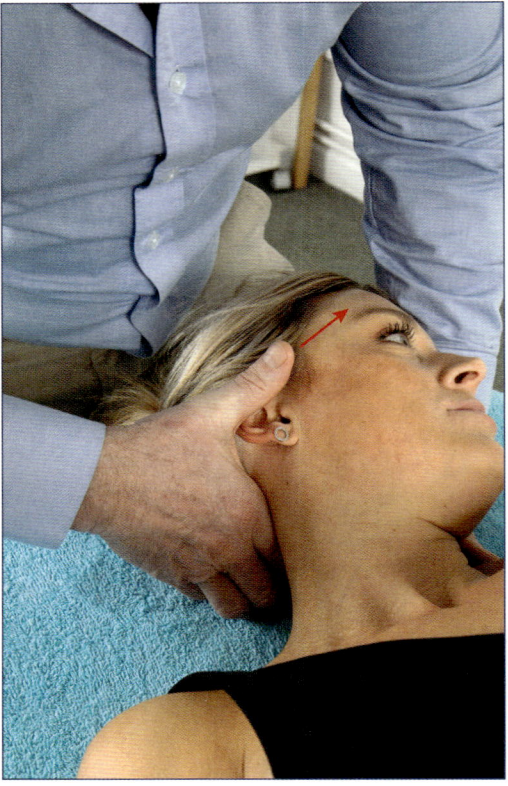

Figure 7.37. From a position of bind the patient is asked to rotate to the right side against a resistance (20%) for 10 seconds.

Figure 7.38. On the relaxation phase, the therapist induces further left rotation.

AAJ Thrust Technique (HVT)

- Begin with the patient supine and you standing at the head of the couch.
- Rotate the cervical spine to the left and apply your second MCP joint to the posterior arch of the patient's atlas, while controlling the left side of their head and neck with your left hand (figure 7.39).
- Bring the cervical spine back into a neutral position and slowly apply flexion to approximately 30°–45°. This will increase the tension to the ligamentum nuchae and will

theoretically resist the motion of the typical cervical vertebra (figure 7.40).

- Next, rotate the cervical spine to the left until you feel a resistance barrier, and from this position, fine-tune other components such as flexion, extension, and side bending until you find the optimal position (figure 7.41).
- Apply a fast rotatory thrust into left rotation mainly through your right hand (second MCP joint) toward the opposite eye (figure 7.42). This will encourage an opening of the C1/C2 facet joint.
- Reassess for restriction.

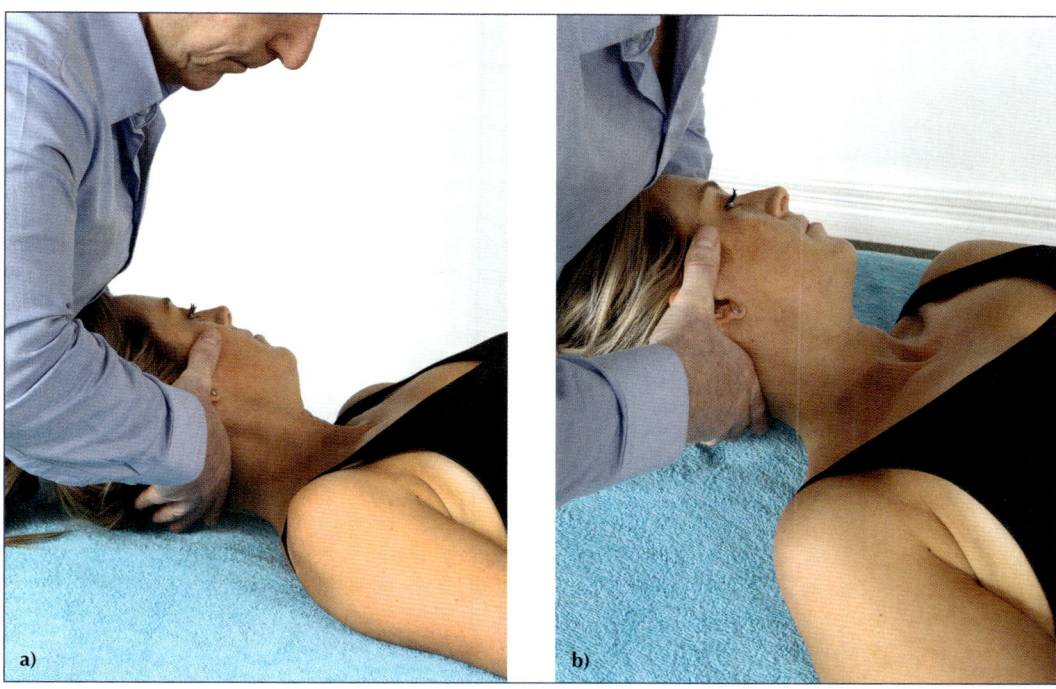

Figure 7.39. (a) Practitioner applies their second MCP joint to the posterior arch of the patient's atlas; (b) close-up of hand position.

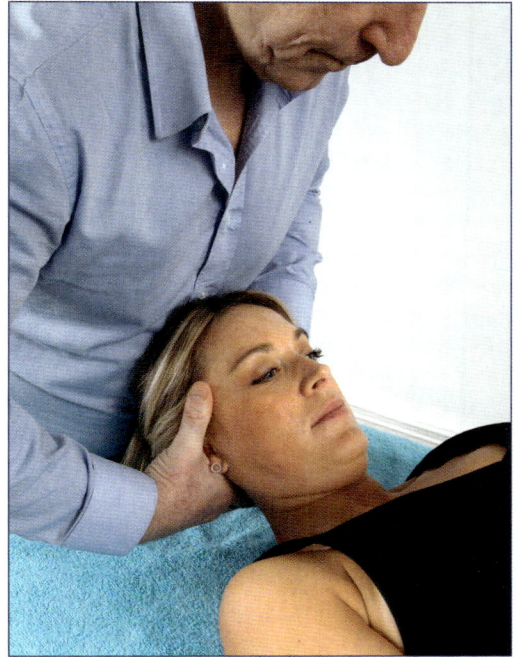

Figure 7.40. Flexion of the cervical spine to 30°–45°.

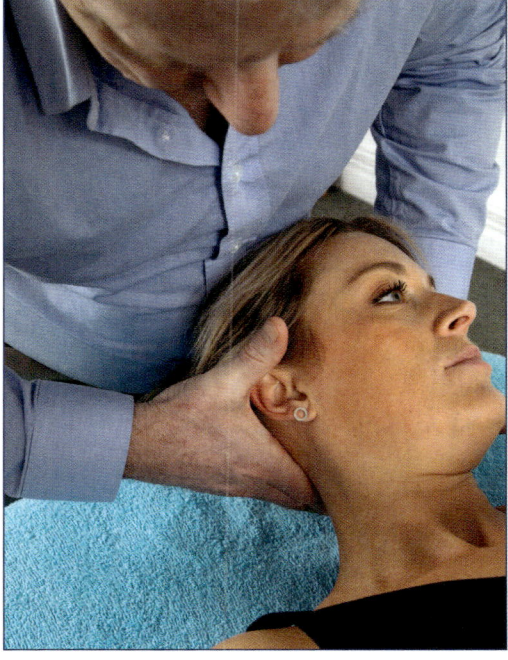

Figure 7.41. Rotation of the cervical spine is applied with fine-tuning.

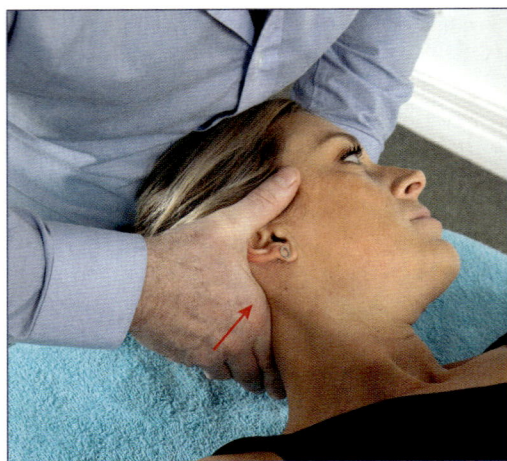

Figure 7.42. From this position a high velocity manipulative thrust is applied.

Manipulation of the AAJ

Treatment Techniques for Typical Cervical Vertebrae (C3–C7)

Diagnosis C4/5 — ERS(r)

Motion restriction: Flexion, left rotation, and left side-bending

- With the patient supine, cradle their head with both hands and gently apply the second MCP joint of your right hand and contact the articular pillar of the right C4—this is the superior vertebra of the dysfunctional vertebral motion segment—while your left hand is controlling the patient's head (figure 7.43).
- Slowly guide the patient's cervical spine into flexion, side bending right, and rotation left (type 1 coupled

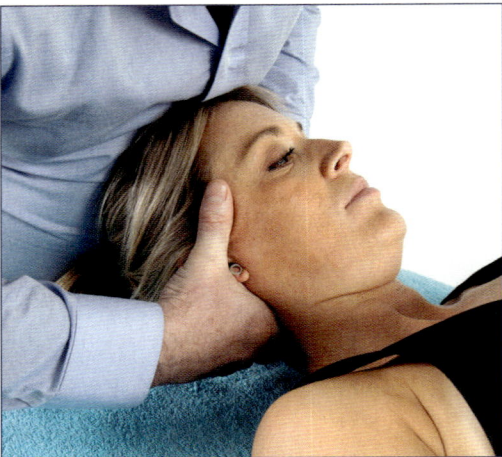

Figure 7.43. Therapist contacts the right C4 articular pillar with their second MCP.

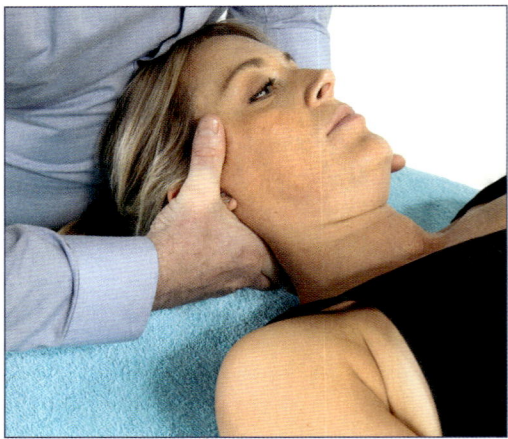

Figure 7.44. The therapist introduces flexion, side bending right, and rotation left until a bind is felt at C4.

motion) until you feel a bind at the second MCP joint (figure 7.44).
- Next, fine-tune the position with a motion of right-side bending, flexion/extension, until there is a feeling of bind.
- Apply an MET or an HVT through your right hand toward the opposite eye (figure 7.45). This will encourage an opening of the C4/5 facet joint.
- Reassess for restriction.

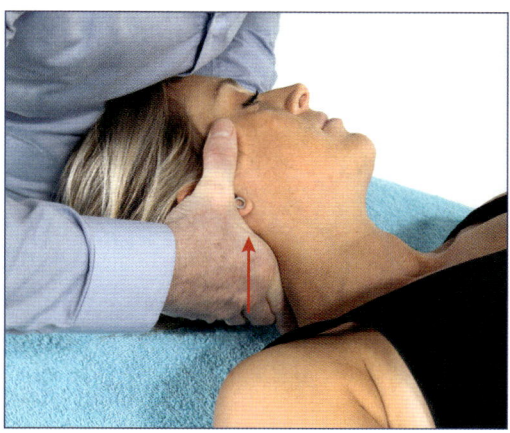

Figure 7.45. An MET or an HVT is performed from this position.

Supine manipulation of middle to lower cervical spine

Supine manipulation of C4/5

Diagnosis C3/4—FRS(r)

Motion restriction: Extension, left rotation, and left side bending

- With the patient supine, cradle their head with both hands and gently apply the second MCP joint of your left hand and contact the articular pillar of the left C3—this is the superior vertebra of the dysfunctional vertebral motion segment—while your right hand is controlling the patient's head (figure 7.46).
- Slowly guide the patient's cervical spine into right rotation, extension

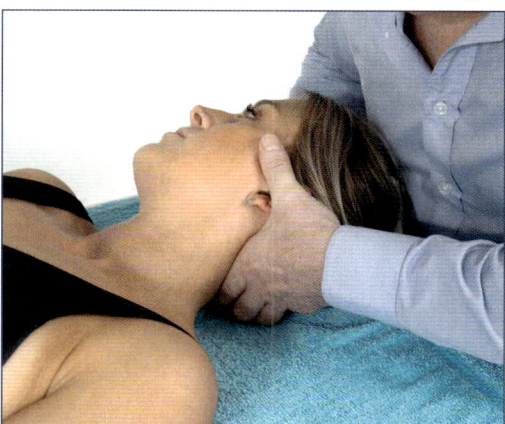

Figure 7.46. The therapist contacts the left C3 articular pillar with their second MCP joint.

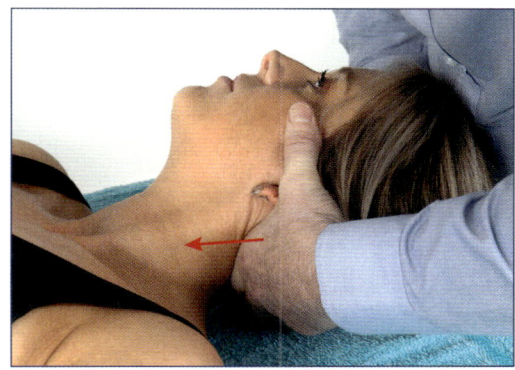

Figure 7.47. A high velocity thrust is performed in a caudal direction to close the facet joint of the left C3/4.

and side bending left, until you feel a bind at the second MCP joint.
- Apply an HVT through your left MCP joint in a caudal direction toward the spinous process of C7. This will encourage a closure of the C3/4 facet joint (figure 7.47).
- Reassess for restriction.

Seated cervical manipulation (male)

Seated cervical manipulation (female)

Diagnosis C4/5—ERS(l)

Motion restriction: Flexion, right rotation, and right side bending

- With the patient seated, cradle their head with both hands and gently apply the middle distal phalanx of your right hand and contact the articular pillar of the left C4—this is the superior vertebra of the dysfunctional vertebral motion segment—while your left hand is controlling the patient's head (figure 7.48).
- Slowly guide the patient's cervical spine into flexion, right rotation and side bending left, until you feel a bind at the distal phalanx of your middle finger (figure 7.49).
- Apply an HVT through your right middle phalanx joint in a rotation motion toward the opposite eye. This will encourage an opening of the C4/5 left facet joint (figure 7.50).
- Reassess for restriction.

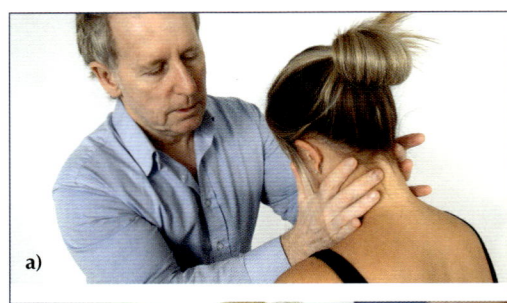

a)

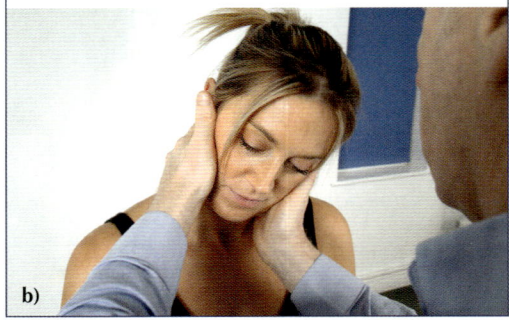

b)

Figure 7.49. (a) The therapist guides the cervical spine into flexion, rotation right, and side bending left; (b) an alternative view.

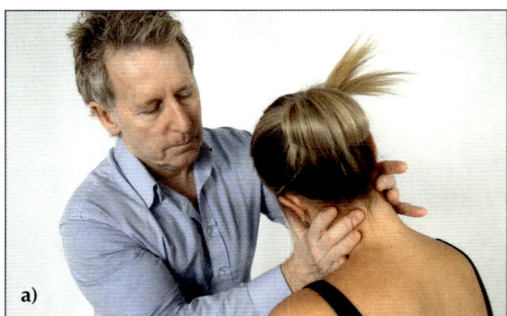

a)

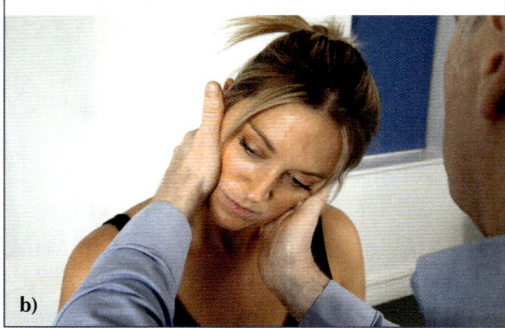

b)

Figure 7.50. (a) A high velocity thrust is performed toward the opposite eye to open the facet joint of the left C4/5; (b) an alternative view.

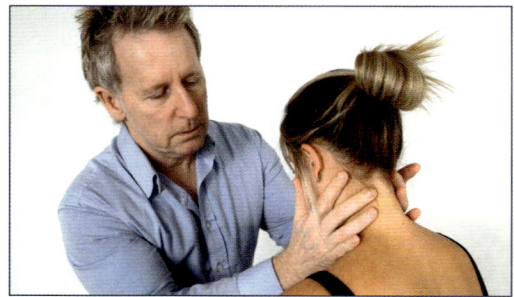

Figure 7.48. The therapist contacts the left C4 articular pillar with their middle distal phalanx.

Techniques for the Atlanto-Occipital Joint

The atlanto-occipital joint (AOJ), or C0–C1 articulation, is a pair of condyloid synovial joints that connect the occipital condyles of the occipital bone (C0) to the superior articular facets of the first cervical vertebra, the atlas (C1), figure 8.1. The superior facets of the atlas face backward, upward, and medially, and are concave. The shape of the occipital condyles is convex, which allows a perfect fit within the concave superior facets of the atlas. The AOJ mainly allows flexion and extension, as in a nodding (nutation and counternutaton) motion.

During flexion (approximately 5°–10°, and resisted by a fibrous capsule) the convex occipital condyles bilaterally roll forward, while at the same time gliding posteriorly on the concave facets of the atlas; in extension (approximately 10°), the occipital condyles roll backward while gliding anteriorly on the atlas. However, during lateral flexion (side bending) of the AOJ, there is a coupled rotation to the opposite side, and this follows the type 1 (neutral) spinal mechanics. For example,

side bending to the left will be coupled with rotation to the right.

During lateral flexion, one occipital condyle will glide superiorly on one side of the atlas and the other will glide inferiorly on the other, coupled with rotation to the opposite side. This range of motion for lateral flexion and rotation is approximately 5°–8° in both planes and is due to the ligamentous attachment, primarily the lateral atlanto-occipital ligament, which attaches from the atlas to the occipital bone, plus the natural slope formed by the superior facets of

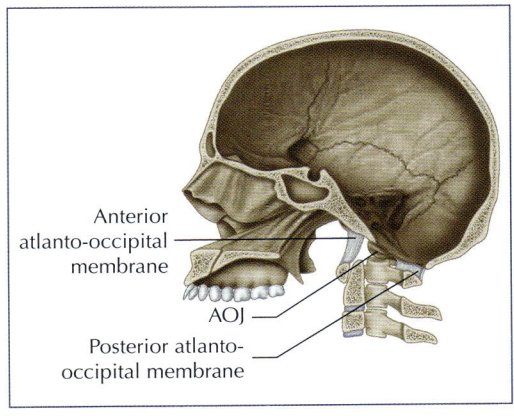

Anterior atlanto-occipital membrane

AOJ

Posterior atlanto-occipital membrane

Figure 8.1. Anatomy of the AOJ.

the C1 (atlas) vertebra. For example, when the occiput rotates to the right on the underlying atlas, the lateral atlanto-occipital ligament causes the occiput to translate to the right, with subsequent side bending to the left.

Assessment of the Atlanto-Occipital Joint

If you remember from earlier, the motion for the AOJ is primarily flexion and extension for approximately 15° within the sagittal plane. The simplest way of thinking about this is a *nodding* type of motion for the head and neck, for example when we say *yes* (we tend to nod forward as we speak this word). The motion of nodding occurs by the occipital bone rolling on the vertebra below, the atlas (C1). The lower cervical spine, especially the interspace of cervical level C5/6, performs most of the full flexion and extension of the cervical spine. There are approximately 5°–8° of lateral flexion at the AOJ with minimal rotation, even though rotation and side bending are coupled to opposite sides (type 1)—for example, rotation of the head to the right will induce side bending to the left of the AOJ.

Motion Testing of the AOJ

When you come to motion testing the AOJ, we can modify the translation test we previously performed for the cervical spine. This time we place our fingertips lightly below the occipital condyles as they articulate with the underlying atlas (figure 8.2).

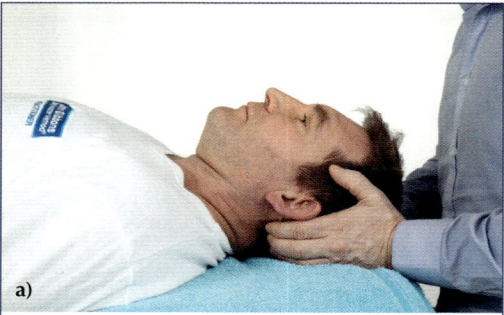

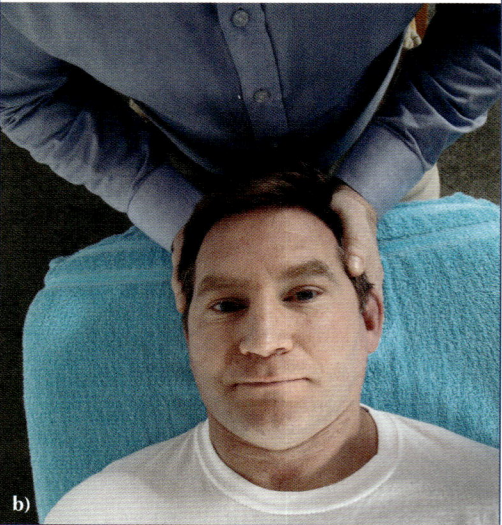

Figure 8.2. (a) Patient is supine and the practitioner palpates the occipital condyles; (b) alternative view.

Apply a translatory motion of the occiput to the left, as this will induce side bending to the right. This is known as *right to left translation*, and when this happens the *right occipital condyle* will extend and glide anteriorly on the atlas (C1), while the *left occipital condyle* is flexing and gliding posteriorly on the atlas (figure 8.3).

To test the opposite side, translate the occiput to the right to induce side bending to the left (*left to right translation*). This motion will cause the left occipital condyle to glide anteriorly (extend)

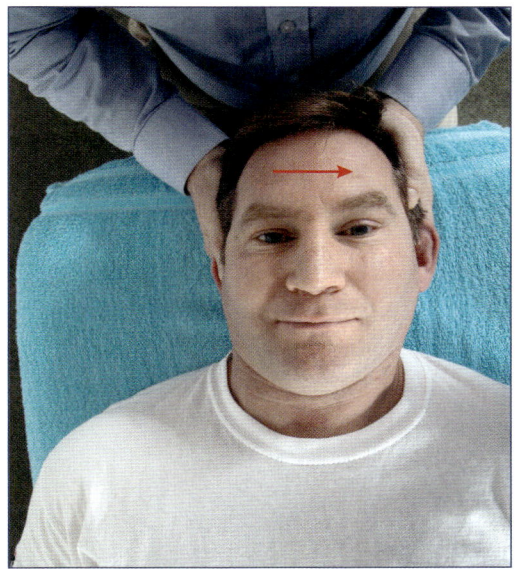

Figure 8.3. The practitioner translates the occiput from right to left.

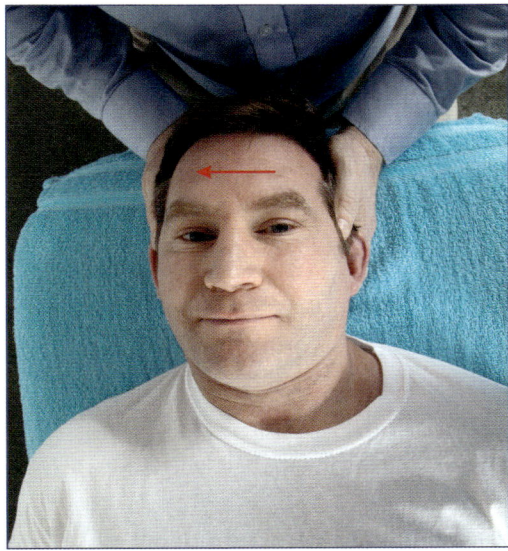

Figure 8.4. The practitioner translates the occiput from left to right.

and the right occipital condyle to glide posteriorly (flex), as in figure 8.4. If you have found a resistance translating from the *right to the left* or from the *left to the right*, you have found a facet restriction within the AOJ.

You will now need to decide which side of the AOJ has the facet restriction. This is simply done by adding an *extension* motion of the occiput and performing the same translation test (from right to left and then from left to right), and then repeating the same motion but this time with *flexion* of the occiput (from right to left and then from left to right).

Extension Testing

Taking the occiput into extension (figure 8.5a and b), gently translate the occiput to the left (right to left translation) as this will further test the ability of the right occipital condyle (same side) to extend and glide anteriorly on the atlas (figure 8.5c).

Note: If you sense a resistance during the right to left translation in extension, the motion restriction is the inability of the right-side occipital condyle to backward bend, right-side bend, and left rotate, so that the right condyle is restricted gliding anteriorly. If the condyle cannot extend, it must be fixed in the opposite direction—flexion—and if the condyle cannot side bend right or rotate to the left side, it must be fixed in the opposite plane (in this case left-side bending and right rotation). The terminology for the fixation is flexion, side bending left, and rotation right, abbreviated as FS(l)R(r).

If you repeat the same translation motion to the right side (left to right translation), this tests the ability of the left occipital condyle (same side) to extend and anteriorly glide on the atlas (figure 8.6).

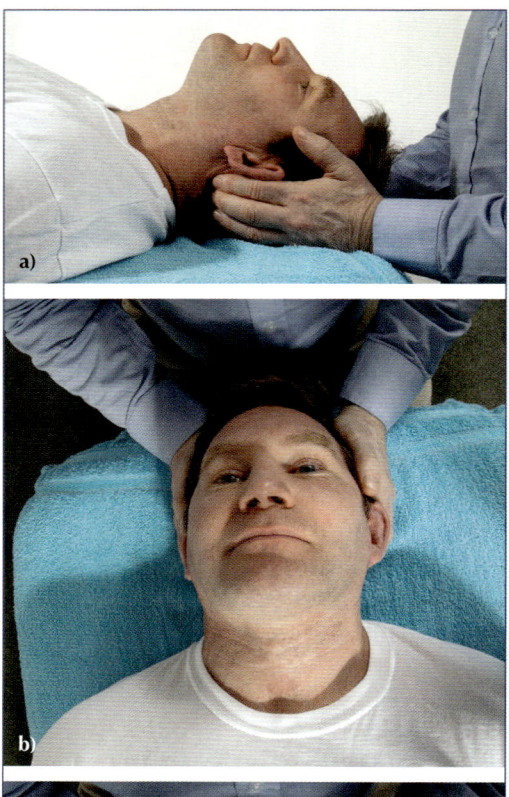

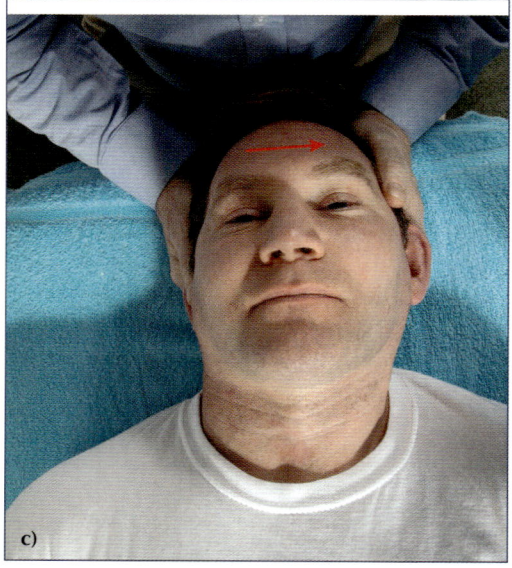

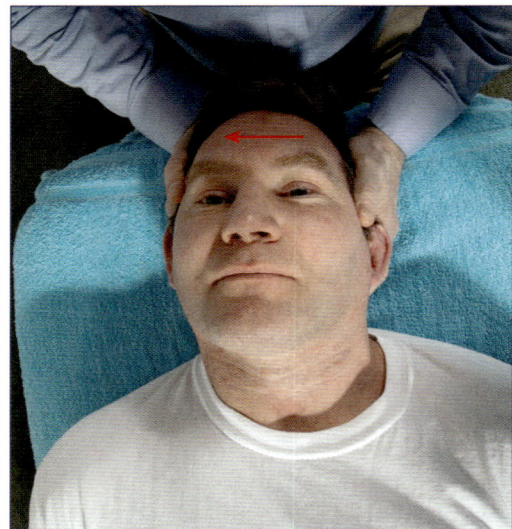

Figure 8.6. The practitioner extends the occiput and translates from left to right to test the ability of the left occipital condyle to extend and glide anteriorly.

Note: If you sense a resistance during the left to right translation in extension, the motion restriction is the inability of the left-side occipital condyle to backward bend, left-side bend, and right rotate, so that the left condyle is restricted gliding anteriorly. If the condyle cannot extend, it must be fixed in the opposite direction—flexion—and if the condyle cannot side bend left or rotate to the right side, it must be fixed in the opposite plane (in this case right-side bending and left rotation). The terminology for the fixation, is flexion, side bending right, and rotation left, abbreviated as FS(r)R(l).

Figure 8.5. (a) The practitioner extends the occiput; (b) alternative view; (c) the practitioner translates from right to left to test the ability of the right occipital condyle to extend and glide anteriorly.

Flexion Testing

In flexion of the occiput (figure 8.7a), you translate it to the left (right to left translation) because this will further test

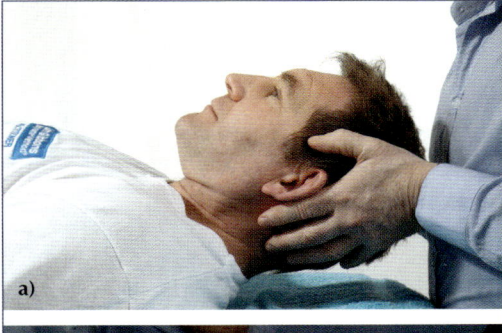

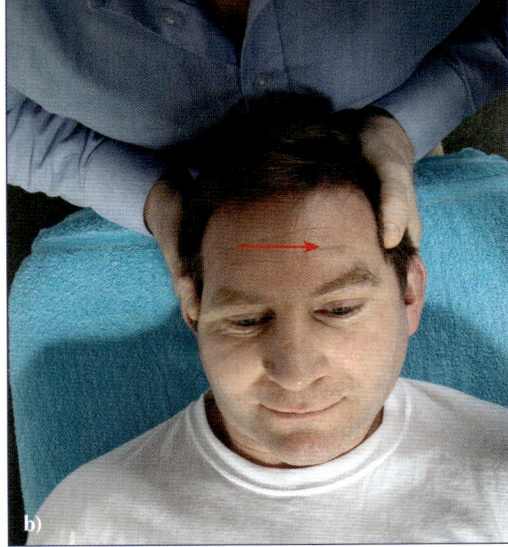

Figure 8.7. (a) The practitioner flexes the occiput, and (b) translates from right to left to test the ability of the left occipital condyle to flex and glide posteriorly.

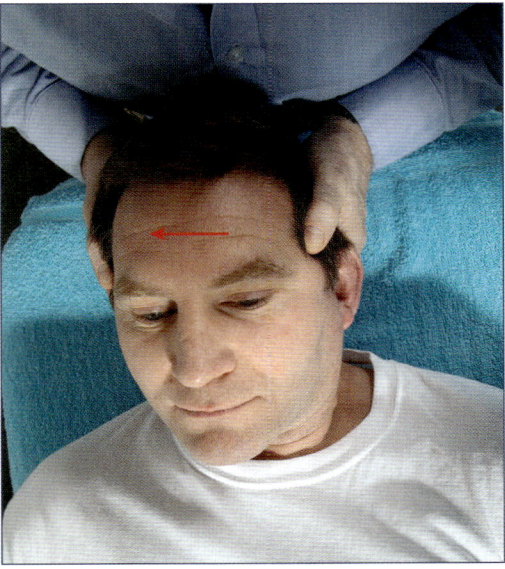

Figure 8.8. The practitioner flexes the occiput and translates from left to right to test the ability of the right occipital condyle to flex and glide posteriorly.

the ability of the left occipital condyle (opposite side) to flex and glide posteriorly on the atlas (figure 8.7b).

Note: If you sense a resistance during the right to left translation in flexion, the motion restriction is the inability of the left-side (opposite this time) occipital condyle to forward bend, right-side bend, and left rotate, so that the left condyle is restricted gliding posteriorly. If the condyle cannot flex it must be fixed in

the opposite direction—extension—and if the condyle cannot side bend right or rotate to the left side, it must be fixed in the opposite plane (in this case left-side bending and right rotation). The terminology for the fixation is extension, side bending left, and rotation right, abbreviated as ES(l)R(r).

If you repeat the same translation motion to the right side (left to right translation), this tests the ability of the right occipital condyle (opposite) to flex and posteriorly glide on the atlas (figure 8.8).

Note: If you sense a resistance during the left to right translation in flexion, the motion restriction is the inability of the right-side (opposite) occipital condyle to forward bend, left-side bend, and right rotate, so that the right condyle is restricted gliding posteriorly. If the condyle cannot flex, it must be fixed in the opposite direction—extension—and if the condyle cannot side bend left or rotate to the right side, it must be fixed in the opposite plane (in this case right-side bending and left rotation). The terminology for the fixation is extension, side bending right, and rotation left, abbreviated as ES(r)R(l).

 Assessment of the AOJ

Alternative Assessment of the Atlanto-Occipital Joint

The following technique is another way of assessing the AOJ and would lead very nicely into an effective treatment protocol, because this time we add in rotation, and the translatory motion is performed from the rotated position.

Rotate the cervical spine to the left approximately 30°, and from this position of rotation, apply a translation motion of the occipital bone, which will induce an anterior glide of the right occipital condyle on C1 (atlas), while simultaneously inducing a posterior glide of the left occipital condyle on C1 (figure 8.9). Feel for any sense of resistance. Repeat on the other side and make a comparison (figure 8.10).

Motion Assessment Technique

With the patient supine, cradle the occipital bone with the left hand and gently stabilize the forehead with the right

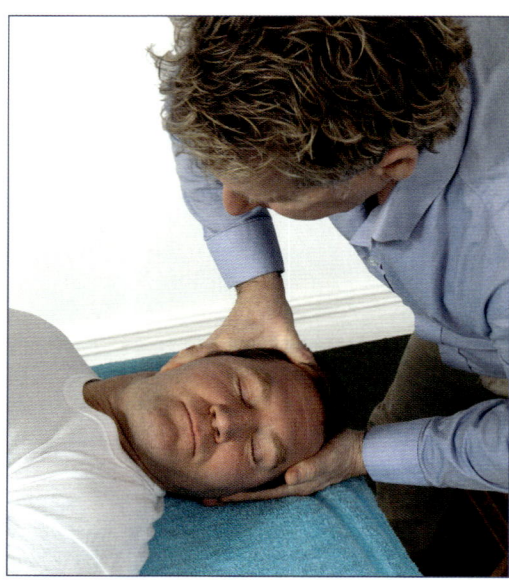

Figure 8.9. Rotation of the cervical spine to the left with translation applied to the occipital condyle.

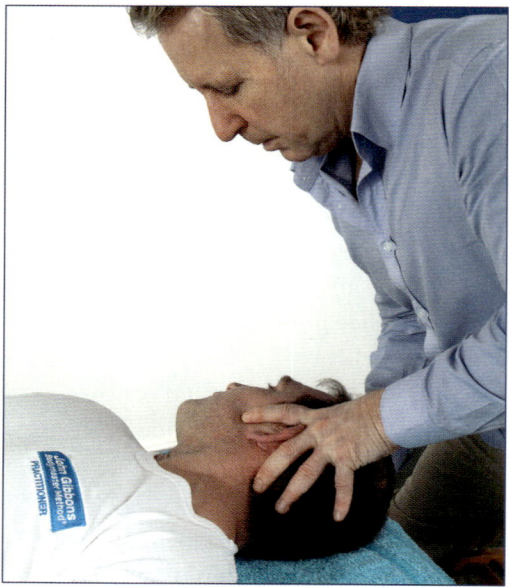

Figure 8.10. Rotation of the cervical spine to the right with translation applied to the occipital condyle.

hand (figure 8.11a). Once the patient is relaxed, apply a nodding type of motion through the use of the left hand guiding

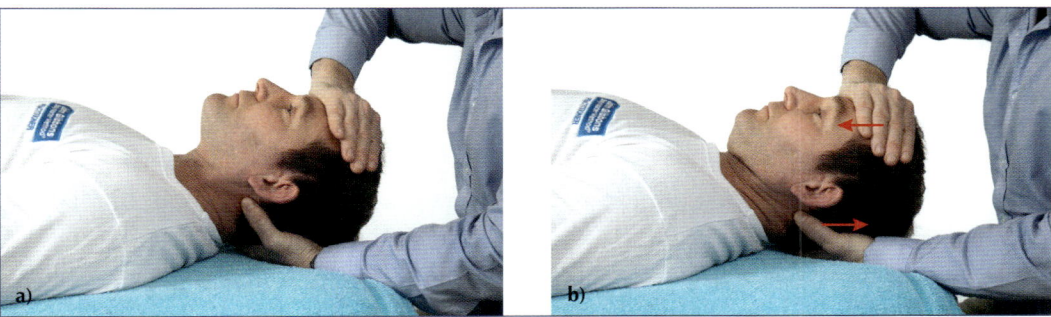

Figure 8.11. (a) The therapist cradles the occipital bone and forehead, and (b) applies a nodding motion to the AOJ.

the occipital bone in a cephalic direction. At the same time, place the right hand on the patient's forehead and apply pressure in a caudal direction. This type of combined movement will ascertain the amount of motion possible for the AOJ (figure 8.11b).

Treatment of the Atlanto-Occipital Joint

In class I often say to the students that when you are assessing you are also treating, and this makes perfect sense for the AOJ because as you are testing the motion of the joint you can utilize these techniques into a continued mobilization.

The following technique will improve the translatory motion of the AOJ using a MET, even though there is no specificity into flexion or extension.

Translation Treatment: PIR Technique

Perform the translation test to either side with the head and cervical spine in a neutral position. If, for example,

the patient has restriction translating from the right to the left side, translate the patient's occiput to the left until you feel bind. From this position, ask the patient to resist by gently pushing their occiput further to the left using approximately 20% muscle strength for 10 seconds (figure 8.12). After the contraction, take the AOJ into further left translation.

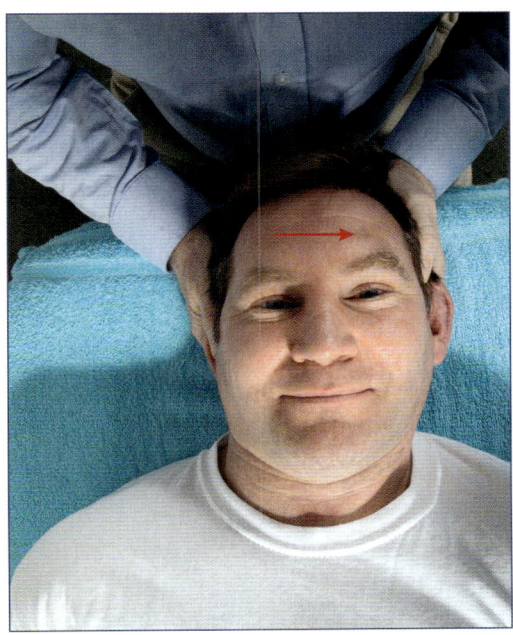

Figure 8.12. PIR for the AOJ—patient pushes to the left side.

Translation Treatment: RI Technique

This technique would be perfect to use if the initial resistance to the left caused some discomfort. Ask the patient to push the occiput to the *right* side, as this will cause a relaxation in the *left* musculature through RI. The patient should still push at 20% effort for 10 seconds; on the relaxation phase, encourage further translation to the left side (figure 8.13).

Flexion and Extension Treatment

From the flexion and extension assessment (nodding motion) of the AOJ, we can simply apply an MET from the point of the bind using either a PIR or an RI technique.

Control the patient's occipital bone with your left hand and place your right hand on top of their forehead. From the bind position of flexion, ask the patient to look toward the ceiling (figure 8.14) while you apply a gentle resistance onto their forehead. This will induce a contraction of the suboccipital muscles.

After the contraction, ask the patient to relax, and take the AOJ into further flexion (figure 8.15).

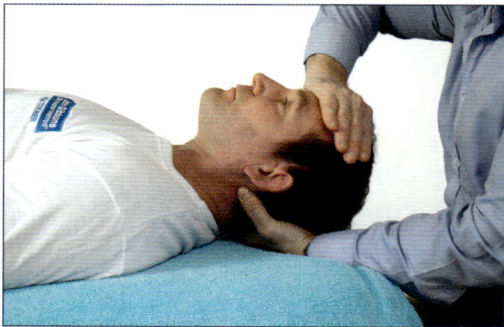

Figure 8.14. From the bind, the patient is asked to look toward the ceiling.

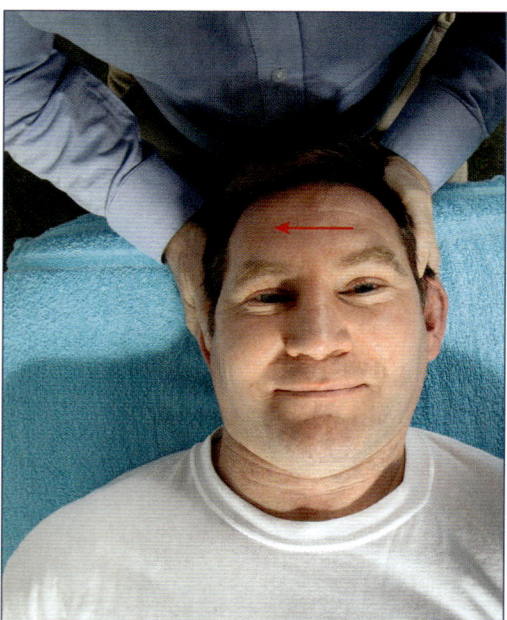

Figure 8.13. RI for the OAJ—patient pushes to the right side, which induces a relaxation of the left muscles.

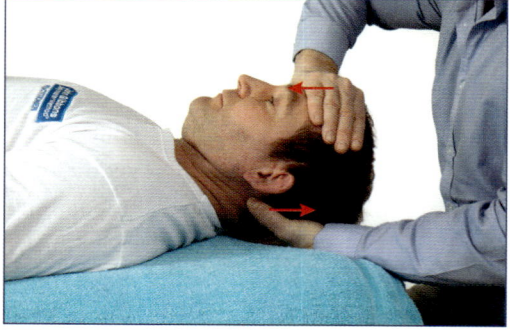

Figure 8.15. After the contraction, the therapist takes the AOJ into further flexion.

If the patient had increased discomfort during this contraction motion of extension of the AOJ, ask them to flex their occiput instead, which will induce an RI effect into the suboccipital muscles (figure 8.16).

After the contraction, still take the patient's occipital bone into flexion.

Mobilization and manipulation of the AOJ

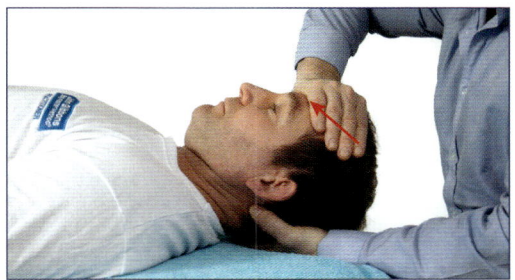

Figure 8.16. The patient is asked to flex their occiput (RI technique), which will induce a relaxation effect in the suboccipital muscles.

Techniques for the Cervicothoracic Junction

W hen I was taught these techniques for this area of the body, located anatomically between the level of C7 and T1, it was described as the cervical-dorsal junction (*dorsal* is the older name for the thoracic spine, so it was known as the CDJ). I still use that term now. However, for this text, I will call it the cervicothoracic junction or the CTJ because this term may make it easier to understand.

C7/T1 is a transitional area where the cervical lordosis comes to its end at C7 and meets the start of the thoracic kyphosis at T1. This junction point is a relatively complex area of the body and is not always an easy region to treat. Dysfunctions found at this level also tend to involve the first rib.

The facet joints of C7 and T1 are found between the inferior articular processes of C7 and the superior articular processes of T1 and are crucial in providing stability, while allowing flexibility in the spine. As the cervical spine at C7 is transitioning to the thoracic spine at T1, the facet joints' orientation is changing to accommodate

the different types of movements and load transfer experienced through the thoracic spine. This part of the spine is involved in supporting the ribcage, and so movements in this region are going to be smaller compared with the wide range of motion possible within the cervical spine.

The nerve root that exits between the levels of C7 and T1 is the C8 nerve root, and in particular this nerve forms part of the branch of the ulnar nerve, which supplies many muscles of the forearm and hand as well as areas of sensation in the hand (figures 9.1 and 9.2).

Assessment of the Cervicothoracic Junction

The following technique is known as *motion testing* or *segmental motion testing* and is very effective at ascertaining motion between vertebral segments. Motion testing of C7 and T1 involves assessing the range of motion and function of these vertebrae in the lower cervical and upper thoracic spine.

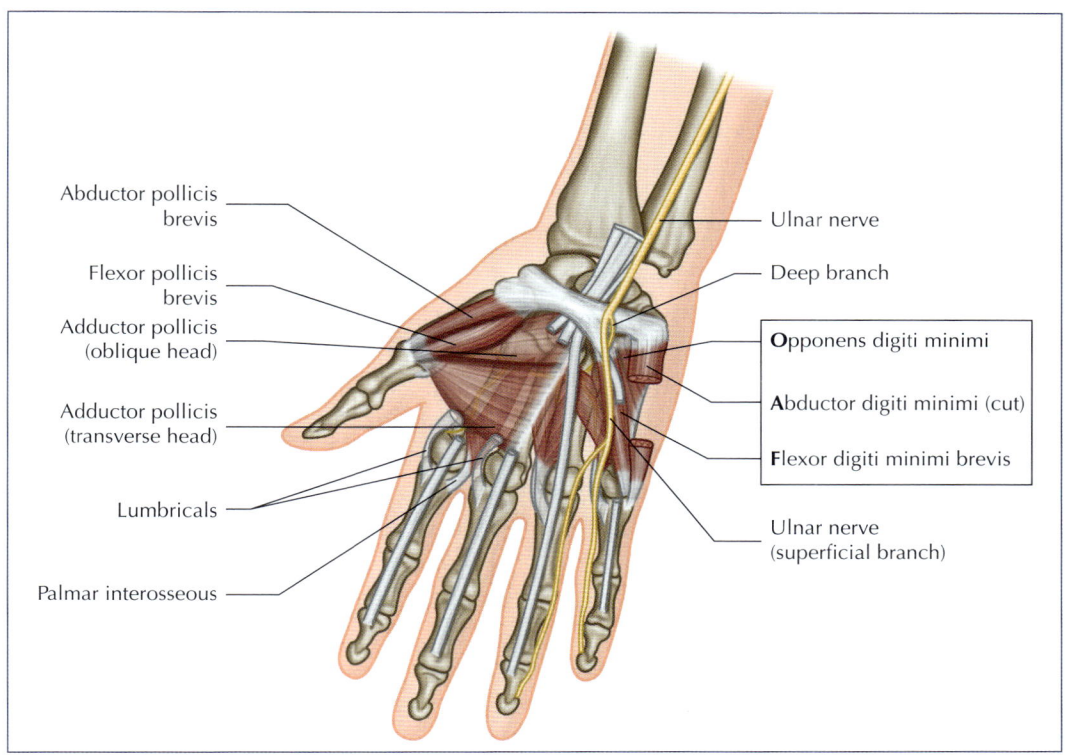

Figure 9.1. Ulnar nerve pathway—motor supply to hand (opponens pollicis, abductor pollicis brevis, flexor pollicis brevis).

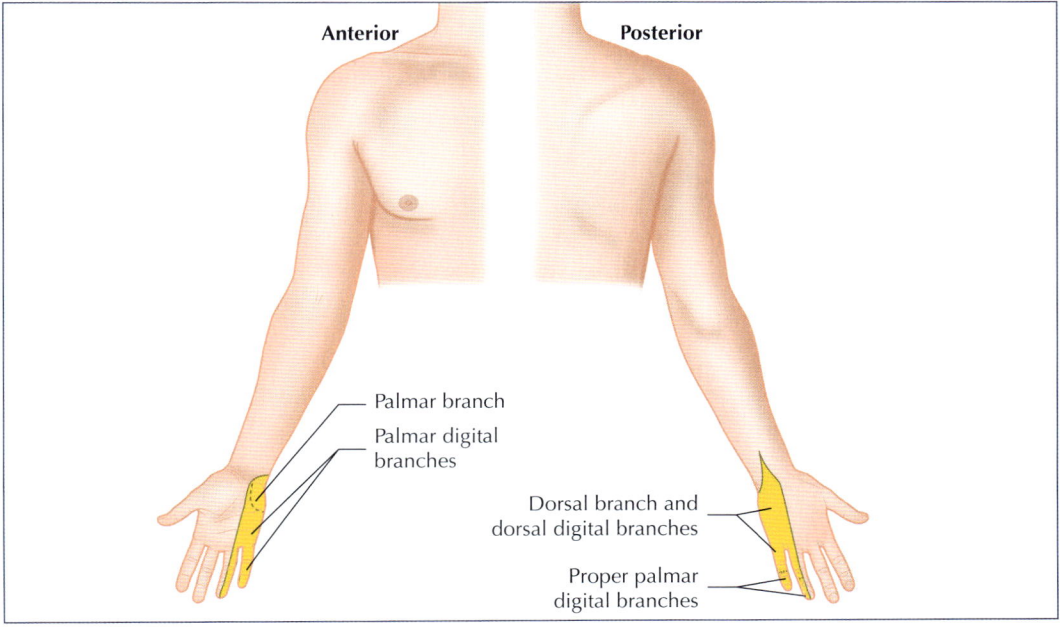

Figure 9.2. Ulnar nerve pathway—sensory supply.

Palpate the spinous processes of C7 and T1 or the interspace between these two levels, and ask the patient to perform active range of motion (AROM) movements of flexion, extension, rotation, and side bending (remember *active* means the patient is performing these motions on their own without assistance), while you feel for any restriction during the range of motion or unusual movement patterns (figure 9.3).

Now, to improve the specificity of the testing procedure, perform passive range of motion (PROM) movements, where you have total control of the motion of the cervical spine.

Use the index finger of your right hand to palpate the interspace between the spinous processes of C7 and T1. Your left hand is controlling the patient's head, and you slowly take the cervical spine into full flexion (figure 9.4), and from there into full extension, while noting the motion at the interspace.

Once you have ascertained motion at C7 and T1, I suggest you continue with your assessment and palpate the levels between T1 and T2 and between T2 and T3, because this will form part of the assessment protocol for motion of the cervical spine also related to other vertebral components, especially the upper thoracic spine.

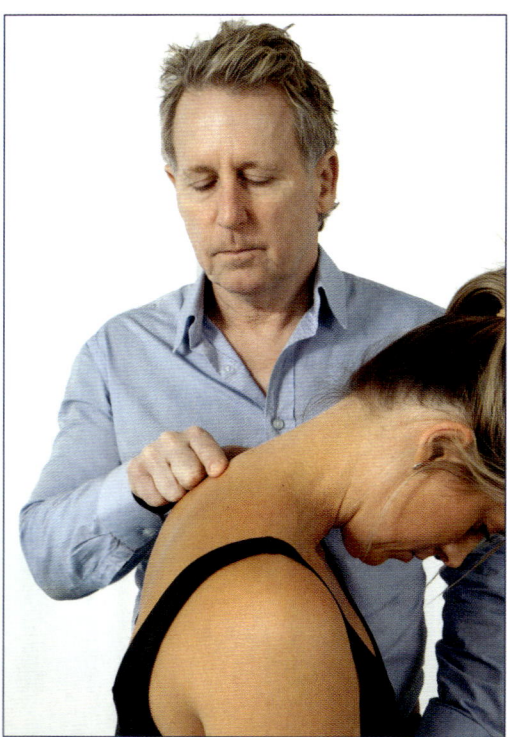

Figure 9.3. Patient is asked to perform AROM movements for the cervical spine as the therapist palpates C7 and T1 spinous processes.

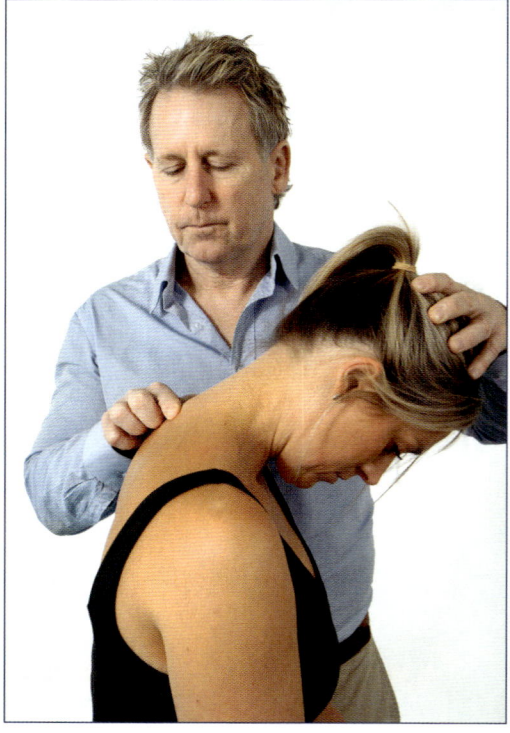

Figure 9.4. The therapist palpates the interspace between C7 and T1 and passively flexes and extends the patient's cervical spine to ascertain motion.

Positional Assessment

The next stage of the assessment is to decide what type of dysfunction is present—an ERS (extension, rotation, and side bending) to the left or the right or an FRS (flexion, rotation, and side bending) to the left or the right. You identify this from your positional palpation with the cervical spine in a neutral, flexion, and extension position (see chapter 6).

 Motion testing and palpation of CT junction

Treatment of the Cervicothoracic Junction

Prior to any form of spinal manipulative techniques, I typically recommend some soft-tissue massage and METs as a standard protocol. These treatments are very effective for encouraging mobilization and subsequent improvement of the patient's restricted joints, especially for the cervical spine. I also suggest that these are done before any type of thrust, as I consider them as a type of *warming up motion*. To perform a spinal manipulative technique without any prior soft-tissue treatment might prove uncomfortable for the patient. Consider that a restricted joint has the potential to make the localized muscles short and consequently tight, and a short/tight muscle can cause the local joint to become restricted.

Therefore, it is important, in my opinion, for the practitioner to have the ability to perform not only soft-tissue techniques but also mobilizations and, if required, spinal manipulation.

MET Treatment of the CTJ

Ask the patient to sit on a couch (or a chair) and passively flex their head with your left hand, while palpating the interspace of C7/T1 with your right index finger until you feel a point of bind (figure 9.5).

From the position of bind, ask the patient to take a breath in, and on the out breath to extend their head against your resistance for 10 seconds at approximately 20% effort (figure 9.6).

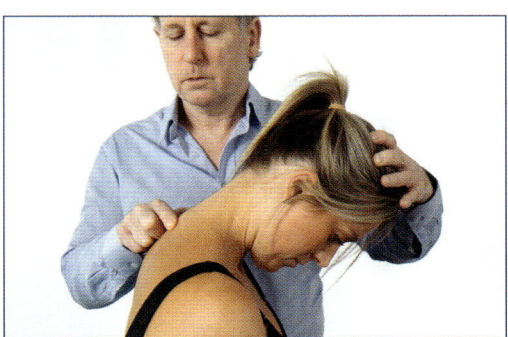

Figure 9.5. The therapist flexes the patient's cervical spine while palpating the interspace of C7/T1.

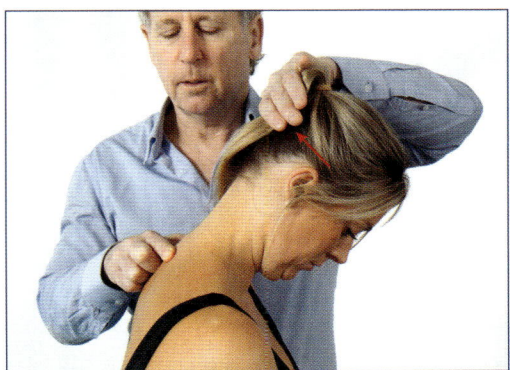

Figure 9.6. Patient is asked to extend their head against a resistance for 10 seconds.

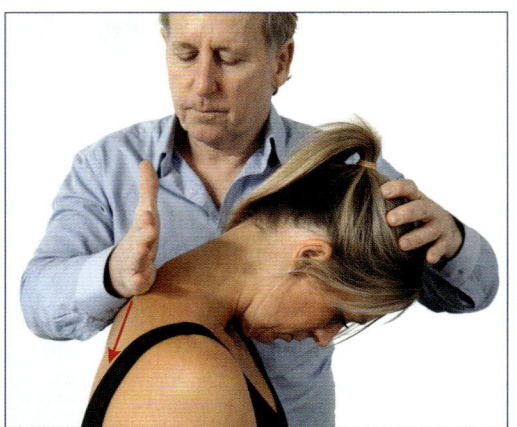

Figure 9.7. After the contraction, the therapist encourages further cervical flexion while stabilizing the T1 vertebra.

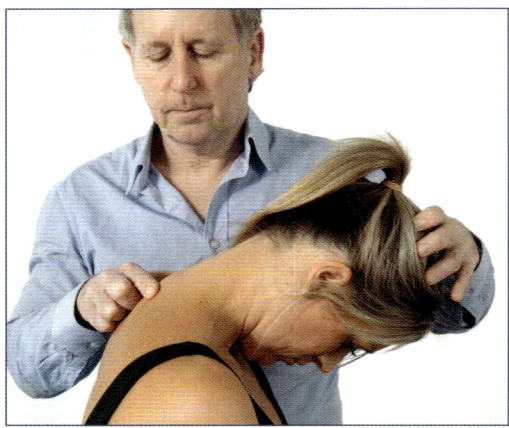

Figure 9.8. The therapist flexes the patient's cervical spine while palpating the interspace of C7/T1.

After the contraction, ask the patient to take a breath in, and on the out breath stabilize the T1 spinous process in a caudal direction using the pisiform bone of your right hand as the fixator, while your left hand encourages further cervical flexion until a new bind is achieved (figure 9.7).

This technique is typically repeated three times, with the last position in cervical flexion being held for approximately 25–30 seconds.

Treatment of C7/T1 ERS(r)

Rather than simply stabilizing T1 and flexing the cervical spine to encourage opening of the facet joint, it makes sense to add in other movements such as rotation and side bending to complement the technique.

For example, let us say that the C7 inferior facet is fixed closed on the right on the superior facet of T1 and has also rotated

and side bent to the right because it has adopted type 2 spinal motion.

Similar to the technique above, ask the patient to sit on either a couch or chair and passively flex their head with your left hand, while palpating the interspace of C7/T1 with your right index finger until you feel a point of bind (figure 9.8).

From the position of bind, ask the patient to take a breath in, and on the out breath to extend their head against your resistance for 10 seconds at approximately 20% effort.

After the contraction, ask the patient to take a breath in, and on the out breath stabilize the T1 spinous process in a caudal direction using the pisiform bone of your right hand, while your left hand encourages further cervical flexion, rotation, and side bending left until a new bind is achieved. This will encourage the right closed fixed facet to open (figure 9.9).

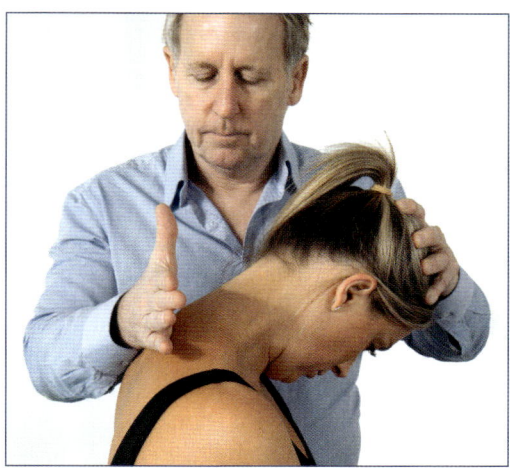

Figure 9.9. After the contraction, the therapist encourages further cervical flexion, rotation, and side bending left, while stabilizing T1.

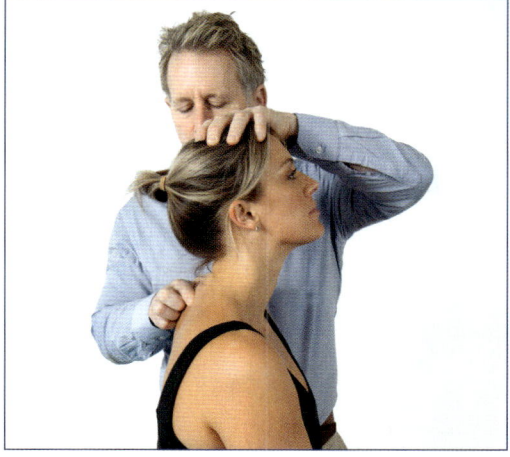

Figure 9.10. The therapist extends the patient's cervical spine while palpating the interspace of C7/T1.

Treatment of C7/T1 FRS(r)

For this dysfunction, we will want to encourage closing of the facet joint. For example, let us say the C7 inferior facet is fixed open on the left on the superior facet of T1, and it has also rotated and side bent to the right because it has adopted type 2 spinal motion.

Remember that with an FRS dysfunction, the open facet is on the opposite side to the side of motion, so with this lesion the vertebra has flexed, rotated, and side bent to the right but the left facet joint is now fixed in an open position. Therefore, treatment this time will be to encourage a closure of the facet joint, compared with the earlier treatment of opening a closed facet joint.

Again, ask the patient to sit either on a couch or chair and passively extend their head with your left hand, while palpating the interspace of C7/T1 with your right

index finger until you feel a point of bind (figure 9.10).

From the position of bind, ask the patient to take a breath in, and on the out breath to flex their head against your resistance for 10 seconds at approximately 20% effort.

After the contraction, ask the patient to take a breath in, and on the out breath stabilize the T1 spinous process in a caudal direction using the pisiform bone of your right hand, while your left hand encourages further cervical extension, rotation, and side bending to the left until a new bind is achieved. This will encourage the left open facet to close (figure 9.11). The following manipulative techniques will be covered for the CTJ:

- **Technique 1:** Sitting—thoracic lift
- **Technique 2:** Standing—thoracic thrust
- **Technique 3:** Prone position (MCP joint)—prone CTJ thrust
- **Technique 4:** Prone position—thumb thrust

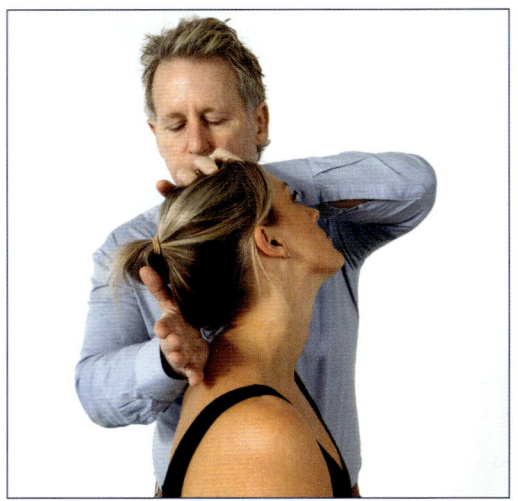

Figure 9.11. After the contraction, the therapist encourages further cervical extension, rotation, and side bending left, while stabilizing T1.

1. Thoracic Lift

With the patient sitting on the couch, place your hands onto their forearms (figure 9.12a), and with your hands in contact with the patient's forearms, ask them to lift their arms and interlink their hands behind their neck (figure 9.12b).

From this position, protect the patient's shoulders by horizontally flexing their arms toward their chest (figure 9.13). This motion will reduce the stress to the shoulder when the thrust is applied.

Next, place the middle or upper part of your chest (use a towel if more

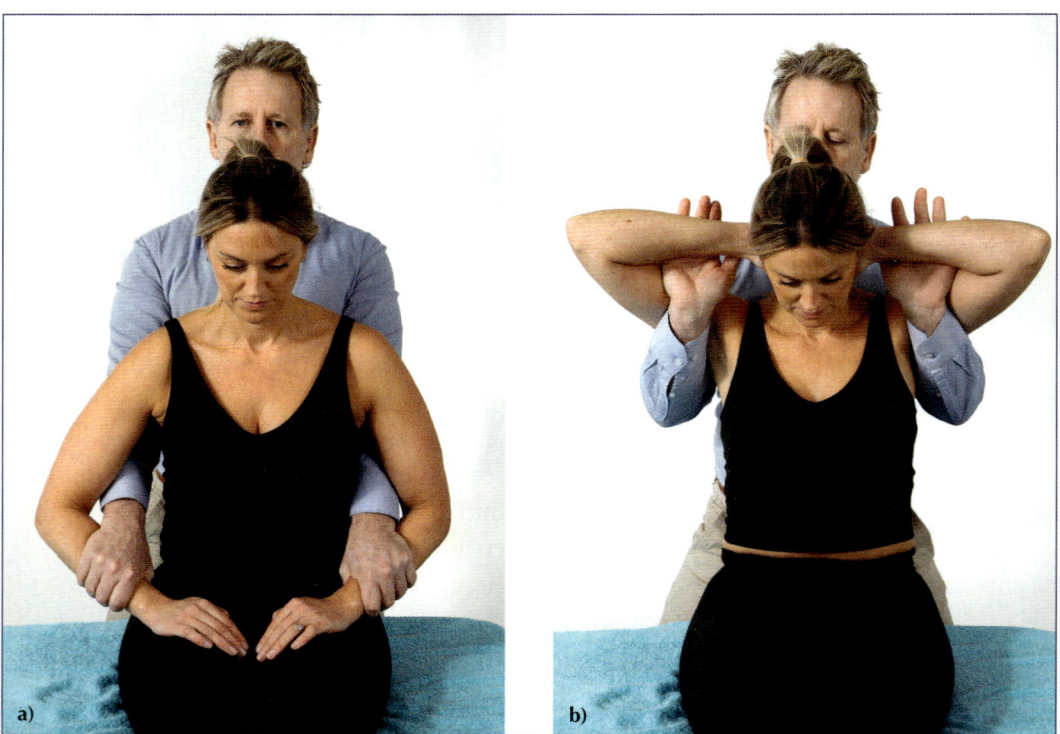

Figure 9.12. (a) Hand placement on the patient's forearms; (b) patient is asked to interlink their fingers and place their hands behind their head.

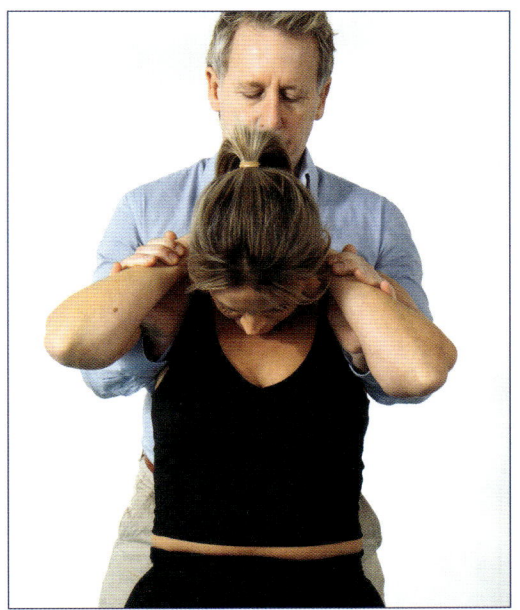

Figure 9.13. The therapist places the patient's arms toward their chest.

appropriate) onto the upper part of the patient's back. From here, slowly bring their arms into horizontal extension while applying an anterior glide from your upper chest to their upper thoracic spine (figure 9.14a). From this position, make any minor adjustments necessary until a bind is felt, prior to the manipulation. When you and the patient are both relaxed, apply the HVT thrust toward you and slightly upward, and simultaneously apply a thrust with your chest directly forward against the thoracic spine (figure 9.14b).

 **Seated CT manipulation**

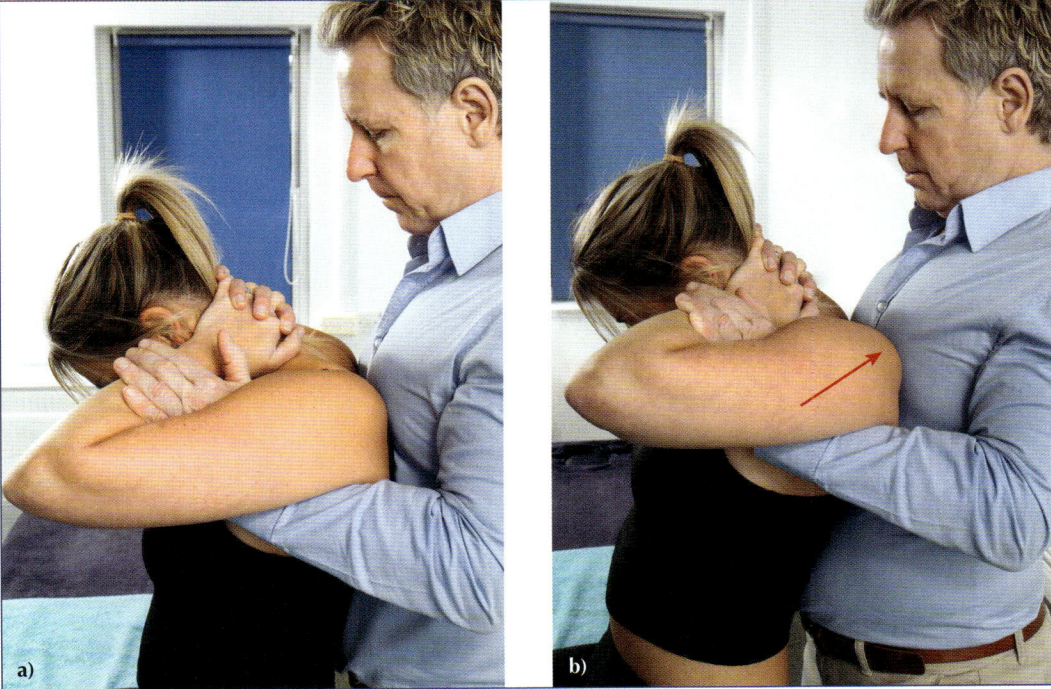

Figure 9.14. (a) Therapist places their chest onto the patient's upper back, and (b) applies a thrust.

2. Standing Thoracic Thrust

This is similar to technique 1 except that the patient is standing (figure 9.15a and b). If there is difficulty in performing this technique safely, for example if the patient is substantially taller than yourself, please bear this in mind when deciding on your choice of technique.

Slowly bring the patient toward you and make any adjustments where necessary prior to the manipulation (figure 9.16a). When you and the patient are both relaxed, apply the HVT thrust toward you and slightly upward, and simultaneously apply a thrust directly forward to the upper part of the thoracic spine (figure 9.16b).

3. Prone CTJ Thrust with MCP

With the patient prone and their arms resting over the couch, place the MCP joint of your index finger down to the level of the transverse process of C7 (figure 9.17). From this position, slowly place the patient's neck into a type 1 mechanic—side bending toward the same side as the MCP joint—and rotate to the opposite side until you feel a tension in your MCP joint.

Make any adjustments where necessary prior to the manipulation. When you and the patient are both relaxed, apply the HVT thrust through the transverse process (TP) of C7 toward the opposite axilla, as shown in figure 9.18a for the left CTJ and figure 9.18b for the right CTJ.

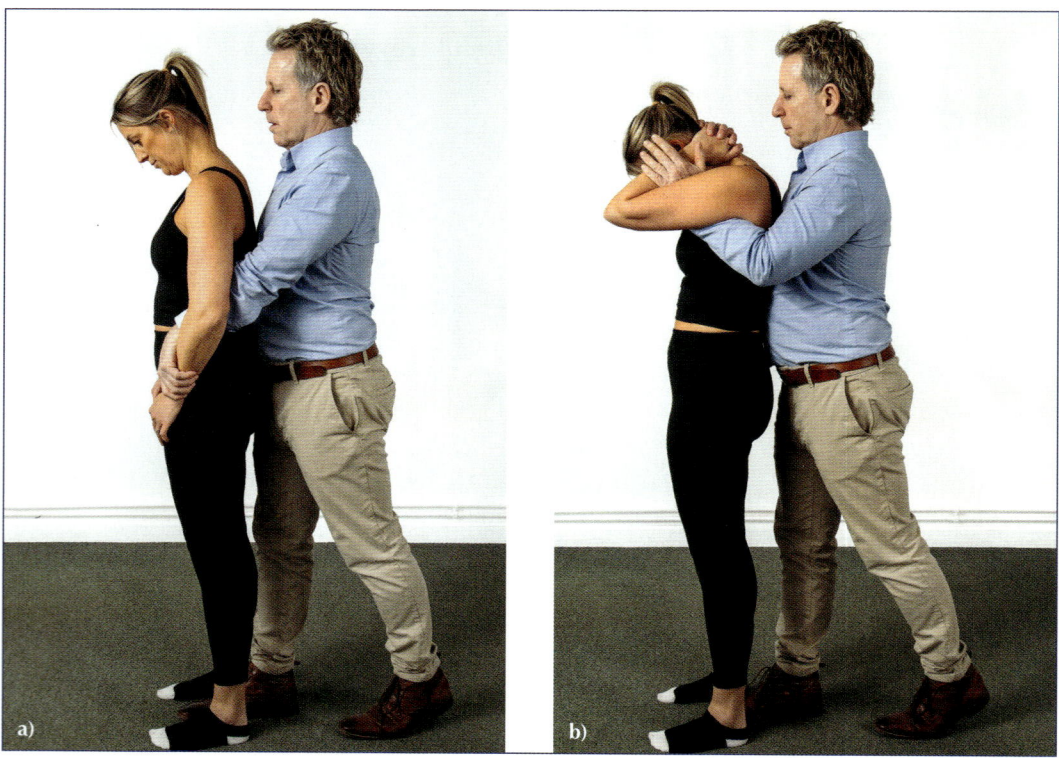

Figure 9.15. (a) Initial hand placement for the standing thoracic thrust; (b) patient interlinks their fingers and places them behind their head.

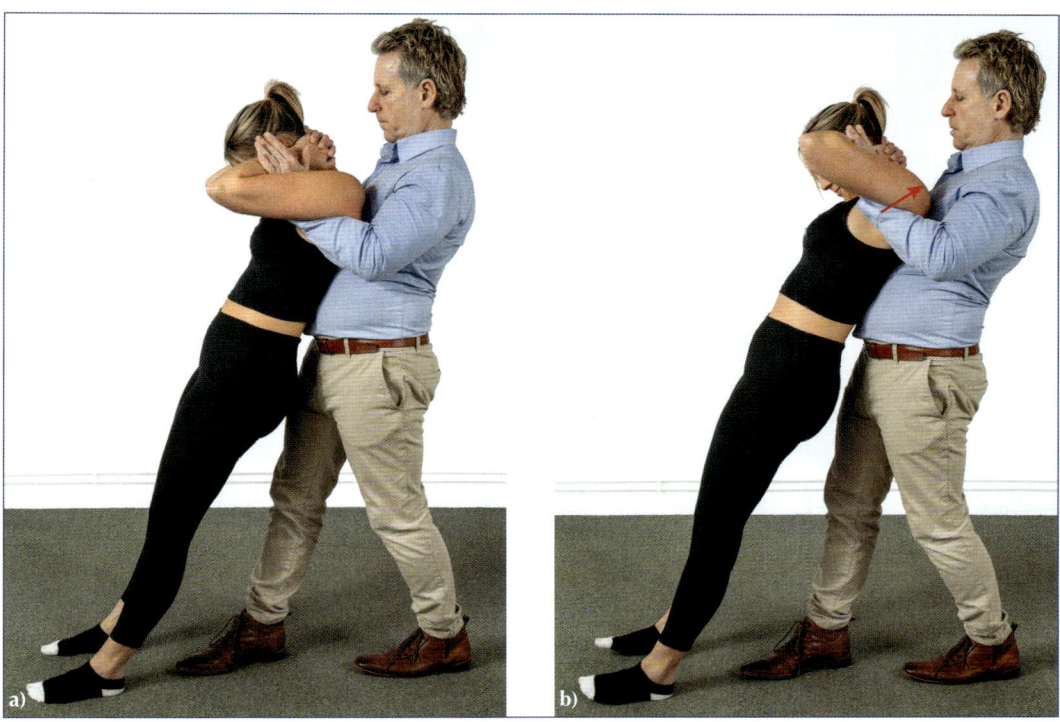

Figure 9.16. (a) The therapist fine-tunes the position. (b) The therapist applies a thrust for the CTJ in standing.

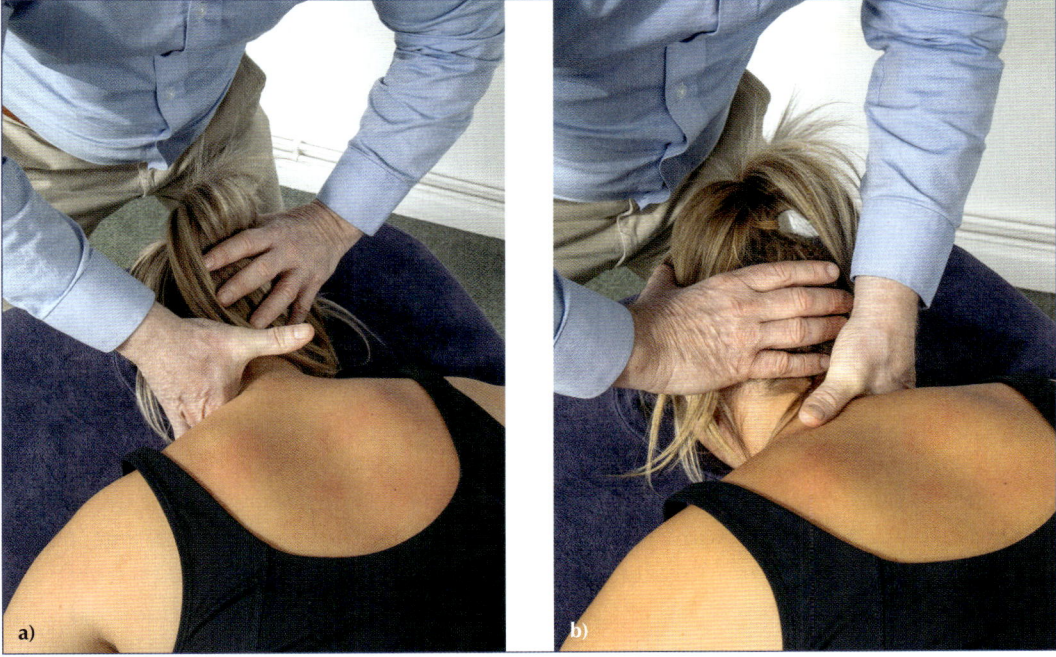

Figure 9.17. Hand placement for the positioning of (a) the left CTJ and (b) the right CTJ prior to the thrust.

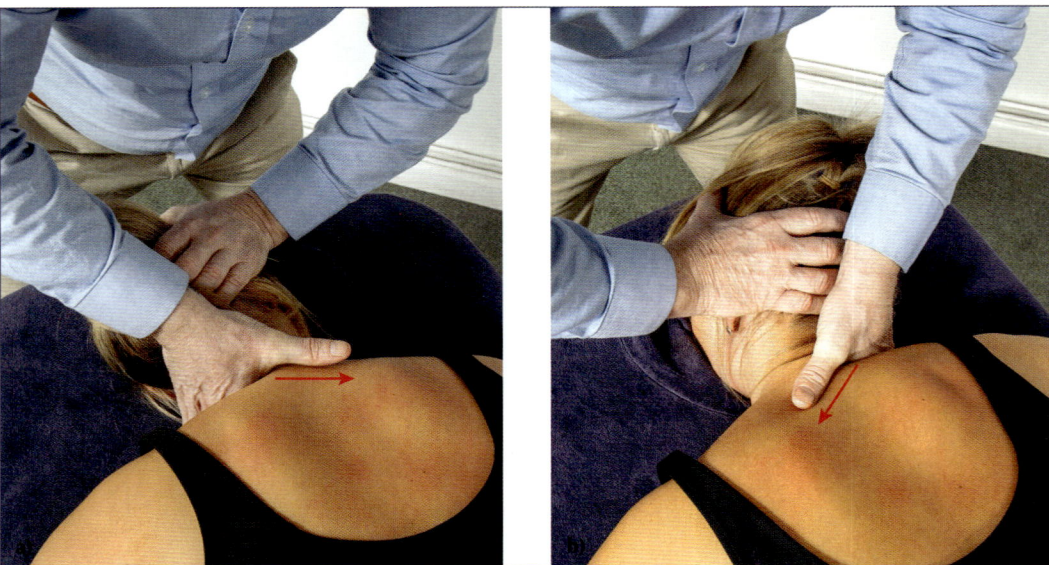

Figure 9.18. The therapist applies the thrust through (a) the left transverse process of C7 or (b) the right transverse process of C7 toward the axilla.

Prone CT manipulation using MCP joint

Prone CT manipulation using thumb

4. Thumb Thrust

This uses the same position as in technique 1, but this time place your thumb (pollux) against the level of the spinous process (SP) of C7 and position the patient's neck into a type 1 mechanic—side bending toward the same side as the thumb—and rotate to the opposite side (figure 9.19a for the left side, figure 9.19b for the right side).

Make any adjustments where necessary prior to the manipulation. When you and the patient are both relaxed, apply the HVT thrust to the spinous process in a horizontal direction (figure 9.20a for the left CTJ, figure 9.20b for the right CTJ).

Note: With the prone thrust techniques where you are using your MCP joint or your thumb, I suggest (for safety reasons) you apply the thrust with only the MCP joint or your thumb, and don't use the cervical spine as a lever during the thrust, (which is very tempting). A chiropractor colleague, Dr. Lewis Watts, said that when he was taught it was a 70/30 split when the thrust is applied; which means 70% thrust is from either the MCP joint or thumb and 30% is from the cervical spine. Personally, I suggest that the thrust is 100% from the MCP joint or thumb, to minimize the chance of exacerbating a preexisting cervical pathology.

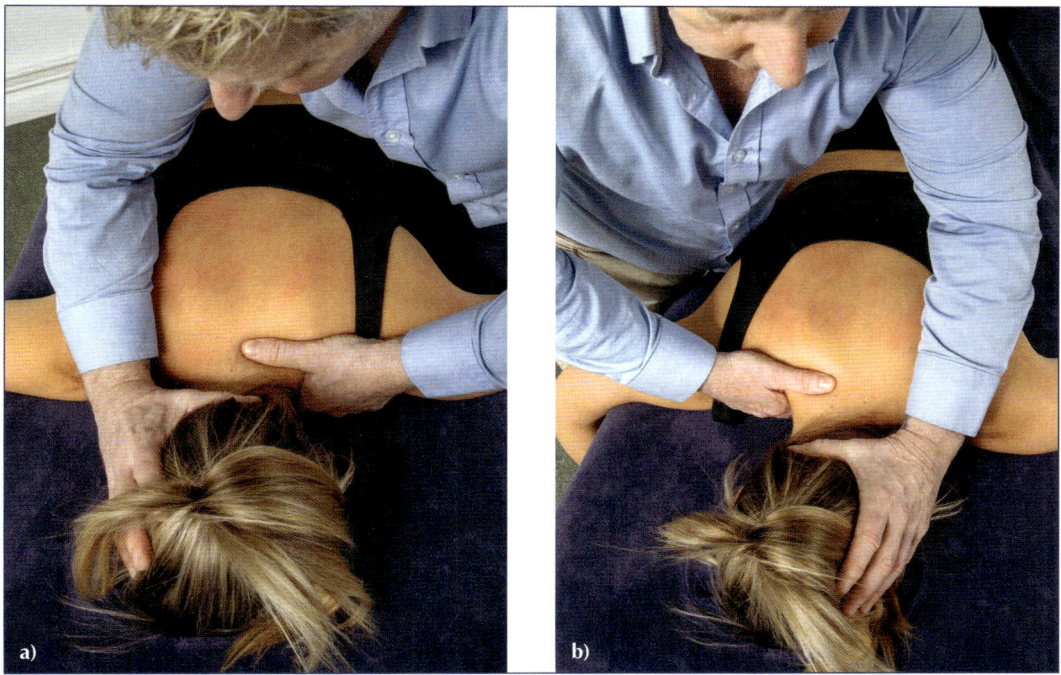

Figure 9.19. Hand placement for (a) the left CTJ and (b) the right CTJ, using the thumb to perform the thrust manipulation.

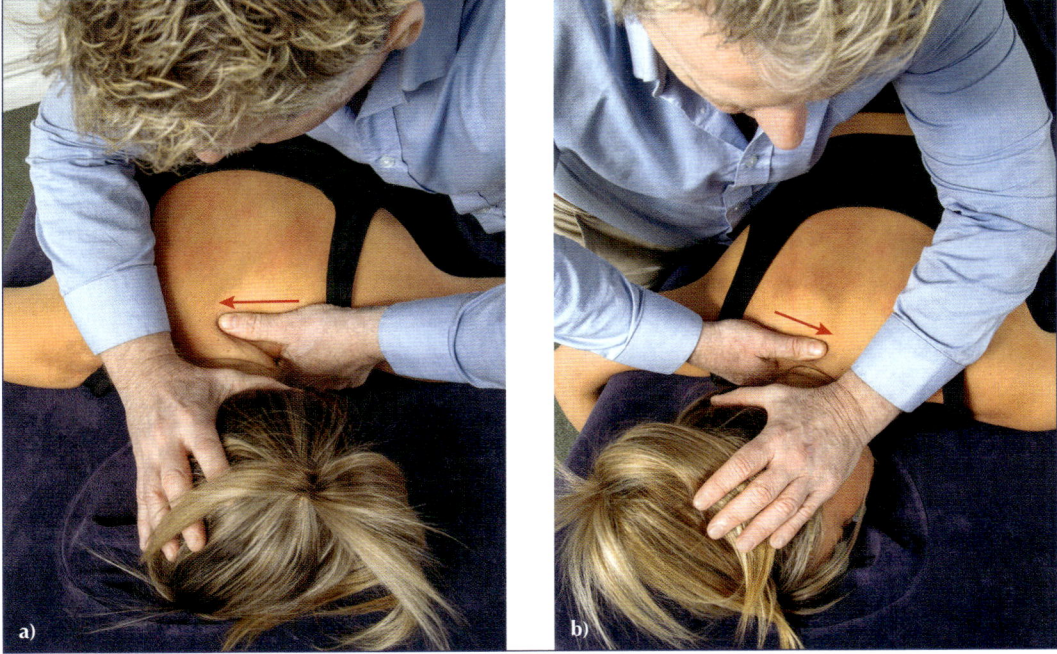

Figure 9.20. The therapist applies the thrust to (a) the left spinous process of C7 or (b) the right spinous process of C7 in a horizontal direction.

Techniques for the Thoracic Spine

Compared with the cervical and lumbar spine, the thoracic spine is relatively immobile, and this immobility is mainly for two anatomical reasons. Firstly, the thoracic spine has a connection to the ribcage and sternum via the costotransverse, costovertebral, and sternocostal articulations, which make this whole structure stable. Secondly, the height ratio of the thoracic intervertebral discs to the vertebral body is approximately 1:5, and this has the effect of reducing intersegmental motion compared with the more mobile segments of the cervical spine where the height ratio of vertebral disc to body is 2:5.

Even the lumbar spine has more mobility, as the ratio of disc height to vertebral body height is approximately 1:3.

Anatomy of the Thoracic Spine

The thoracic spine (TSp) consists of 12 vertebrae—T1–T12—and is known for its natural kyphosis (primary) curvature, which is mainly due to the wedge shape of the vertebral bodies. The ribs are attached

to the thoracic spine, so therefore the ribs and thoracic spine are considered as a single unit.

The functions of the thoracic spine are to provide protection for the spinal cord; to provide stability for the attachment of soft tissues like muscles, tendons, and ligaments; to allow the attachment of the associated ribs to form the ribcage; and to allow for the motions of inspiration and expiration. The thoracic spine is also designed for movement of the rest of the body—for example, bending forward and backward, rotation, and bending to the side—as well as facilitating movement of the shoulders and arms through its unique shape and design.

Because the thoracic region has a flexion primary curvature, it forms two transitional areas: one with the extension secondary curvature of the lumbar spine (LSp) below and one with the extension curve of the cervical spine (CSp) above. These two transitional areas are called the thoracolumbar junction, or TLJ, and the cervicothoracic junction, or CTJ, and treatments to these areas will be discussed and demonstrated here.

The thoracic facet joints are orientated in a more vertical plane, which limits flexion and extension but allows for some rotation and side bending. The superior facets face backward, upward, and laterally, while the inferior facets face forward, downward, and medially.

Manual therapy techniques like mobilizations and manipulations that are applied to the TSp have been proven to benefit many patients presenting with all types of thoracic and spinal pathologies— for example, thoracic stiffness, rib dysfunction, T4 syndrome, cervical/lumbar spine, and even shoulder girdle pain.

I always teach that if you have a problem with the TSp, more than likely an issue will eventually develop within the LSp or CSp or even both. Edmondston and Singer (1997) discussed the interactions between thoracic spine posture and mobility, and they believed that the position of the thoracic spine plays a role in the development of spinal pain syndromes.

Furthermore, Harrison et al. (2002) discussed how an anterior/posterior translation of the thoracic spine affects the lumbar spine, pelvis tilt, and thoracic kyphosis, resulting in patients' presenting symptoms.

To palpate the transverse processes (TPs) of the TSp is a challenging task because of their anatomical location: they are relatively deep compared with the superficial tissues associated to the TSp. However, Mitchell et al. (1979) have described a method to accurately predict the location of each of the levels of the thoracic TPs from their corresponding

spinous processes (SPs), which they called the "rule of threes." This method of palpation and location has been an invaluable tool for the physical therapist (figure 10.1).

Anatomy of the thoracic spine

The Rule of Threes Explained

T1–T3

The palpable tips of the SPs are in the same plane as their associated TPs, so the SP of T2 will be in line with the TPs of T2.

T4–T6

These SPs project more caudally (inferiorly), so are halfway between their own TPs and the TPs of the vertebra below, so the SP of T5 is located halfway between the TPs of T5 and T6.

T7–T9

These SPs project even more caudally, so now the SPs are in line with the TPs from the vertebral level below, so the SP of T8 will be in line with the TPs of T9.

T10–T12

These have similar characteristics to *all* of the three previous methods described. T10 is like T7–T9, so its SP is in line with

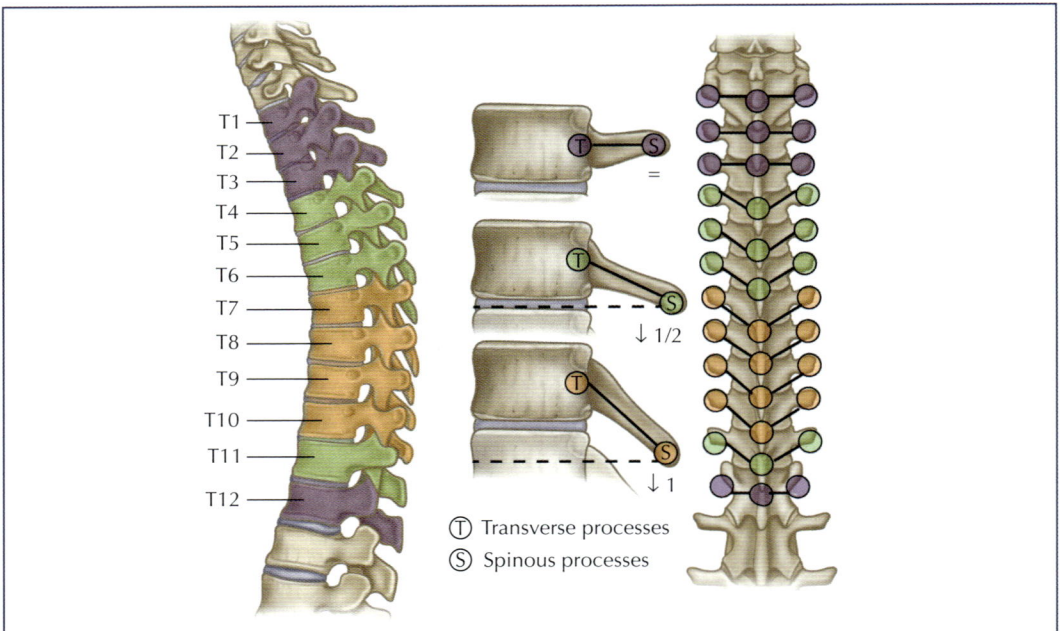

Figure 10.1. The rule of threes.

the TPs of T11 below. T11 follows the halfway rule as for T4–T6, and T12 follows the first method, for T1–T3: its SP is in line with its corresponding TPs.

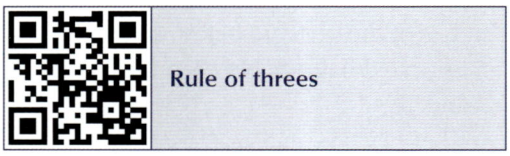

Rule of threes

Anatomy of the Ribcage

See chapter 11 for details of ribcage anatomy and true and false ribs.

Assessment and Treatment Protocols

In chapter 6 I discussed how to assess the thoracic spine through palpation of

your thumbs onto the TPs of the thoracic spine in three anatomical positions: neutral, flexion, and extension. From these positions you would then decide which position the facet is fixed in: extension dysfunction coupled with rotation and side bending (ERS) or flexion dysfunction coupled with rotation and side bending (FRS). In terms of treatment, we are going to encourage either an *opening* or a *closure* of the dysfunctional facet joint.

Motion Testing

The following technique (we can use this as a simple reminder from the previous chapter) is used to ascertain motion of the lower cervical spine where it articulates with the upper thoracic region, plus we can continue with motion testing for the remainder of the upper thoracic spine.

From the technique demonstrated, it is also a great way to then treat any dysfunctions found using METs, mobilizations, and manipulations.

With the patient sitting at the end of a couch, initially palpate the SP of C7 using the tip of your index or middle finger, because this is an easy landmark to locate—vertebra prominens—due to its larger size. Next, lightly place the tip of your finger to the interspace between C7 and T1, and then slowly guide the patient's head passively into flexion and extension to ascertain motion between these two vertebrae.

It is difficult to say what is normal because you have nothing to compare it with, hence you should now palpate the interspace between T1 and T2 (figure 10.2), then T2 and T3, and so on. If you find a restriction and lack of obvious

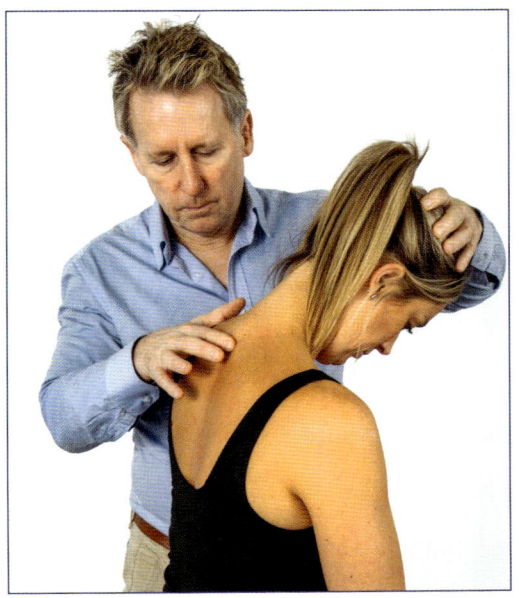

Figure 10.2. Motion testing of the interspace between T1 and T2.

separation between the two vertebrae into flexion, then you have found a fixed *closed* facet (ERS). You would now palpate the TPs as already explained in the three positions to decide if the closed facet joint is on the left or right side.

For a fixed *open* facet joint, then the interspinous space will remain wider (open) and unable to approximate on the extension movement of the cervical and thoracic spine (FRS). If you consider there is a fixed open facet, then again you would palpate the three positions to decide if the dysfunction is on the left or right side.

To palpate below the level of T3/T4, it is unrealistic to use the cervical spine passively, so you would need to use the patient's arms as a lever to assist in the flexion (figure 10.3a) and extension of the thoracic spine (figure 10.3b).

Diagnosis T1/T2 ERS(r)

Treatment: MET. The facet joint is fixed *closed* on the *right* side between the levels of T1 and T2, so the treatment will be to open the facet joint using an MET.

Technique 1

With the patient sitting, palpate the interspace level between T1 and T2 and slowly passively flex the patient's head until you feel motion at your finger. From this position ask the patient to extend against your resistance (20% effort) for 10 seconds (figure 10.4).

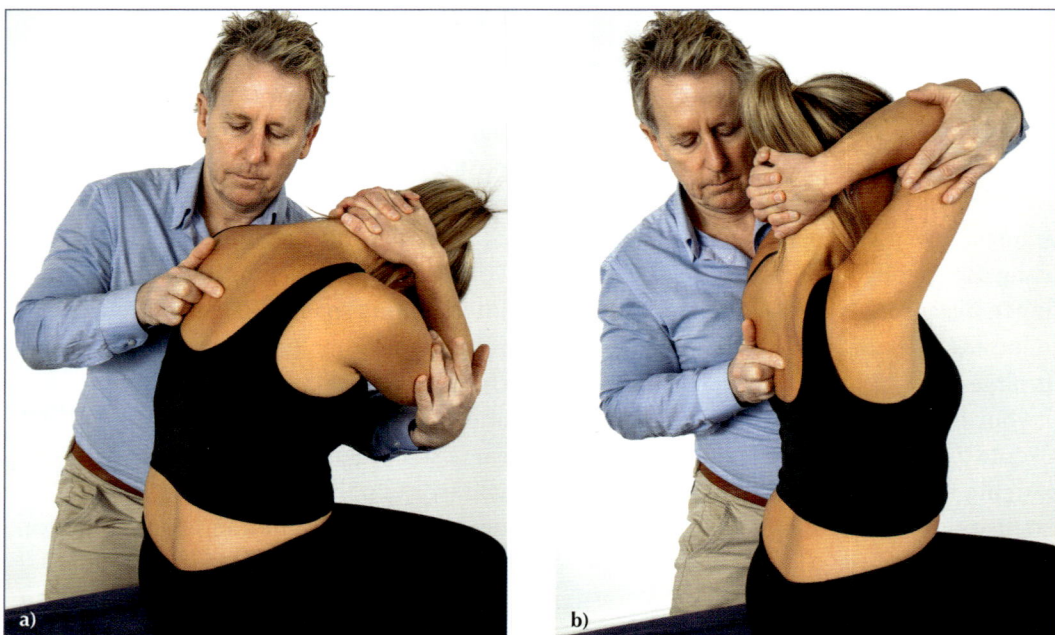

Figure 10.3. (a) Motion testing for flexion of the thoracic spine below T4 by using the patient's arms as a lever; (b) motion testing into extension of the thoracic spine.

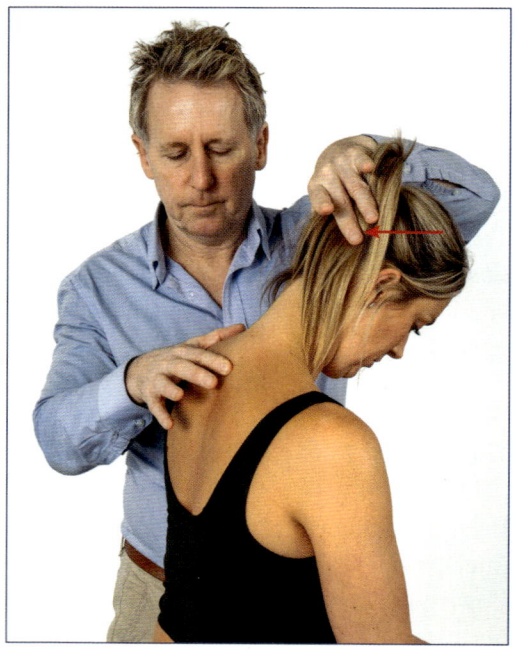

Figure 10.4. The patient is asked to extend their head against a resistance for 10 seconds.

After the contraction, ask the patient to breathe in, and then take the head into further flexion while you apply caudal pressure through your index finger to the SP of T2 (figure 10.5a), or you might find it easier to use your pisiform bone (figure 10.5b), because this gives the T1 vertebra the chance for the facet joint to open on the level below.

Technique 2

You can also take the patient's head from the flexed position and combine it with rotation and side bending left (figure 10.6), because this motion will encourage further opening of the facet joint that is fixed on the right side (you still apply caudal pressure to T2).

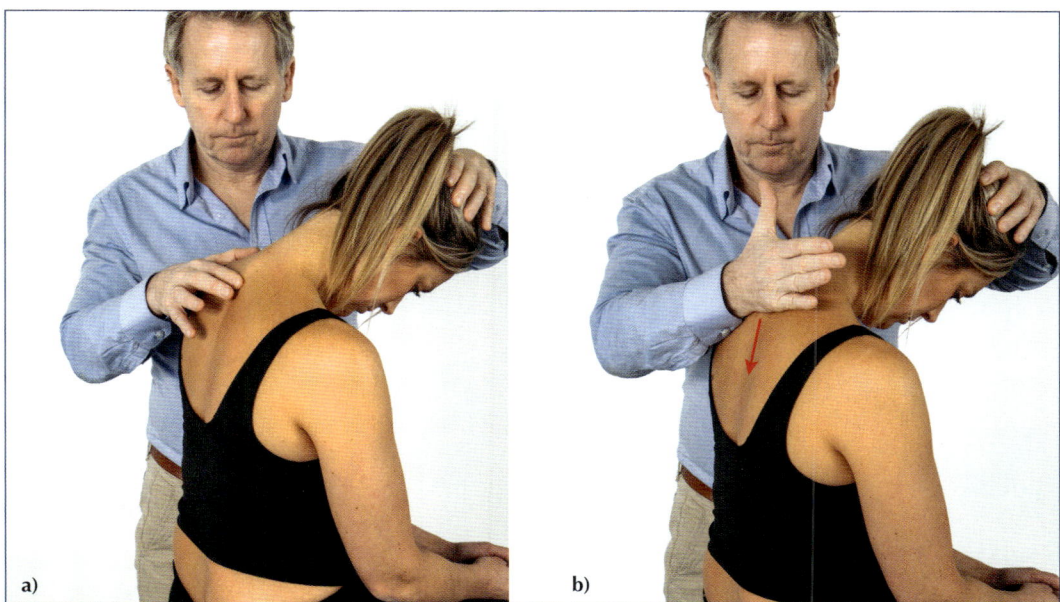

Figure 10.5. (a) The therapist now guides the patient's head into further flexion, while applying caudal pressure to T2 through their finger; (b) caudal pressure to T2 through use of the pisiform bone.

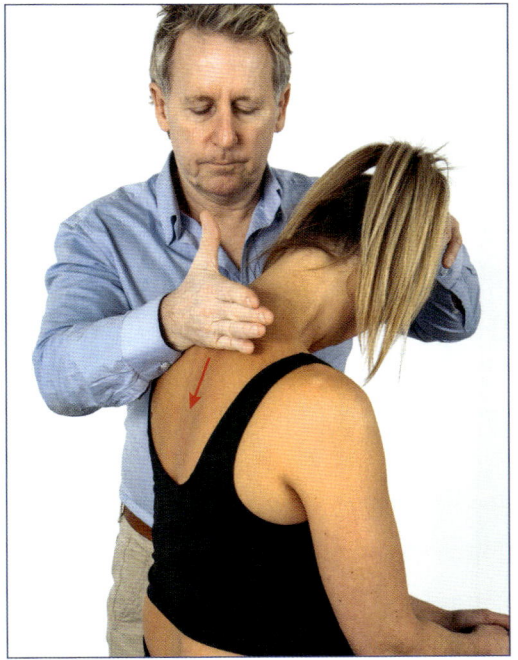

Figure 10.6. The therapist now guides the patient's head into further flexion, with rotation and side bending left, while still applying caudal pressure to T2.

MET of T1/T2 for an ERS(L)

Diagnosis T2/T3 FRS(l)

Treatment: MET. The facet joint is fixed *open*, and remember it is on the opposite side, so the facet joint is flexed, rotated, and side bent to the left. However, it is the *right*-side facet joint that is fixed *open* between the levels of T2 and T3, so the treatment will be to assist closure of the facet joint using an MET.

Technique 1

With the patient sitting, palpate the interspace level between T2 and T3, and slowly passively extend the patient's

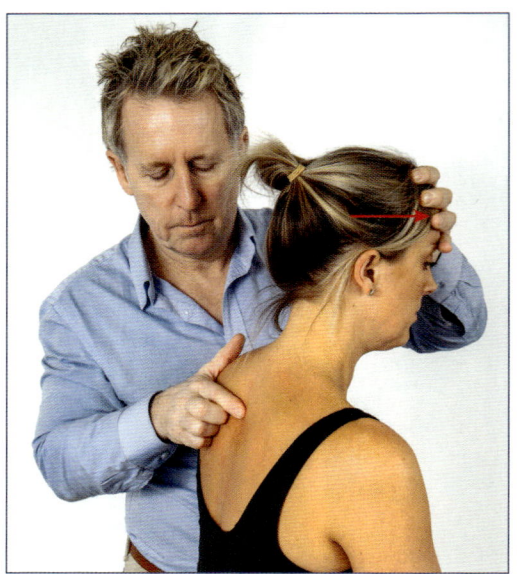

Figure 10.7. The patient is asked to flex their head against a resistance for 10 seconds.

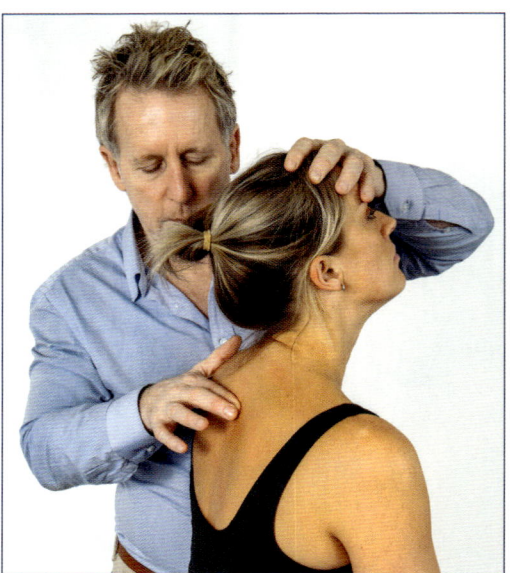

Figure 10.8. The therapist now guides the patient's head into further extension.

head until you feel motion at your finger. From this position, ask the patient to flex their head against your resistance (20% effort) for 10 seconds (figure 10.7).

After the contraction, ask the patient to breathe in, and then take the head into further extension (figure 10.8).

Technique 2

You can also take the head of the patient from the position of extension and combine it with rotation and side bending right (figure 10.9), because this motion will encourage further closing of the facet joint that is fixed open on the right side.

Diagnosis T6/T7 ERS(r)

Treatment: MET. The facet joint is fixed *closed* on the *right* side between the levels

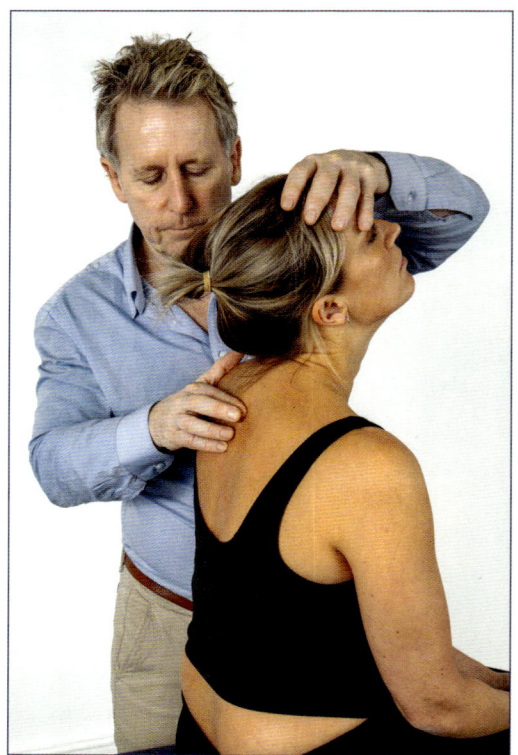

Figure 10.9. The therapist now guides the patient's head into further extension, with rotation and side bending right.

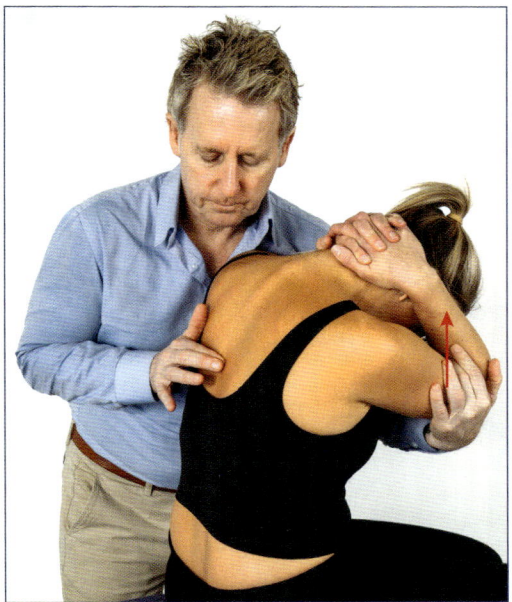

Figure 10.10. The patient is asked to extend their thoracic spine against a resistance for 10 seconds.

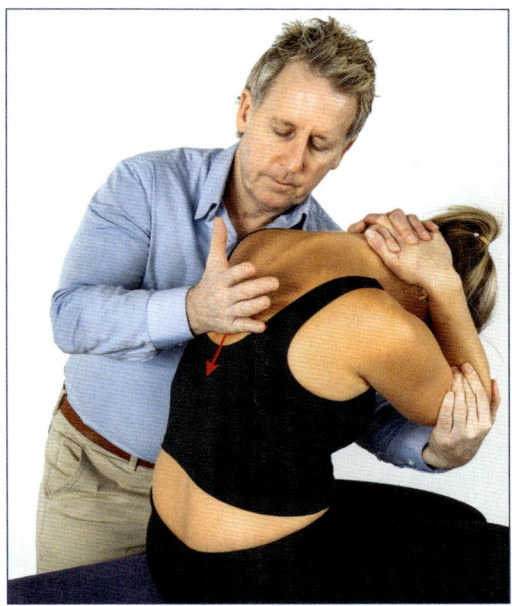

Figure 10.11. The therapist now guides the patient's thoracic spine into further flexion, while applying caudal pressure to T7.

of T6 and T7, so the treatment will be to open the facet joint using an MET.

Technique 1

With the patient sitting, palpate the interspace level between T6 and T7, ask the patient to interlock their fingers behind their neck, and using their arms as a lever passively flex the thoracic spine until you feel motion at your finger. From this position, ask the patient to extend against your resistance (20% effort) for 10 seconds (figure 10.10).

After the contraction, ask the patient to breathe in, and then take their thoracic spine into further flexion while applying caudal pressure to the SP of T7 (figure 10.11), because this gives T6 the chance for the facet joint to open on the level below.

Technique 2

You can also take the patient's thoracic spine from the flexed position and combine it with rotation and side bending left (figure 10.12). This motion will encourage further opening of the facet joint that is fixed on the right side (you still apply caudal pressure to T7).

Diagnosis T5/T6 FRS(r)

Treatment: MET. The facet joint is fixed *open*, and remember it is on the opposite side to the motion, so the facet joint is flexed, rotated, and side bent to the right; however it is the *left*-side facet joint that is fixed *open* between the levels of T5 and T6, so an MET treatment will be used to assist closure of the facet joint.

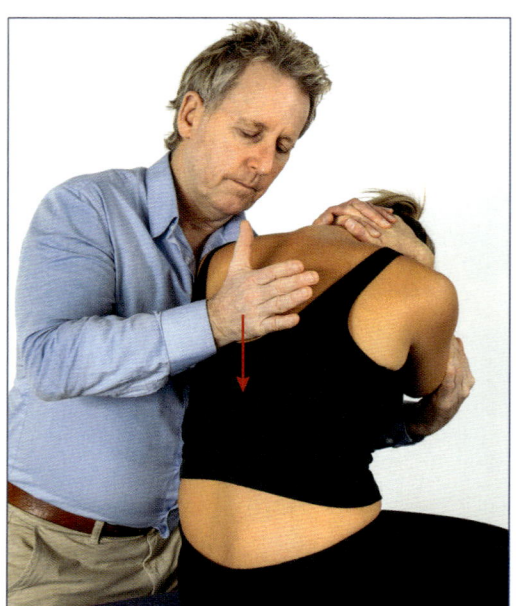

Figure 10.12. The therapist now guides the patient's thoracic spine into further flexion, with rotation and side bending left, while still applying caudal pressure to T7.

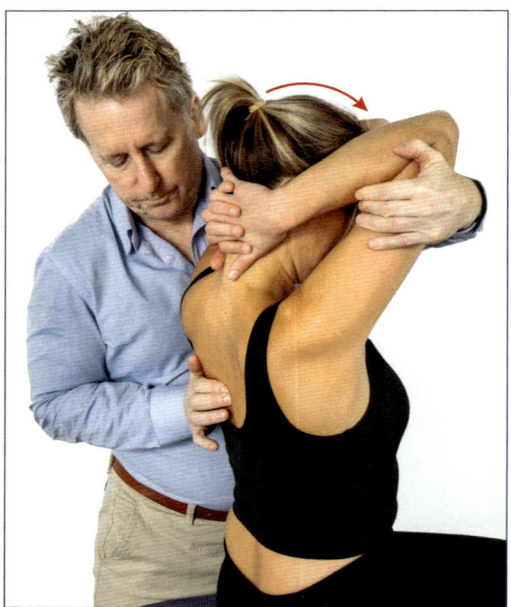

Figure 10.13. The patient is asked to flex their trunk against a resistance for 10 seconds.

Technique 1

With the patient sitting, palpate the interspace level between T5 and T6, and slowly passively extend the patient's thoracic spine until you feel motion at your finger. From this position, ask the patient to flex their trunk against your resistance (20% effort) for 10 seconds (figure 10.13).

After the contraction ask the patient to breathe in, and then take the trunk into further extension (figure 10.14).

Technique 2

You can also take the patient's trunk from the position of extension and combine

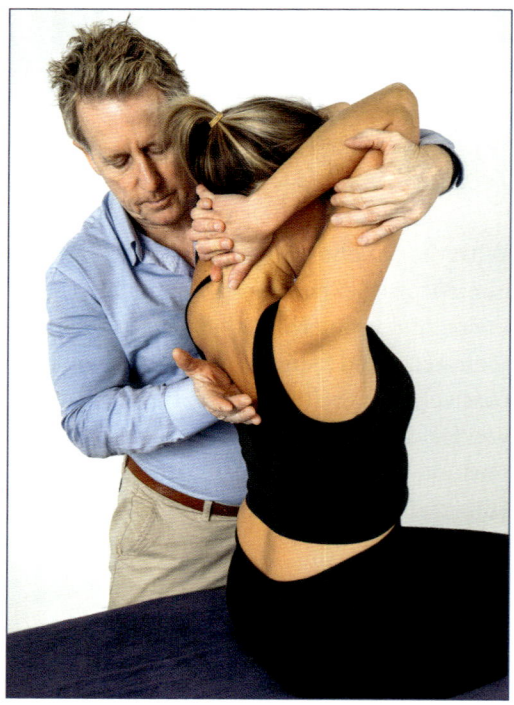

Figure 10.14. The therapist now guides the patient's thoracic spine into further extension.

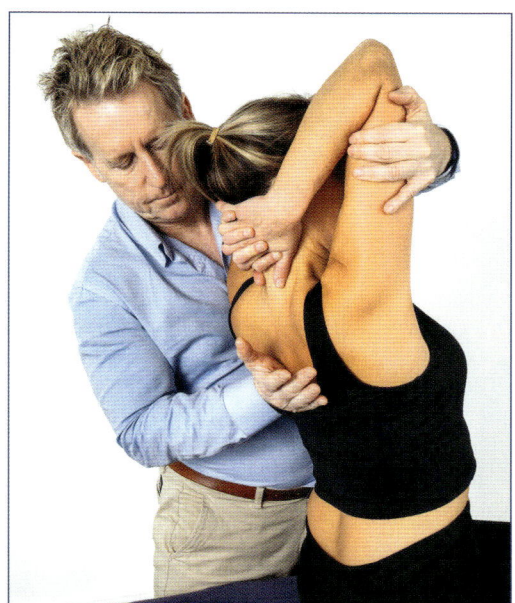

Figure 10.15. The therapist now guides the patient's thoracic spine into further extension, with rotation and side bending left, while monitoring T6.

it with rotation and side bending left (figure 10.15), because this motion will encourage further closing of the facet joint that is fixed open on the left side.

General Mobilization Techniques

The following mobilizing techniques are suitable for anybody who has general stiffness to the thoracic region, because they are all effective mobilizations that will assist in improving the mobility of the thoracic spine and the associated and attached ribcage. I also suggest that the following six mobilizations are included in your overall treatment protocol, not just for the thoracic spine but for the whole of the spine.

Remember that a restricted thoracic spine can be the cause of pain within the lumbar

or cervical spine, so it makes sense to include this area as part of the treatment modality.

For all the following mobilizations, the patient is sitting at the end of a couch, and in a chair for the last technique.

Technique 1a—Rotation

Ask the patient to sit in a neutral position and cross their arms over their chest. Place your left arm over the patient's arms to stabilize their torso, and place the heel or fingers of your right hand onto the opposite erector spinae muscles (right side of spine). Passively guide the patient into left rotation while you apply pressure to the erector spinae to increase the rotation (figure 10.16).

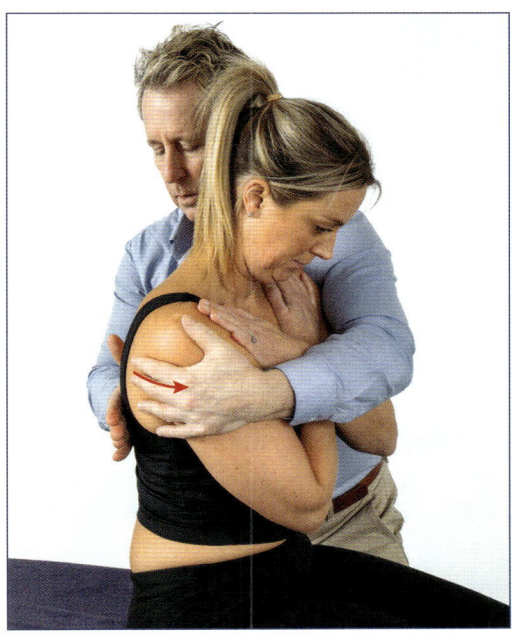

Figure 10.16. The therapist passively rotates the patient to the left while applying pressure to the erector spinae muscles.

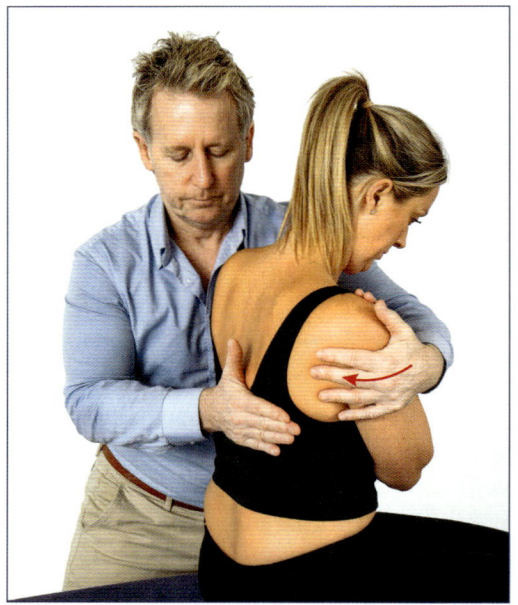

Figure 10.17. The patient is contracting by rotating to the right.

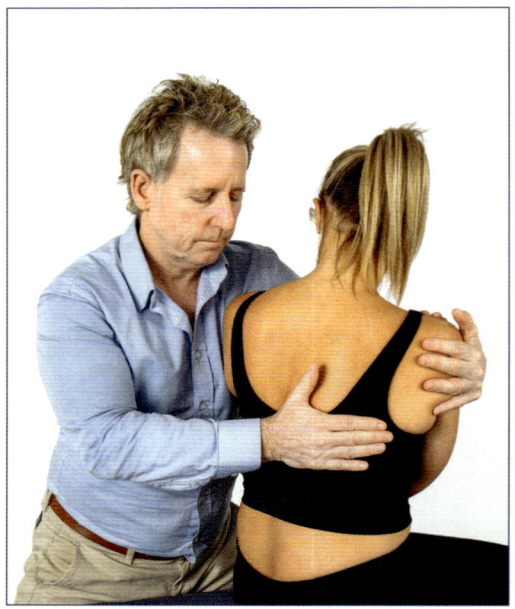

Figure 10.18. After the relaxation, the therapist encourages further left rotation.

Technique 1b—Rotation with MET

An MET can also be applied from the position of bind: ask the patient to rotate to the right for 10 seconds (figure 10.17), and on the relaxation phase passively encourage further left rotation (figure 10.18).

Technique 2a—Side Bending

With the patient in the same position as above, place your left arm over their arms to stabilize their torso, and place the heel or fingers of your right hand onto the same-side ribcage (left side of spine). Passively guide the patient into left side bending while applying pressure to the ribcage to increase the motion (figure 10.19).

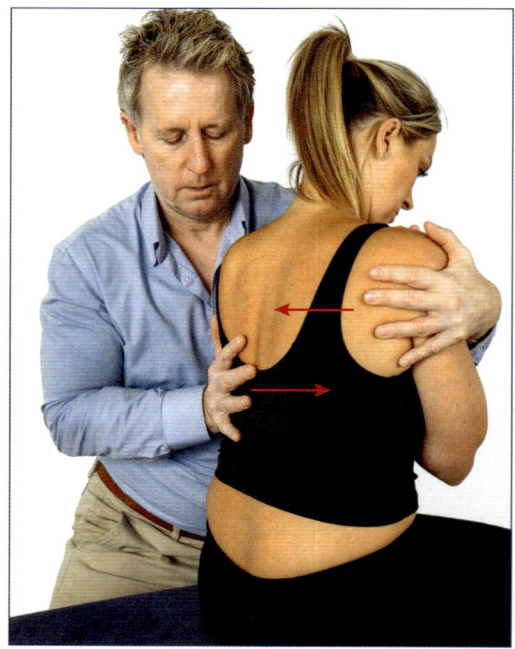

Figure 10.19. The therapist is passively side bending the patient to the left while applying pressure to the ribcage.

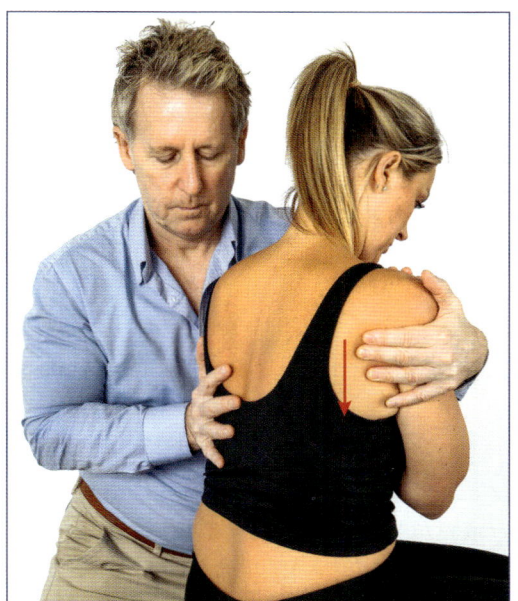

Figure 10.20. The patient is contracting by side bending to the right.

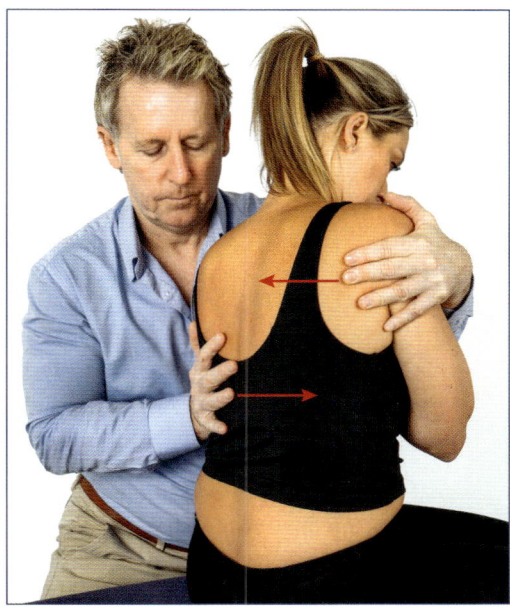

Figure 10.21. After the relaxation, the therapist encourages further left side bending.

Technique 2b—Side Bending with MET

An MET can also be applied from the position of bind. Ask the patient to side bend to the right for 10 seconds (figure 10.20), and on the relaxation phase, passively encourage further left side bending (figure 10.21).

Technique 3a—Flexion and Extension

In the same position as above, either place your left arm over the patient's arms to stabilize their torso, or ask the patient to interlock their fingers behind their neck. Support the patient's elbow and use this as a lever, and place the heel of your right hand directly onto the SPs. Passively guide the patient into flexion (figure 10.22) and extension (figure 10.23) while you

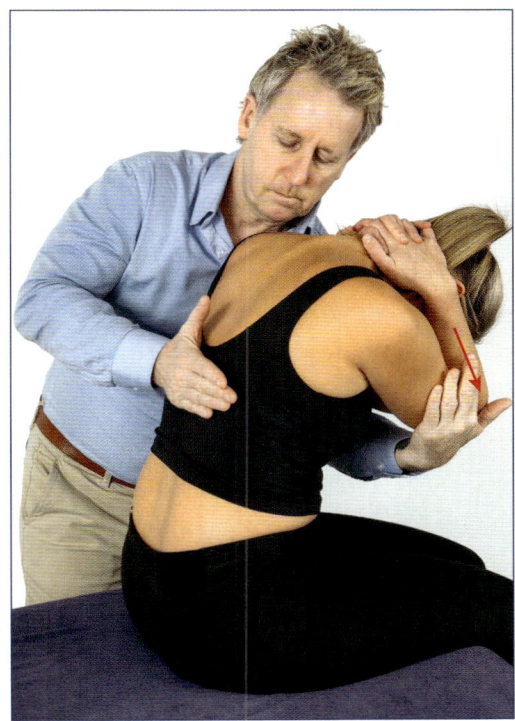

Figure 10.22. The therapist is passively flexing the patient's thoracic spine, with pressure applied to the spinous processes.

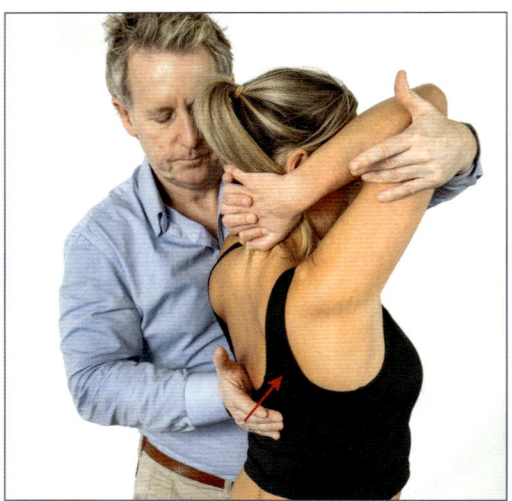

Figure 10.23. The therapist is passively extending the patient's thoracic spine, with pressure applied to the spinous processes.

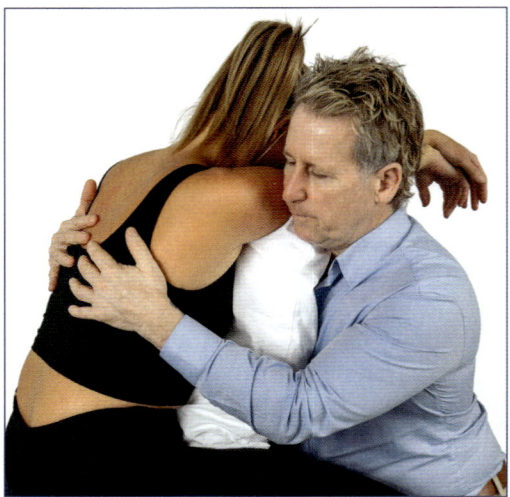

Figure 10.24. The therapist is passively flexing the patient's thoracic spine, with pressure applied to the erector spinae muscles.

apply pressure to specific SPs to increase the motion.

Technique 3b—Flexion and Extension with MET

An MET can also be applied from the position of bind. Ask the patient to either extend or flex their spine against your resistance for 10 seconds, and on the relaxation phase, encourage further flexion or extension.

 General mobilizations of thoracic spine and ribcage

Technique 4—Flexion and Extension with a Pillow

Ask the patient to place both of their arms over one of your shoulders, and

place a pillow between you for privacy and comfort. Place your fingers adjacent to the spinal column and apply a flexion (figure 10.24) and extension motion (figure 10.25) using your hands, whilst at the same time using your legs to assist the motion by slowly standing up and down.

Technique 5—Rotation and Side Bending with a Pillow

In the same position as above, place your fingers adjacent to the spinal column, enabling you to apply a rotation motion through the use of your hands (figure 10.26), and then to change the technique to assist in side bending (figure 10.27).

Note: Once one side of the thoracic spine is mobilized, ask the patient to place their arms over your other shoulder so that the opposite side of their thoracic spine can also be mobilized.

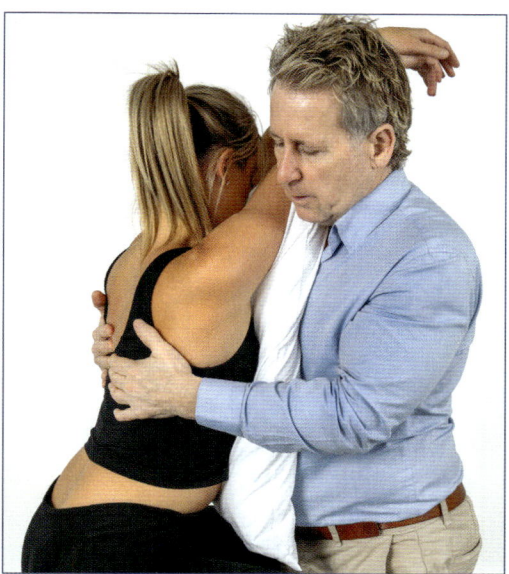

Figure 10.25. The therapist is passively extending the patient's thoracic spine, with pressure applied to the erector spinae muscles as they stand up.

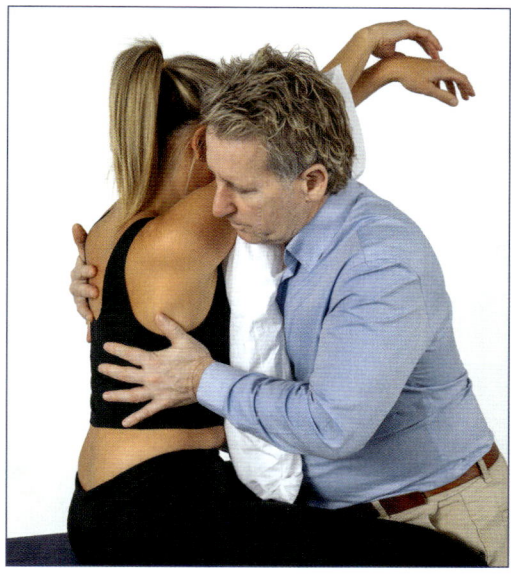

Figure 10.27. The therapist is passively side bending the patient's thoracic spine.

Mobilizations of the thoracic spine using a pillow

Technique 6a—Upper Thoracic Flexion and Extension

Ask the patient to place their arms parallel to each other at 90°, with their elbows flexed at shoulder height, and to place their forehead on their forearms. Interlock your arms through the patient's arms and head, and contact the upper thoracic spine (figure 10.28a). From this position, slowly bring the patient forward so that they are flexed through their lumbar spine (figure 10.28b).

You are now able to apply a flexion (figure 10.29a) and extension motion (figure 10.29b) to the area of the upper thoracic spine using your fingers.

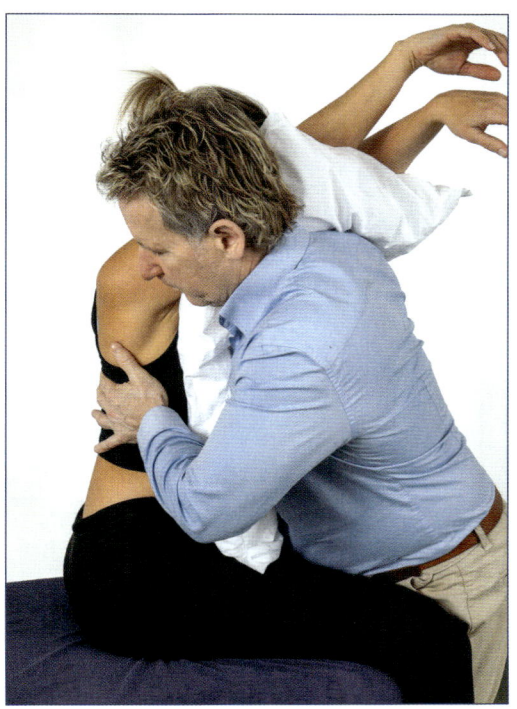

Figure 10.26. The therapist is passively rotating the patient's thoracic spine.

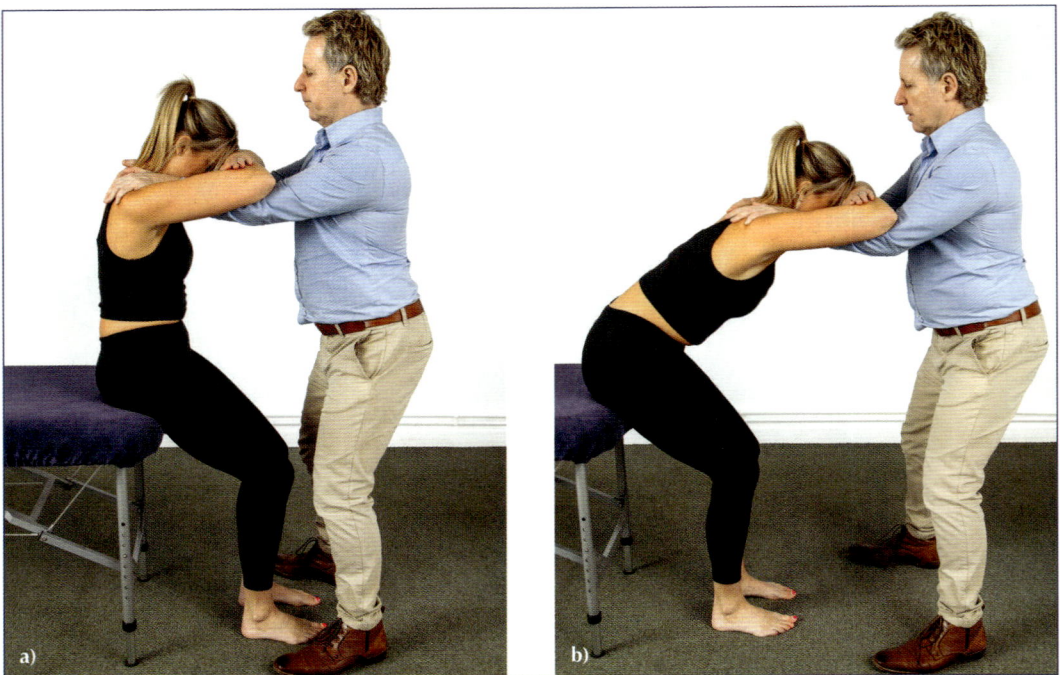

Figure 10.28. (a) The therapist interlocks through the patient's arms and contacts their upper thoracic spine, and (b) slowly brings them forward into flexion.

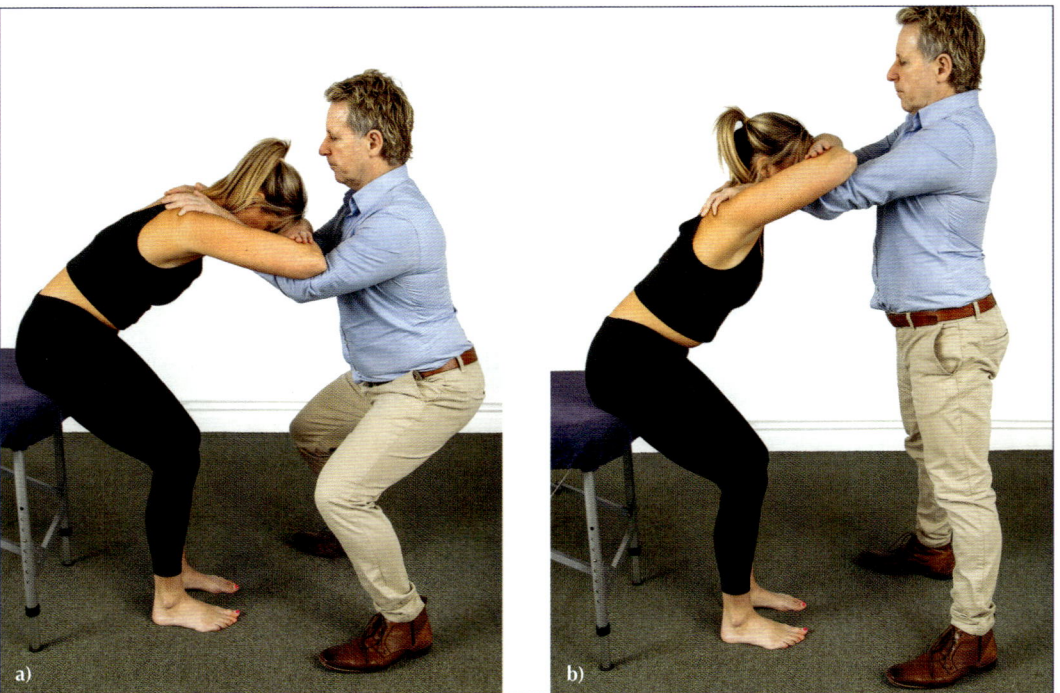

Figure 10.29. The therapist is passively (a) flexing and (b) extending the patient's upper thoracic spine.

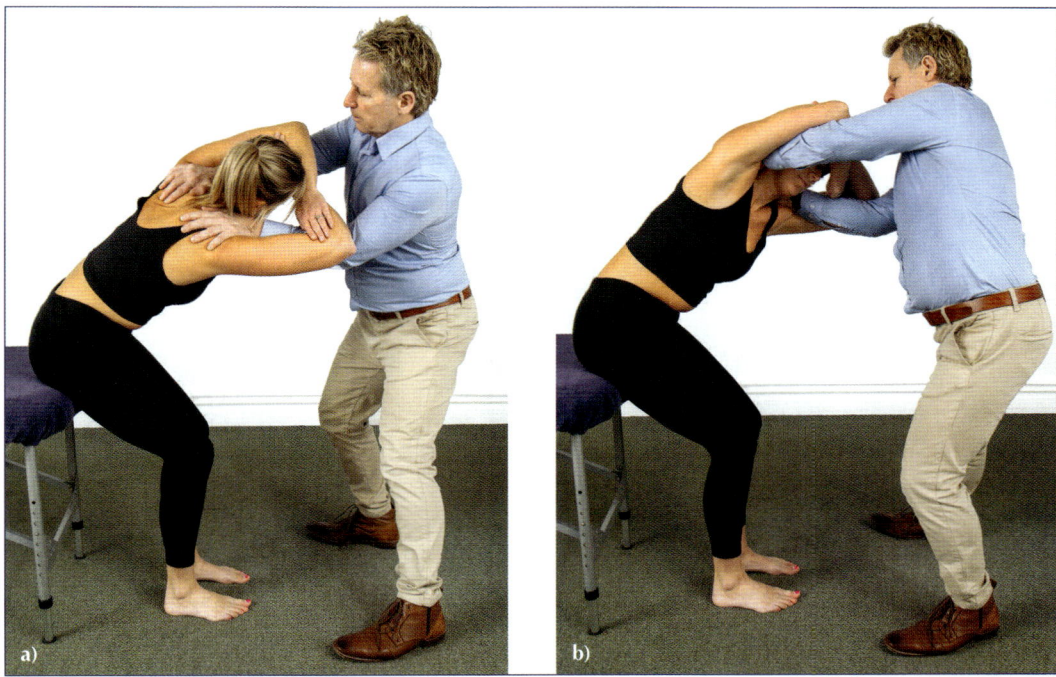

Figure 10.30. The therapist is passively rotating the thoracic spine (a) to the left and (b) to the right.

Technique 6b—Thoracic Rotation and Side Bending

This technique is identical to the one above except this time you induce a rotation left (figure 10.30a) and right (figure 10.30b) of the thoracic spine, and then introduce a side bending motion of the thoracic spine to the left (figure 10.31a) and right side (figure 10.31b). You can see for the side bending techniques that the therapist is performing a type of lunge motion through their legs, which will protect their own spine.

Mobilizations of upper thoracic spine

Mobilizations of middle thoracic spine

Spinal Manipulations (HVT)

The following treatments for the thoracic region are mainly manipulative techniques. However, one doesn't physically have to perform the motion with a *thrust* at the point of bind— from this position you may choose a mobilization technique instead of a manipulation. Some techniques may be more appropriate for some patients, and even for the therapist.

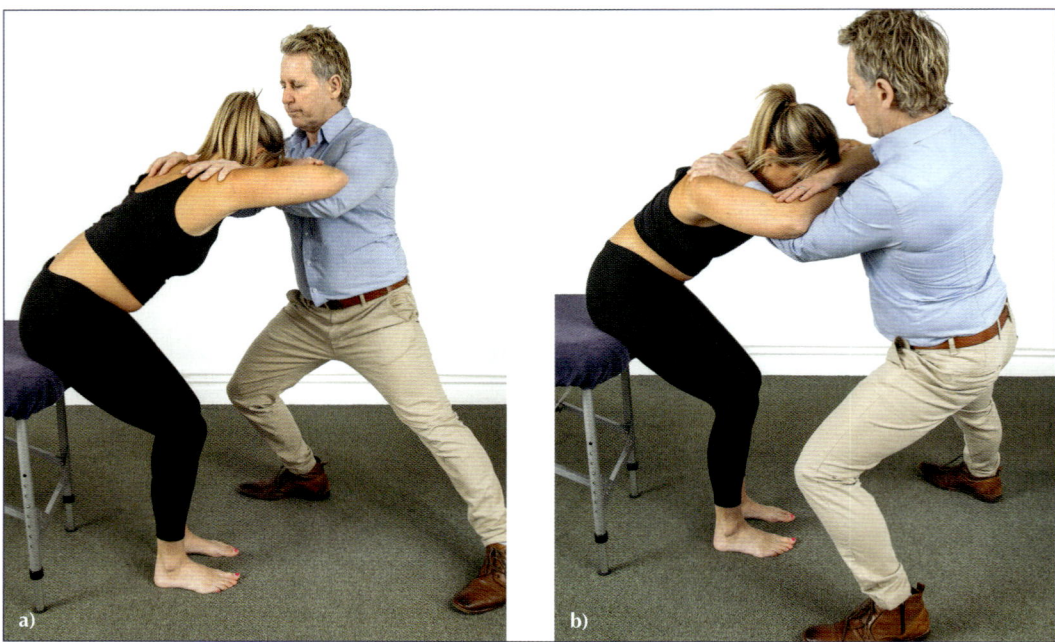

Figure 10.31. The therapist is passively side bending the thoracic spine (a) to the left and (b) to the right.

Seated Thoracic Thrust: Diagnosis T6/7 ERS(r)

Motion restriction: Flexion, left rotation, and left-side bending

Position: Patient seated

Note: This technique will also work for an ERS(l) because when the thrust is applied, the facet joints on both sides will open, rather than the technique specifying just the right side.

With the patient seated on the couch, ask them to sit as far back as is comfortable. A bolster under the knee can be used for comfort if required. Roll up a small hand towel as tightly as you can and place it against your sternum, and then make contact to their thoracic spine, and specifically to the level of the spinous process of T7 (figure 10.32).

Place the patient's right arm under their left arm, so that their arms are crossed

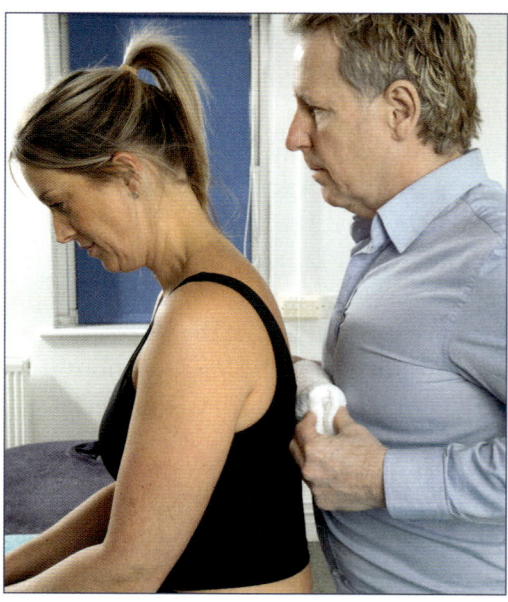

Figure 10.32. The patient is sitting near to the end of the couch with a bolster under their knee, and the therapist applies a towel to the level of T7.

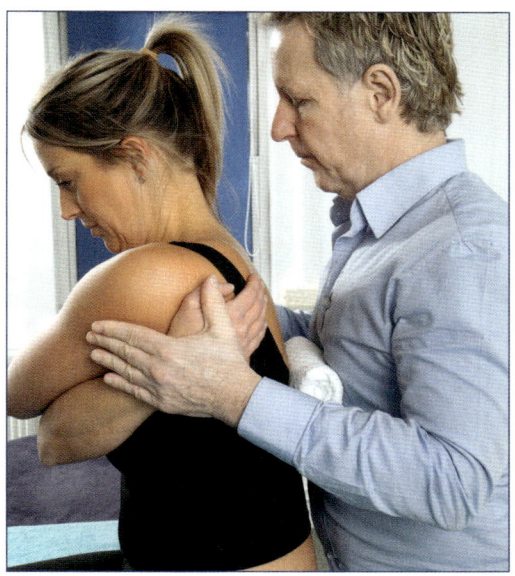

Figure 10.33. The patient's arms are crossed over in front of their chest.

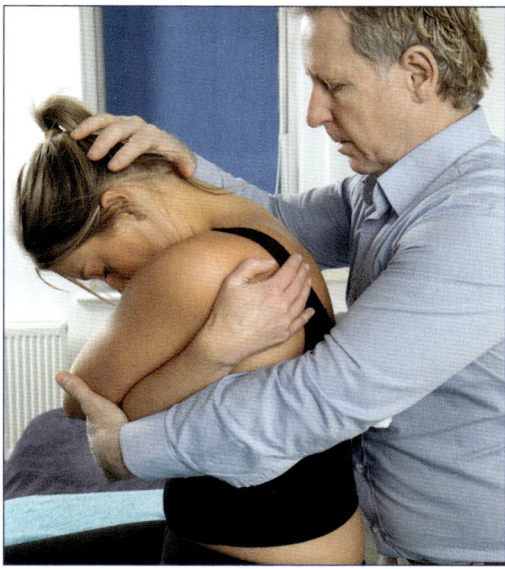

Figure 10.34. The patient is passively flexed until the therapist feels a bind to their sternum.

over their chest and their hands around the back of their shoulders (figure 10.33).

Place your left hand onto the elbows of the patient, and with your right hand slowly apply flexion to the patient's head and trunk until you feel a bind at the sternum (figure 10.34)

From this position, place both your arms around the patient's elbows, and slowly apply a pulling type of motion to their elbows. At the same time, push your chest forward against the towel (figure 10.35). The idea of these two movements is that the pulling motion from the patient's elbows causes a *posterior* glide of the T6 level (above), and the pushing motion from your chest causes an *anterior* glide of the T7 vertebra below (one might also call it an anterior–posterior [AP] glide technique).

Make any adjustments where necessary prior to the manipulation, and when

you and the patient are both relaxed, ask them to take a deep breath in, and on the relaxation phase, apply the HVT thrust through their elbows directed toward you and slightly upward. Simultaneously

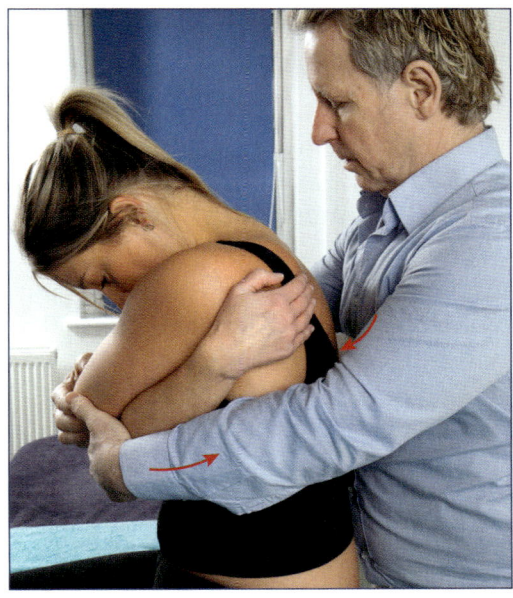

Figure 10.35. Anterior/posterior gliding motion of T6/T7 with a technique using a towel.

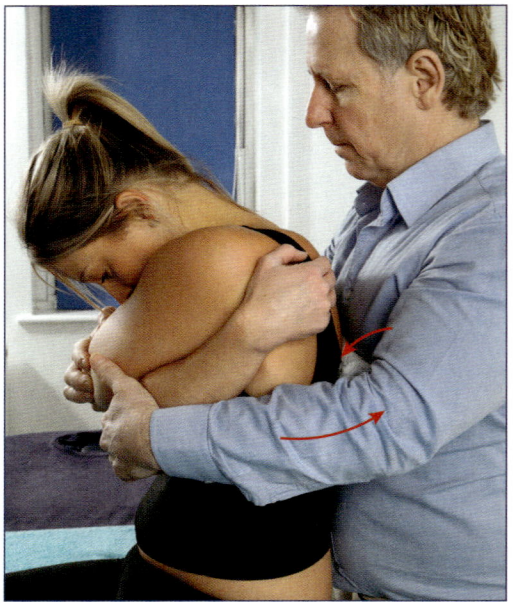

Figure 10.36. A thrust is applied toward the therapist and slightly upward.

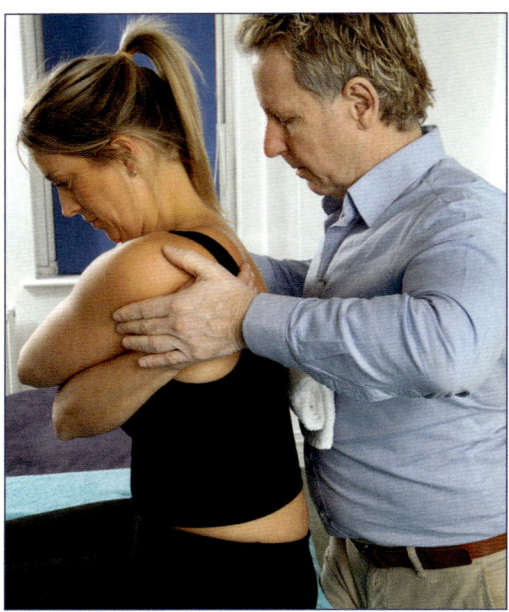

Figure 10.37. The therapist applies the towel at the level of T10.

apply a thrust directly forward against the spinous process of T7 with your sternum through the towel (figure 10.36).

 Middle thoracic spine manipulation

Seated Thoracic Thrust: Diagnosis T9/10 ERS(l)

Motion restriction: Flexion, right rotation and right-side bending

Position: Patient seated

Adopt the same position as with technique 1 above. However, in this case take the patient into slightly more flexion because the target area is the lower thoracic spine, and the technique performed is more

of a lift with a thrusting motion (a thoracic *lift* rather than a thoracic *thrust*).

Roll up a small towel and place it against your sternum, and then make contact to the patient's thoracic spine, and specifically to the level of the spinous process of T10 (figure 10.37). Apply more flexion to the patient's head and trunk until you feel a bind at the sternum (figure 10.38).

From this position, place both your arms around the patient's elbows and apply a tension motion (explained above) to encourage T9 to glide posteriorly and T10 to glide anteriorly (figure 10.39).

Make any adjustments where necessary prior to the manipulation, and when you and the patient are both relaxed, ask them to take a deep breath in, and on the relaxation phase, apply the HVT thrust through their elbows directed toward you

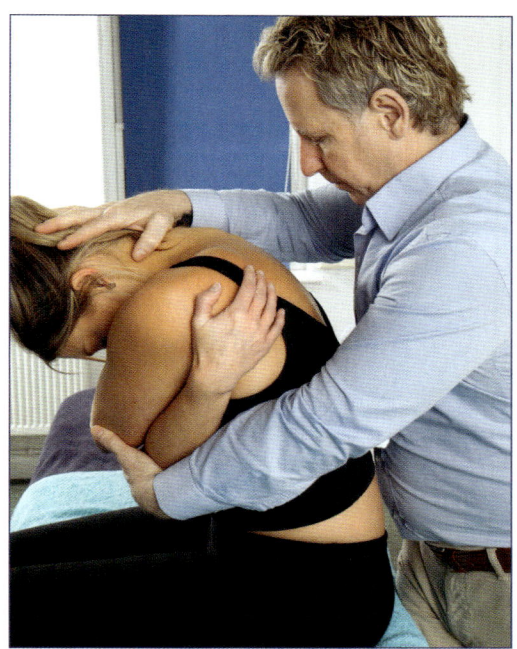

Figure 10.38. The patient is passively flexed until the therapist feels a bind to their sternum.

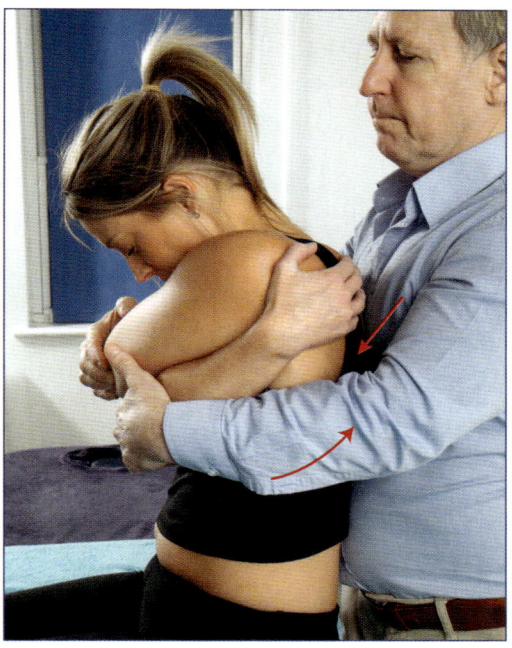

Figure 10.40. A thrust is applied toward the therapist and upward.

and upward. Simultaneously apply a thrust directly forward with your sternum against the spinous process of T10 (figure 10.40).

 Lower thoracic spine manipulation

Standing Thoracic Thrust: Diagnosis T6/7 ERS(l)

Motion restriction: Flexion, right rotation, and right-side bending

Position: Patient standing

Ask the patient to stand and place a small towel between your sternum and the spinous process of T7 (figure 10.41).

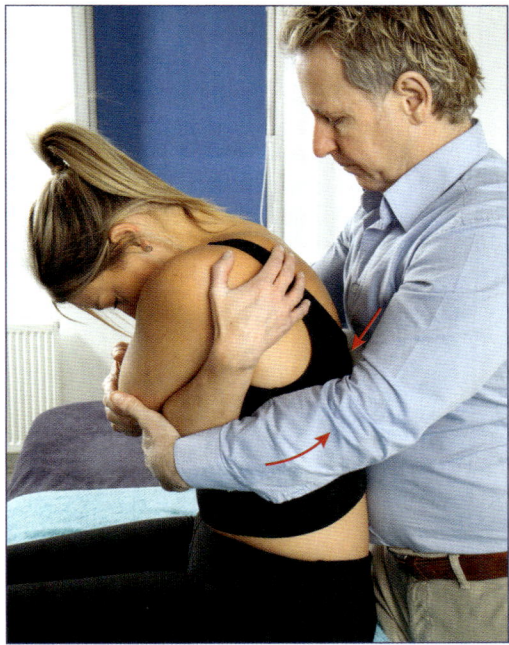

Figure 10.39. Anterior/posterior gliding motion of T9/10 through use of a technique using a towel.

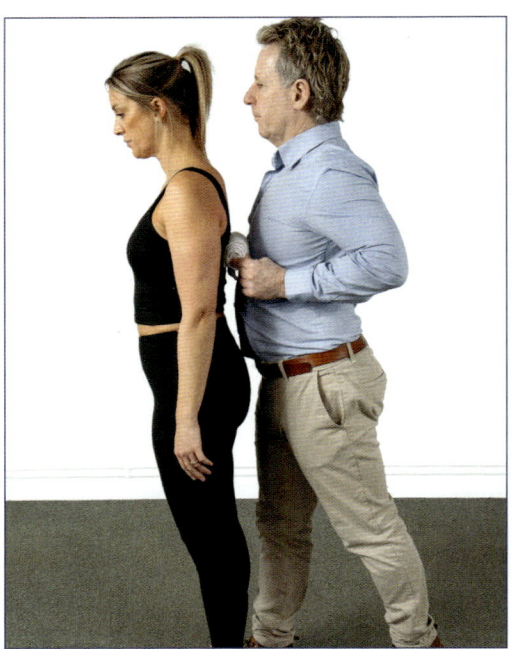

Figure 10.41. The therapist applies the towel at the level of T7.

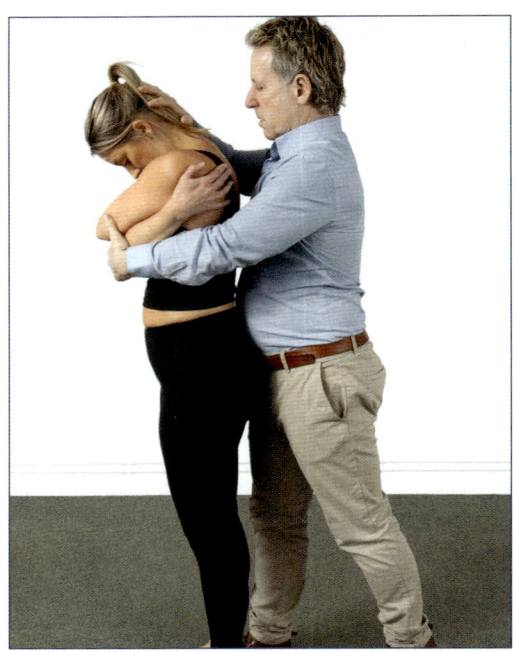

Figure 10.42. The patient is passively flexed until the therapist feels a bind to their sternum.

Ask the patient to cross their arms over their chest and wrap their hands around their shoulders. Apply more flexion to the patient's head and trunk until you feel a bind at the sternum (figure 10.42).

From this position, place both your arms around the patient's elbows and slowly bring them back toward you, whilst providing support through your back leg. Next, apply a tension motion (explained above) to encourage T6 to glide posteriorly and T7 to glide anteriorly (figure 10.43).

Make any adjustments where necessary prior to the manipulation. When you and the patient are both relaxed, apply the HVT thrust toward you and slightly upward. Simultaneously apply a thrust directly forward with your sternum against the towel onto their SP at T7 (figure 10.44).

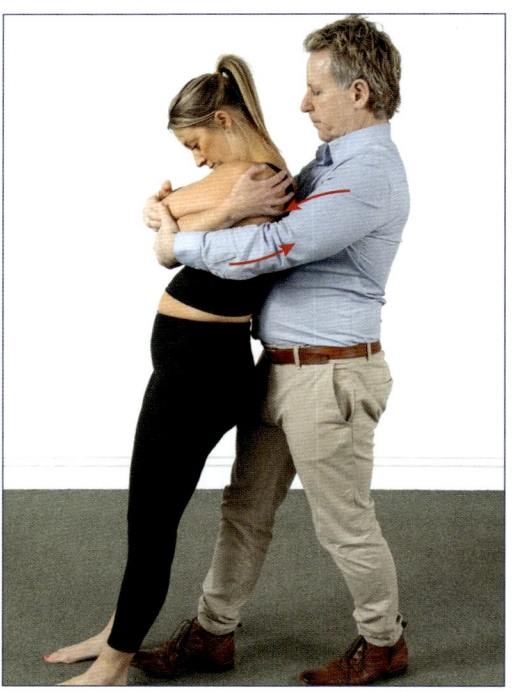

Figure 10.43. Anterior/posterior gliding motion of T6/7 through a technique using a towel.

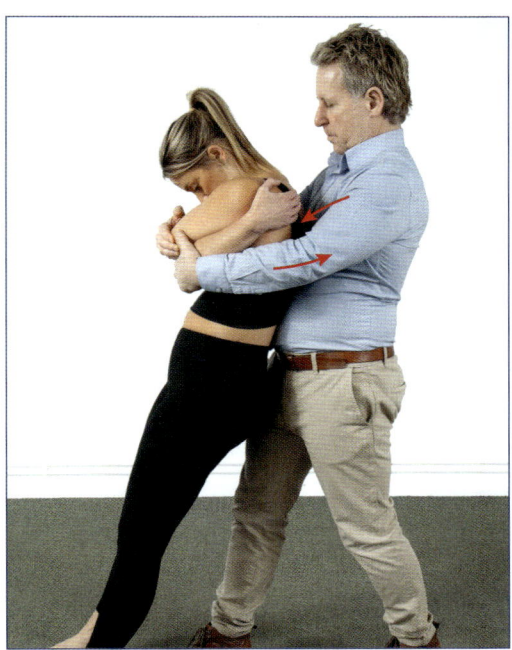

Figure 10.44. A thrust is applied toward the therapist and slightly upward.

 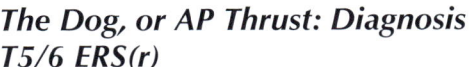
Standing thoracic spine manipulation

The Dog, or AP Thrust: Diagnosis T5/6 ERS(r)

Motion restriction: Flexion, left rotation, and left-side bending

Position: Patient supine

Ask the patient to lie supine on the couch, with arms crossed over their chest and hands wrapped around their shoulders (figure 10.45). Place your elbow onto the patient's hip (figure 10.46), and roll the patient toward you.

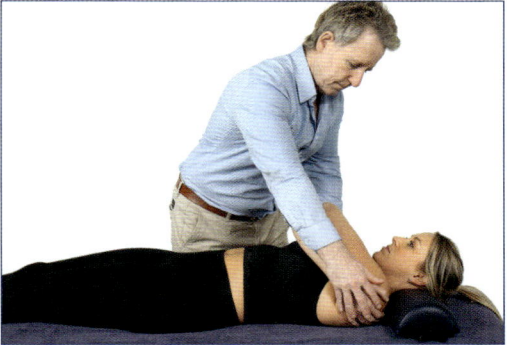

Figure 10.45. The patient is asked to place their arms across their chest and to hold the backs of their shoulders.

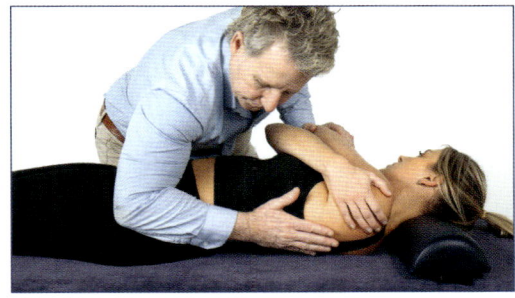

Figure 10.46. The therapist places their elbow on the patient's hip.

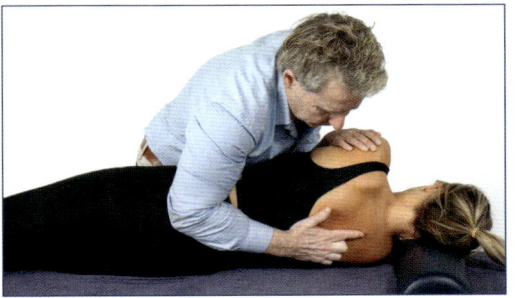

Figure 10.47. The patient is rolled toward the therapist and the manipulating hand is in contact with the thoracic spine.

Next, place your right hand (if right handed) onto the area of the thoracic spine to be manipulated. I personally use a pistol-type of grip (figure 10.47).

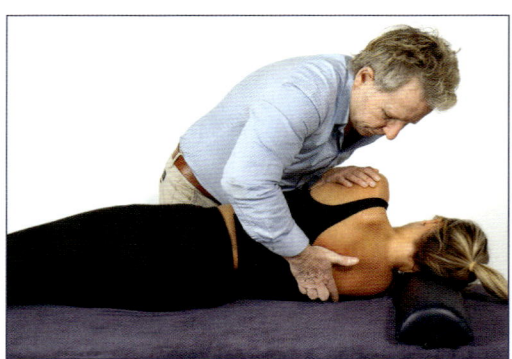

Figure 10.48. The therapist rotates their hand 90° so that the patient's SP is in contact with their second MCP joint.

From this position, I typically rotate my hand 90° so that the relevant SP is in contact with my second MCP joint (figure 10.48).

The hand position can be varied according to your personal preference. Position one is the standard way, whereby you flex your distal phalanges to be level with your metacarpals (figure 10.49).

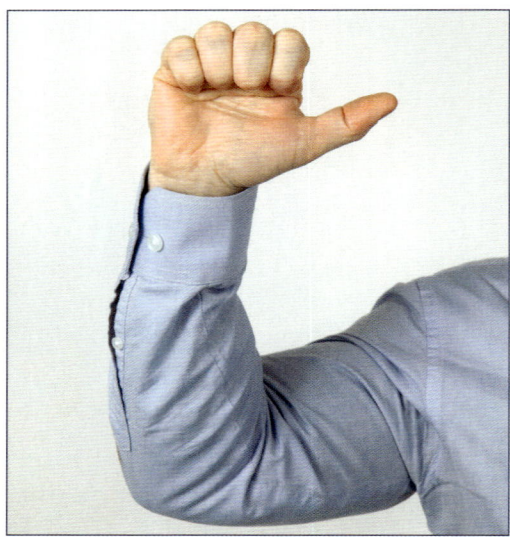

Figure 10.50. Hand position two.

Position two is where you flex your middle phalanges (figure 10.50), and position three is a typical cupping of the hand position (figure 10.51).

I have my own unique hand position (figure 10.52), which I call a *pistol hand* position as the hand shape is reminiscent

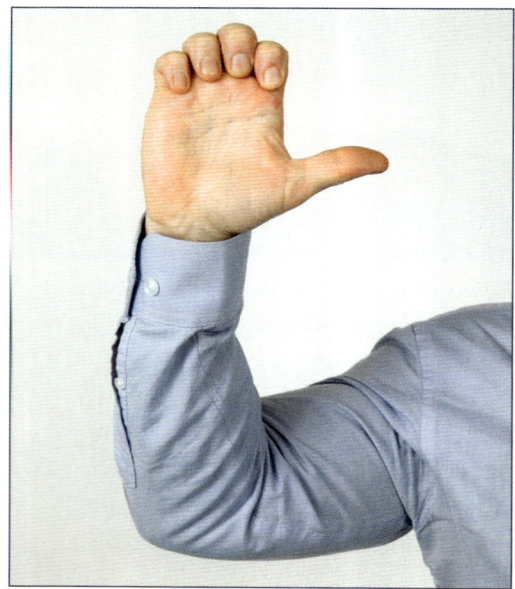

Figure 10.49. Hand position one.

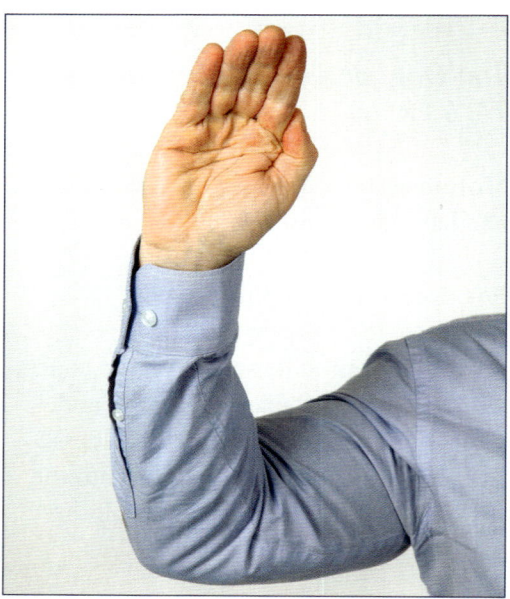

Figure 10.51. Hand position three.

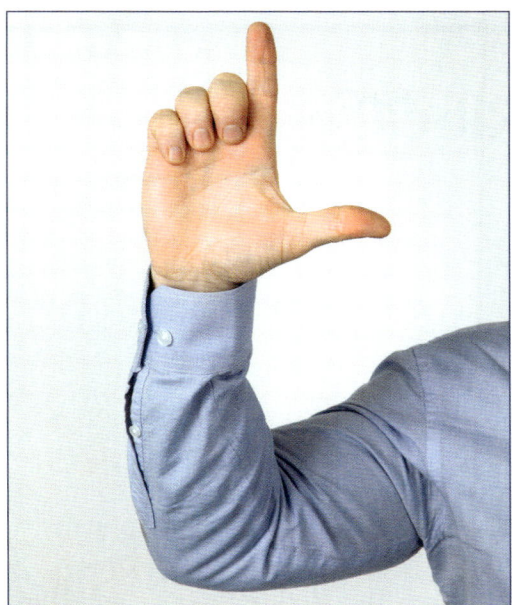

Figure 10.52. Pistol hand position.

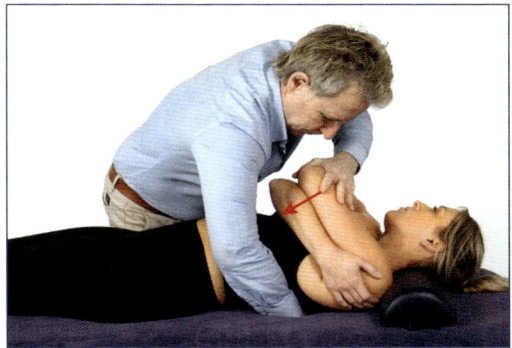

Figure 10.53. The therapist rotates the patient onto their back and adds in flexion to the specific level requiring treatment.

of a pistol. When I contact the patient, my index finger is parallel to the SPs and I rotate the hand 90°, which increases the leverage to the underlying tissue, and then I continue as normal with the technique.

The reason I show all four positions is because not all therapists are capable of position one, or even my hand position (depending on the mobility of their finger joints), so if they want to perform this type of technique, they must be able to adapt their hand position.

Maintain contact with the patient's elbows as they are rotated back onto the couch. At the same time, introduce flexion or extension (but rarely), depending on what is required at that specific level (figure 10.53).

Ask the patient to take a deep breath in, and on the out breath apply the HVT

thrust (using your bodyweight, through the patient's elbows to your hand located on the spinous process) downward toward the couch (figure 10.54).

Please note: Some female therapists might find the use of a towel or pillow more appropriate. This is applied between the patient and the therapist to give more privacy and potentially make the technique more comfortable for both patient and therapist.

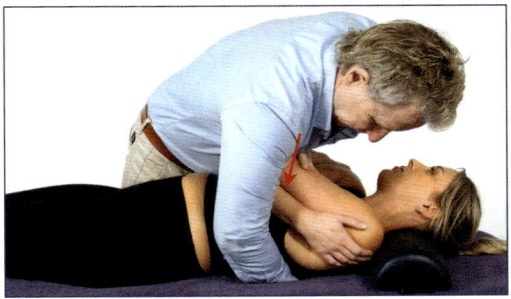

Figure 10.54. The thrust is applied (using bodyweight) downward toward the couch.

Manipulation of thoracic spine using dog technique

Techniques for the Ribcage

In this chapter the focus will be on the treatment of the ribs, but before we dive into the mobilization and manipulation techniques, we need to look at the functional anatomy of the ribs and their relationship to other anatomical structures.

Anatomy of the Ribcage

The sternum, thoracic spine, and the ribs form the ribcage, also known as the thoracic cage. Their function is to provide protection for the heart and lungs and allow the movements of inhalation and exhalation. Typically, there are 24 ribs formed in 12 pairs, which anteriorly attach to the sternum, xiphoid process, and costal cartilages, and posteriorly to the 12 thoracic vertebrae (figure 11.1).

True and False Ribs

The first seven pairs of ribs—classified as *true* ribs—attach directly to the sternum. The next five pairs (8–12) are classified as *false* ribs because they do not directly attach to the sternum, and rib pairs 8–10 attach indirectly to the sternum via the costal cartilages. The last two pairs (11 and 12) are known as *floating* ribs because they have an attachment only to the thoracic spine, and anteriorly have a cartilaginous tip but no *direct* attachment to the costal cartilage.

To recap, the ribs consist of 12 pairs, comprising true, false, and floating ribs:

- **True ribs:** The first seven pairs, which attach by costal cartilage directly to the sternum
- **False ribs:** Pairs 8–10, which attach to costal cartilage, but not directly to the sternum
- **Floating ribs:** Pairs 11–12, which lack attachments either to costal cartilage or to the sternum

Costovertebral (Capitular) and Costotransverse Joints

Type of Joint

The *costovertebral* (*capitular*) and *costotransverse* joints are both classified

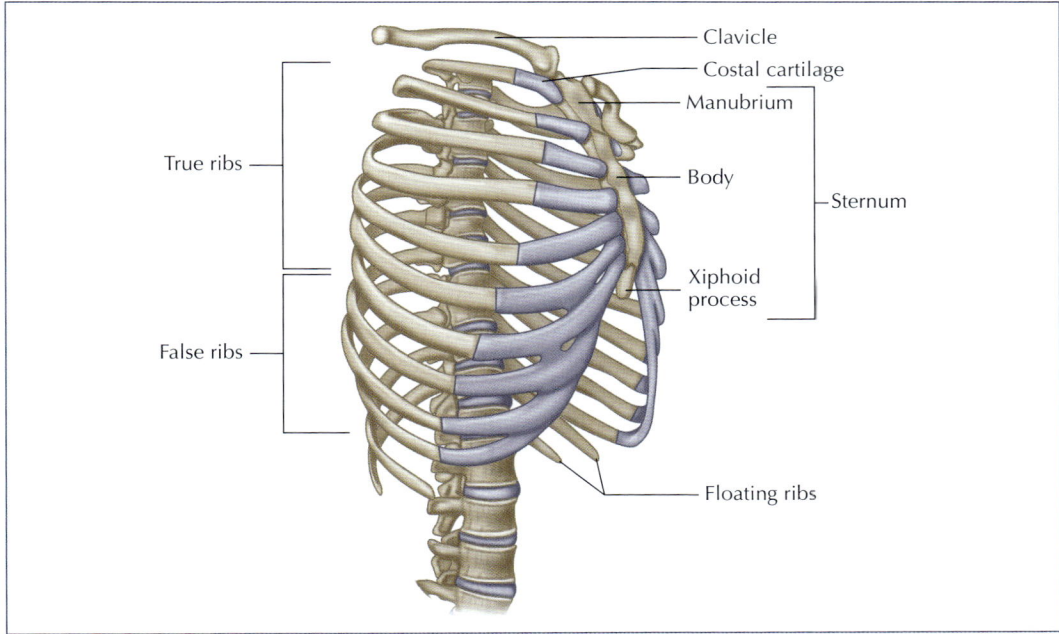

Figure 11.1. Anatomy of the ribcage.

as synovial plane joints and connect the heads of the ribs to the thoracic vertebrae.

Articulations

The superior and inferior articular facets of the costovertebral joints on the head of a typical rib articulate with the facets on the two adjacent vertebral bodies. This means that the rib's head sits between two vertebral bodies and against a shallow depression on the intervertebral disc.

The costotransverse joints are where the tubercle of a typical rib articulates with the transverse process of the lower of the two vertebrae to which its head is joined, with associated ligaments attaching it to the transverse processes of both vertebrae.

Note: The first rib and the last two or three ribs have atypical vertebral connections, because the heads of these ribs have only one facet, not two; they therefore articulate with one vertebral body rather than two. The tubercles of the lowest ribs do not form synovial joints with the transverse processes.

Movements

The costovertebral and costotransverse joints of each rib together form a hinge, causing the anterior part of the rib to be raised (with some lateral expansion) during inspiration and to be lowered (with some medial contraction) during expiration (figure 11.2). This effectively increases and decreases the anteroposterior and transverse diameters of the thorax with each in breath and out breath. (Bucket handle and pump handle rib motion is explained later in this chapter.)

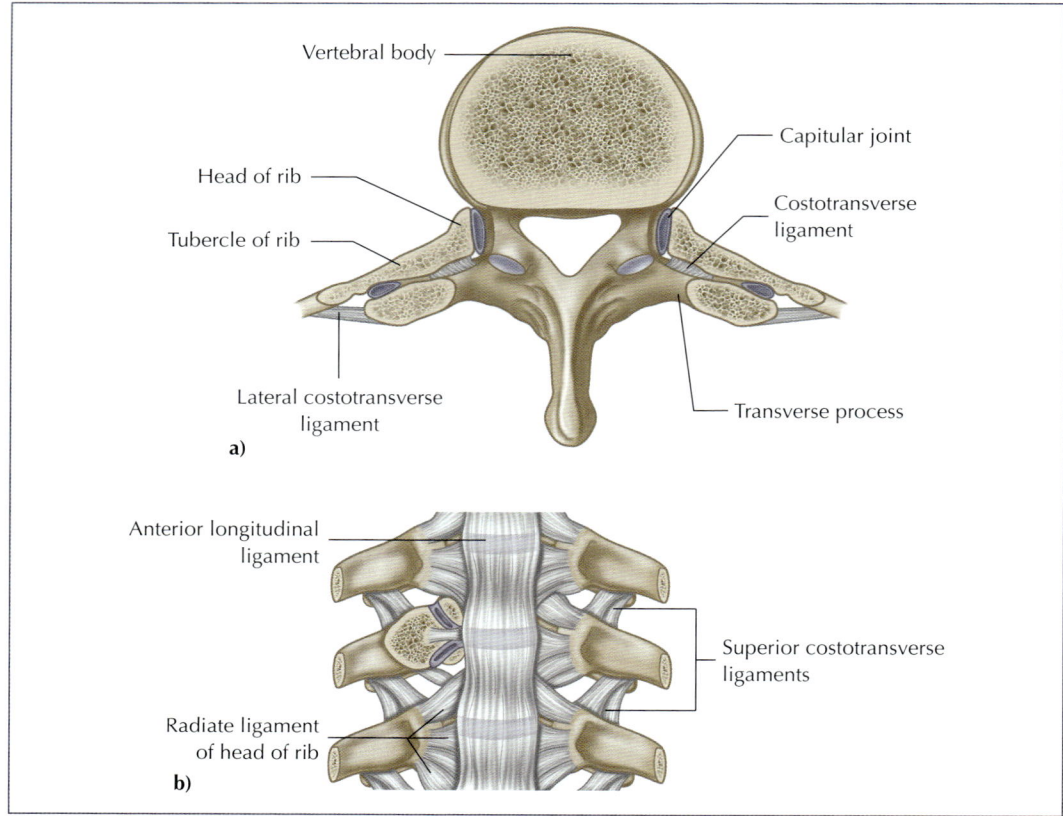

Figure 11.2. Costovertebral and costotransverse joints: (a) transverse section; (b) anterior view.

Sternocostal Joints

The hyaline cartilage that is continuous with the anterior end of each rib is called the *costal cartilage* (figure 11.3).

Types of Joint

- **First rib:** Cartilaginous immovable (synchondrosis)
- **Ribs 2–7:** Simple synovial plane
- **Ribs 8–10:** Simple synovial plane articulations at the interchondral joints

Articulations

- **First rib:** Via costal cartilage to the body of the sternum
- **Ribs 2–7:** Via costal cartilages to facets on the sides of the body of the sternum; the joint cavities are divided into two by an intra-articular ligament (until cavities disappear in old age)
- **Ribs 8–10:** Costal cartilages unite with the costal cartilage of rib 7
- **Ribs 11–12:** Do not articulate anteriorly, but end freely in the muscles of the flank; they are therefore called floating ribs

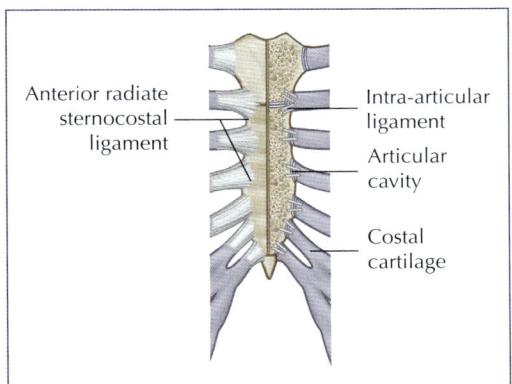

Figure 11.3. The sternocostal joint (anterior view).

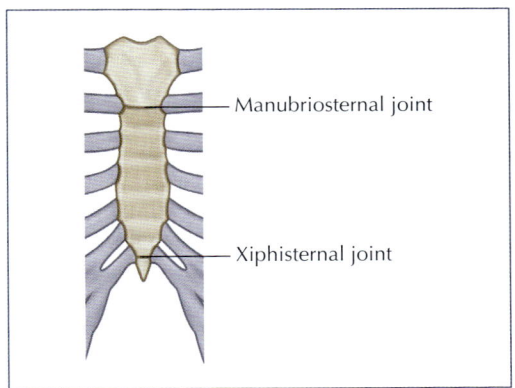

Figure 11.4. The sternal joints (anterior view).

Movements

The sternocostal joints enable expansion and contraction of the ribcage (as described under "Costovertebral and costotransverse joints").

Sternal Joints

Types of Joint

- The *manubriosternal joint* is similar in appearance to a cartilaginous symphysis (slightly movable) joint.
- The *xiphisternal joint* is cartilaginous and immovable (synchondrosis), and typically becomes ossified as we approach old age.

The sternal joints are shown in figure 11.4.

Articulations

- The manubriosternal joint is located between the manubrium and the body of the sternum, adjacent to the second costal cartilage.

- The xiphisternal joint is located between the body of the sternum and the xiphoid process. This joint marks the inferior extent of the thoracic cavity.

The Abdomen and its Relationship to the Ribs

The entire ventral cavity is concerned mostly with chemical exchange with the outside world. To move, grow, and sustain life, living creatures must bring *matter* in from the outside world and make it their own, and export other matter out as waste.

There is a large opening in the upper half of this cavity. Located here is a central pump that helps to move this matter to and from the cells, and special bellows that filter out gases that require a faster exchange than the alimentary canal allows—these are the heart and lungs.

The heart requires protection and a steady base from which to work, and the lungs require a constantly varying pressure, raised and lowered. The structures that have evolved to meet those contrasting needs are the ribs and sternum, bent and sprung into the truss of the thoracic spine. The heart sits in a tough set of bags slung between the more fixed points of the posterior breastbone and the anterior part of the spine. The sponges of the lungs sit on either side, slung vertically between the neck and lower back, being alternately stretched and compressed by the highly mobile ribs.

The individual and collective mobility of the ribs suggests that, while the word rib*cage* might be a useful concept with regard to protecting the heart, the image of your mother's old wicker laundry basket might be more appropriate for the way the ribs surround the lungs.

The Ribs in Four Sections (Rib Basket)

This rib basket can be usefully divided into four sections (figure 11.5). Taking it from the bottom, the lowest three ribs form a useful section that relates the ribs to the hips. At least two, and sometimes all three, of these ribs are floating ribs, with free distal ends.

This extra freedom permits more movement, which is of great benefit because the abdominal muscles, especially the two obliques, link these ribs to the pelvis, allowing or restraining the twisting and leaning motions that take place between these two large blocks.

These *pelvic* ribs surround the kidneys and are associated with them and the adrenal

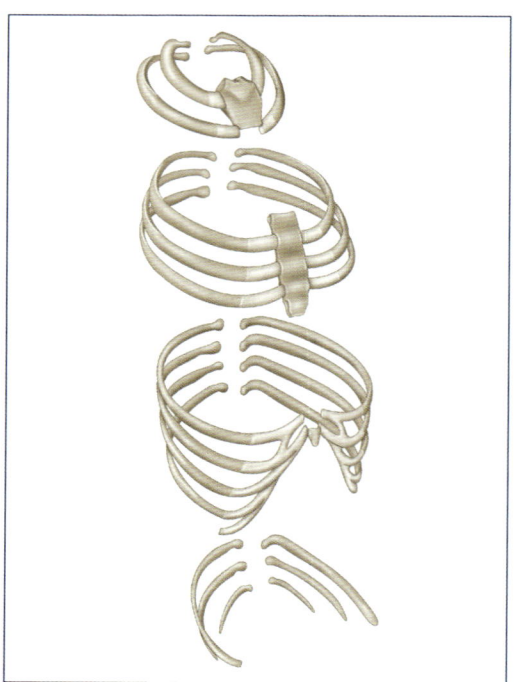

Figure 11.5. The rib basket has four major sections, with different functions: the first two neck ribs, the three chest ribs, the four abdominal ribs, and the final three pelvic ribs.

glands that sit atop the kidneys. Their movement in breathing is mostly neither up nor down but opening posteriorly on the inhale.

The next functional division of the rib basket consists of a set of four ribs—all connected to the subcostal cartilage—which we will term the *abdominal* ribs. While these ribs are not as free as the floating ribs, the large cartilage breastplate allows a lot of movement. These ribs exhibit a strong *bucket handle* effect, expanding out to the side on the inhalation. These ribs surround the stomach and spleen on the left and the liver on the right and are associated with the glands of the pancreas and liver and with the small xiphoid point of the sternal dagger.

The next section is ribs 3–5, the *chest* ribs, all of which tie directly into the body of the sternum, thus making these ribs more stable. They surround the heart (and are thus associated with the thymus) and make a strong connection between the mediastinum and the shoulders. The pectoralis minor—the major tether for scapular movement—attaches to these ribs. While still mobile, these ribs have more stabilizing duties than the ribs below them.

The final section of the ribs is the upper two. These ribs are flatter, smaller, and even more stable than the other ribs below. Both attach into the handle of the sternal dagger, the manubrium. They are known here as the *neck* ribs, since, via the scalene muscles, they provide a stable base for neck movements and for controlling the heavy head atop the delicate neck. In practice, they also provide a stable platform for the shoulders. These ribs are associated with the thyroid gland.

Ribs and the Spine

In humans and many other vertebrates, the ribs are attached to the spine (vertebral column). The ribs curve around the torso, naturally forming a protective cage for the thoracic organs (heart and lungs).

Evolutionary Perspective

It has been suggested that early ancestors of vertebrates had a simpler rib structure, possibly with only three pairs of ribs and in different orientations.

If we take a look around the back to see how the ribs are attached to the spine, we find a very interesting pattern. At one point in our ancestry, similar in form to a six-rayed starfish, ribs lay in an anterior, transverse, and posterior orientation from a central spine or notochord (a flexible rodlike structure found in all chordate embryos, which is a precursor to the vertebral column of vertebrates), as shown in figure 11.6.

The posterior ribs bent together at the back to form the neural arch and the spinous processes. The transverse ribs became the transverse processes.

Six-Rayed Star Fish Analogy

The pattern described is like the radial symmetry found in starfish, which have arms (rays) extending from a central point.

In our early ancestors, there may have been a similar radial arrangement around the notochord, but with ribs instead of arms.

Theoretically, the ancient anterior ribs remain with us today as our ribs, but, reflecting the old pattern, they bend at the angle of the ribs (clearly palpable as the ribs change angle at about the outer edge of the erector spinae group) to pass under the back muscles, in front of the transverse process (with a costotransverse joint), to put the arrowhead-like rib heads up against the discs—at least, in ribs 2 to 9 (figure 11.7).

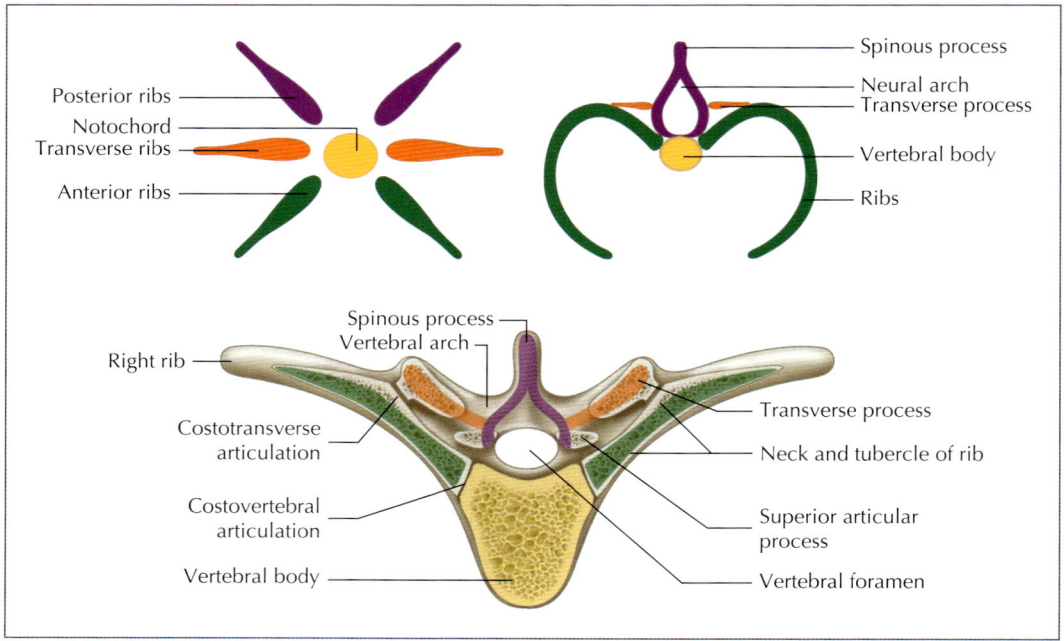

Figure 11.6. Two of the original three sets of ribs have converged to form the neural arch, the spinous processes, and the transverse processes that form the principal places of muscle attachment in the spine.

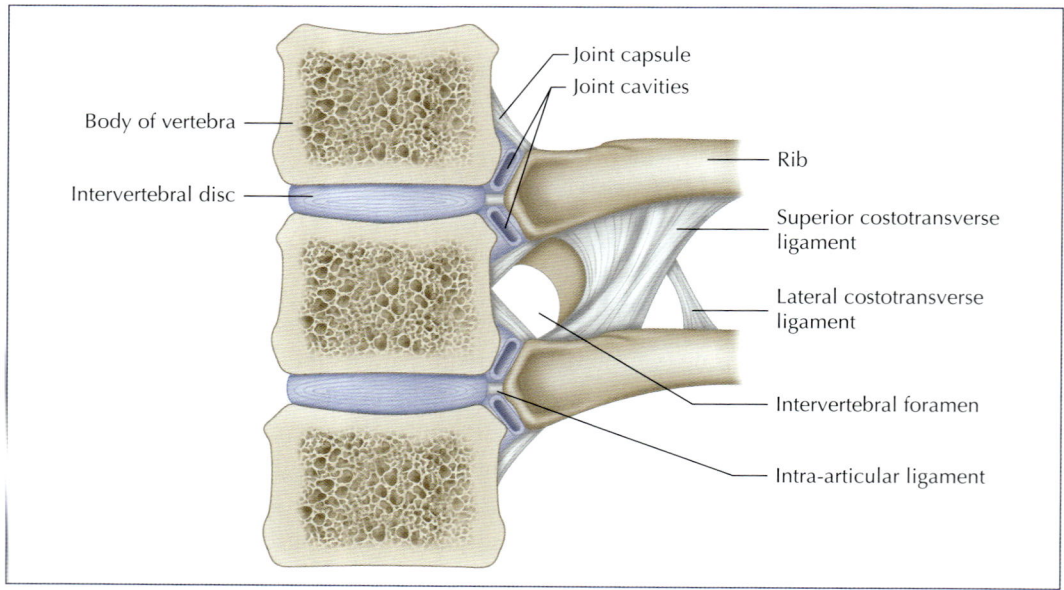

Figure 11.7. The rib heads attach to the transverse processes on their way to a complex and interesting joint with the corresponding disc, and the two vertebral bodies on either side of it.

This means that a complete movement of the ribs in breathing acts also to *hydrate* the discs and keep them healthy. For many of us, our perception of the ribs stops somewhere around the sides, and does not extend into the back, where the complete movement of the ribs really contributes to our long-term health, especially as age dries out and thins the thoracic discs.

Muscles for Breathing

Accessory Muscles of Breathing

The principal muscle for breathing is the *diaphragm*, to which we will turn our attention in a moment. Several other muscles surround the rib basket and help (or hinder) breathing. Let us look at those first (figure 11.8).

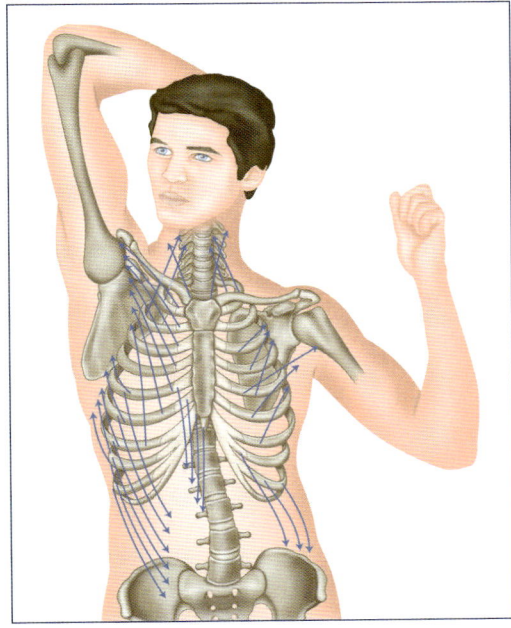

Figure 11.8. The many muscles around the ribcage can assist with breathing when required or inhibit breathing if they are too tight and short.

The abdominal obliques hold the pelvic and abdominal ribs to the pelvis, and thus they provide a steady base for the initial part of diaphragmatic movement, though they must relent in the latter stage to allow the ribs to rise. In my opinion, standing tension in the rectus abdominis runs counter to easy and complete breathing, but there are as many theories of the "proper breath" as there are people to espouse them.

The quadratus lumborum provides a direct extension of the diaphragm from the twelfth rib to the pelvis and can inhibit deep breathing in the back if is too tight or, more often, too fascially short.

The serratus posterior superior and the serratus posterior inferior are often listed as breathing assistants. The muscular elements of these fascial retinacula are so diminutive as to leave us wondering whether they really have much effect on breathing.

Of course, other accessory muscles can be used in breathing if it is for some reason difficult: the SCM, the pectoral muscles, and the erector muscles of the back can all help in extremis. The principal muscles assisting the diaphragm, though, are the scalenes and the intercostals.

The accessory muscles of breathing are most often considered as accessories to a difficult inhalation, but in holding isometric tension they can act to prevent an easy exhalation. The reverse is also true—standing tension in the muscles of forced exhalation can prevent a full inhalation.

The intercostals are commonly thought to draw the ribs together on inhalation, but putting your fingertips between the ribs and performing a strong inhale will soon dispel that idea. The ribs really do not get closer to each other—even in a strong inhale— nor do they spread during the exhale. If the intercostals are active in breathing, it is to slide the ribs obliquely along each other. The intercostals primarily are used as muscles of walking—winding and unwinding the torso's rotation with each step.

The scalenes are often seen these days as the secondary muscles of breathing, leaving the intercostals as tertiary (figure 11.9). The scalenes surround the transverse processes of the second through the sixth cervical vertebra, coming down to the first and second ribs like a skirt around the neck. In breathing, they lift

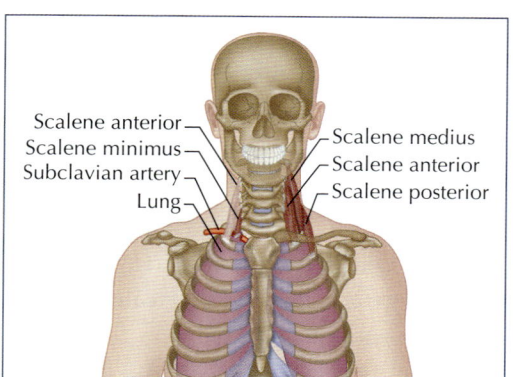

Scalene anterior
Scalene minimus
Subclavian artery
Lung
Scalene medius
Scalene anterior
Scalene posterior

Figure 11.9. The scalenes form a skirt around the neck from the first and second ribs; the middle and posterior scalenes moderate side-to-side movement of the head, as well as assisting in breathing; the anterior scalene can really pull the cervical vertebrae down and forward in dysfunction.

the upper two ribs, or prevent them from being pulled down.

In dysfunction, we should divide the middle and posterior scalenes from the anterior (a group of three separate pairs of muscles). The middle and posterior muscles are paravertebral, and therefore act as the *quadratus lumborum of the neck*, creating—or more often preventing/ stabilizing—lateral flexion of the neck.

The anterior scalene runs more anteriorly from the anterior tubercles of the third through the sixth cervical vertebra down and forward to the first rib—acting more as the *psoas of the neck*. It is designed to use the neck as an origin and the ribs as an insertion, pulling up on the ribs during inhalation. If you push your SCM out of the way medially and place your finger pads on the slick, dense muscle beneath it and breathe in, you will feel the anterior scalene tighten, either all the way through the breath, or right at the top of the breath at least.

Unfortunately, our neck is not the most stable part of the spine, especially if the suboccipital muscles start to shorten (as they often do in sustained fear patterns). Too often, the anterior scalene shortens to pull the neck down to the ribs; it should be opened in cases of head-forward posture, or its variant, a posteriorly tilted ribcage.

The Diaphragm

The diaphragm is the undisputed primary muscle of breathing. One only has to get the *wind knocked out* by a blow to the xiphoid area to realize how useless the other muscles of breathing are without the diaphragm.

The diaphragm is a thin but remarkably strong muscle that lies poised between the digestive organs of the abdominal cavity and the heart and lungs of the thoracic cavity. The word "poised" is appropriate. In a four-legged creature, the diaphragm pumps backward and forward, perpendicularly to gravity. In humans, it pumps up and down more or less in line with gravity. Nevertheless, at the bottom of the breath, the positive pressure from the lower cavity (which is there no matter how you starve or purge yourself) is balanced by the suction and negative pressure from the spongy lungs (which always want to collapse, no matter how far you breathe in or out). The diaphragm lives in the neutral space between.

The diaphragm is a large umbrella whose stem comprises two crura, which attach to the front of the lumbar spine, much closer to the middle of the body than most people visualize (figure 11.10). The edges of the umbrella are attached to the xiphoid and all the way around the lower margins of the ribs, creating two large domes under the lungs. The movement of these domes in respiration is remarkably similar to that of a jellyfish.

The diaphragm is thus a double dome with a central tendon running from the center of one dome to the other under the heart. This central portion develops with the heart essentially *above the head* in the embryo's septum transversum and is folded

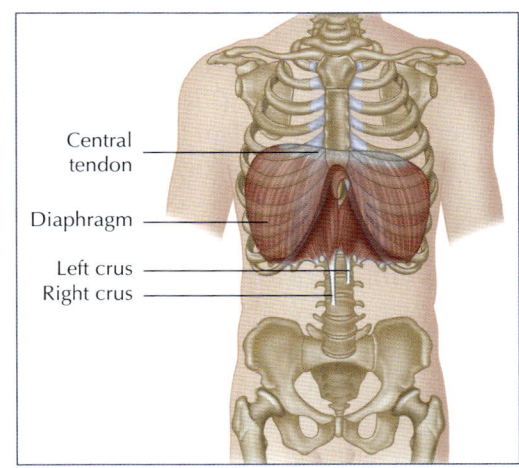

Figure 11.10. The diaphragm is a double dome—one dome under each lung—that moves down on the inhalation and recoils back up on the out breath; the pressure is always positive below it and negative above it.

down into the chest in a unique piece of developmental origami. Therefore, the diaphragm cannot move down very far without pulling on the pericardial bag around the heart, so this center point only moves down about half an inch (1.25 cm) in most people, though it can be trained by singers, divers, and pranayama practitioners to move four times that distance.

The two domes under the lungs, however, move down several inches (again, dependent on activity and training), pulling air into the lungs above each dome, and acting like a piston in the middle of the ventral cavity to move all the organs. While the heart—safe in its triangular housing and attached to the sternum and thoracic spine—escapes being moved much, the liver and stomach both move down and, together, the kidneys ride up and down the psoas, while the intestines roll and unroll in the wake of the diaphragmatic pulse. Even the lungs themselves rotate within the ribs as we breathe, turning medially to *embrace* the heart as they expand on the inhale, and returning laterally on the exhale.

Diaphragmatic Movement

It is essential to understand that the diaphragmatic fibers are mostly vertical. Most of the muscle fibers of the body run either directly along the line of the body or slightly obliquely to it. The diaphragm is widely thought of as a horizontal muscle, but in fact the only horizontal part is the central tendon, the connective tissue under the lungs and heart. Most of the muscle fibers are on the sides of the domes, and therefore—for the most part—act vertically.

This puts the diaphragm in the unique position of being a muscle that regularly switches its origin for its insertion in the middle of its movement. At the beginning of the inhale, when the diaphragmatic fibers contract, the lower rim of the ribs and the lumbar spine are the stable origin, and the central tendon is the insertion (figure 11.11a). The central tendon is pulled down on either side, also stretching the lungs down and pulling air into them. As the tops of the domes move down, the organs of the abdominal balloon move down with them, compressing the abdomen. Fluid-filled organs can compress only a little, and soon the central tendon is pulled down snugly against the resistant, fluid-filled balloon.

Since it cannot go any farther down, at this point in the breath the diaphragm's

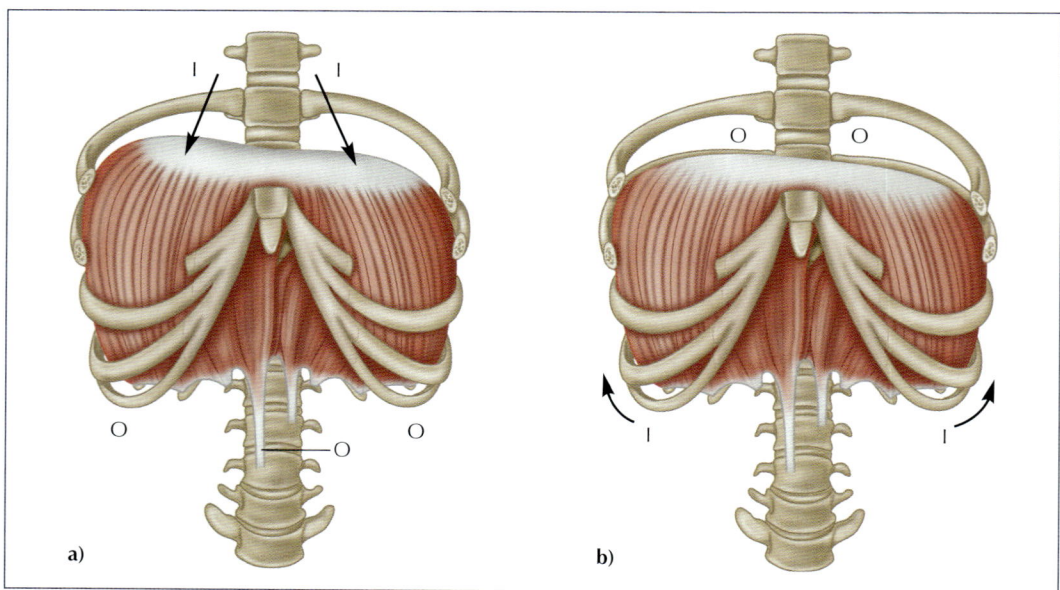

Figure 11.11. The diaphragm switches its origin and insertion in the middle of its contraction: (a) at first the ribs form the origin, and the centers of the domes are pulled down; (b) in the second half of the inhalation, the central tendon becomes the origin, and the contraction of the diaphragm lifts the ribs.

origin and insertion reverse. The central tendon, resting on the abdominal balloon, becomes the origin, and the vertical fibers—continuing to contract—act to pull the lower rim of the rib basket up. In most breathing patterns, the scalenes assist from above to lift the upper ribs (figure 11.11b).

You can feel this shift in yourself or in others by putting your hands on ribs 6 to 9 (the easiest place for your hands is on the sides) and listening to a few breath cycles. Breathing patterns differ, but in most people, there will be two distinct phases of the inhale. The early part will have the ribs more still, and in the second half they will move up more strongly. The transition may be more gradual or even indiscernible

in those with a trained breath for singing or yoga, but nevertheless you will realize that they are moving differently at the end of the breath than at the beginning.

This second movement of the diaphragm, pulling up on the ribs, is primarily and paradoxically responsible for the expansion of the rib basket, both from side to side and from front to back—both the "bucket handle" movement of the ribs out to the side and the "pump handle" movement of the ribs away from the thoracic spine in front (figure 11.12a and b). The diaphragm itself is pulling up and in on the ribs; yet the box expands in these two ways because of the way the ribs are shaped and sprung, not because the ribs are

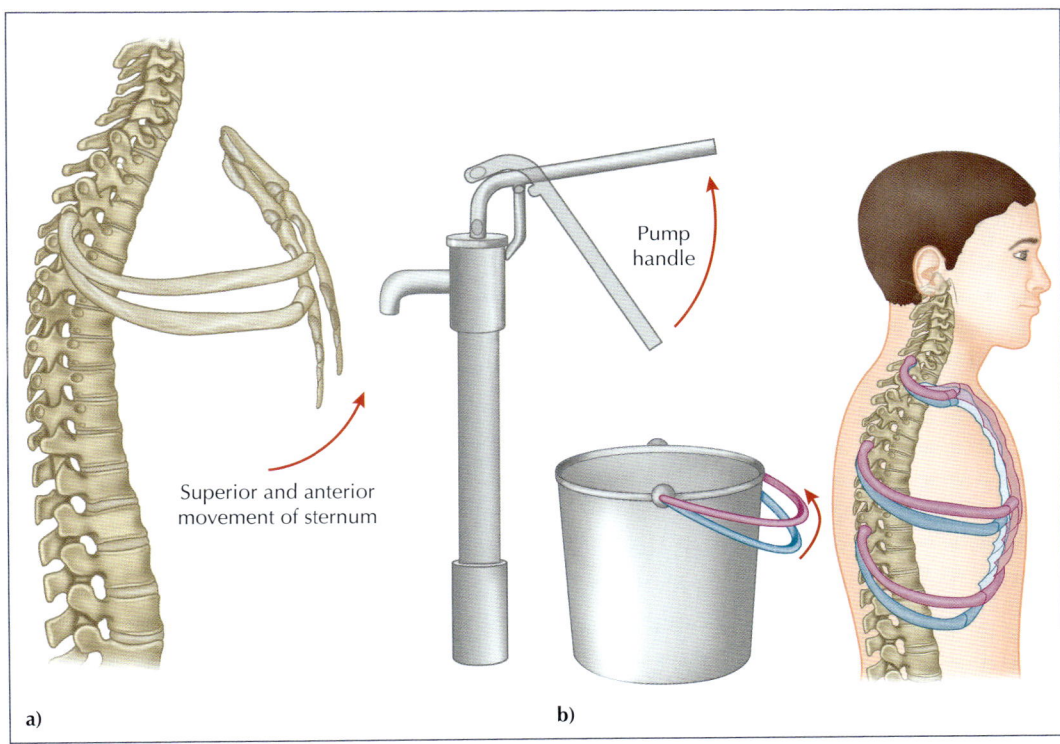

a)

Superior and anterior movement of sternum

Pump handle

b)

Figure 11.12. Rib motion. (a) Pump-handle, and (b) bucket-handle movements.

being pulled out and up by muscles outside the ribs, even though they may help. The primary movement that powers the inhalation is the diaphragm.

The exhalation is said to be a natural process of elastic recoil in the lungs, requiring no action at all, but very few people have a contraction-free exhale in our speeded-up Western society. Who can wait that long for the natural exhalation to happen? Assess your clients for excess contraction on the exhale, and do what you can to make it lighter and less effortful.

The other exhalation problem frequently encountered but difficult to see is that the diaphragm fails to fully relax at the bottom of the exhale. Many people—especially if they are anxious—tend to retain some tension in the diaphragm all the time, so it never fully relaxes, and never fully expels the air in the lungs. Tracking the out breath and using your hands to assist a full relaxation of the diaphragm is a service to all the regulatory systems of your client's body—neural and organic, as well as musculoskeletal.

Breath flows in and out of the body around 17,000 times per day. To call it the *river of life* is no exaggeration, though it more resembles the tide, ebbing and flowing. In any case, it is the essential and central movement on which so many others are built. Small aberrations in the breathing pattern—repeated so many times per day, so many days in a row—can lead to many imbalances.

The converse is also true: getting the breathing to take a more balanced path can make diverse problems disappear as the body rights itself.

Assessment and Treatment

It is rare to have dysfunctional rib articulations, unless you have had direct trauma to them—like a kick from a horse or a fall from a bike—where some ribs have been fractured. The thoracic spine should be addressed before the assessment and subsequent treatment of the ribcage, because the thoracic spine is the base foundation for the attachment of the 12 pairs of ribs. Typically, if a primary dysfunction is present within the thoracic spine, there will probably be some form of compensatory dysfunction present within the ribcage. We have already addressed a lot of mobilization work for the thoracic spine in chapter 10, and usually you will find that mobilizations to that area of the spine will promote motion of the associated rib attachments and will only have a positive effect in those terms.

Most of the mobilization and manipulative techniques I demonstrate within this chapter are used as part of my ongoing assessment of the ribcage, rather than having lots of separate assessment procedures.

However, it makes sense to discuss some assessment procedures, as this will help you to formulate a treatment plan.

Assessment of the Ribcage

Anterior Assessment

Palpation assessment is typically used, and we can palpate the motion of the ribcage with the patient sitting, supine, or prone.

Initially, palpate the middle and lower ribs for asymmetry, and move your hands onto the lateral side of the ribs to continue the assessment.

Ask the patient to take a deep breath in (inhalation) and then to continue to take a full breath out (exhalation), while you palpate for motion of the upper, middle, and lower ribs (figure 11.13a to d).

Remember you are looking and feeling for any asymmetry and whether there is equal expansion of the paired ribs on the in breath.

Next, ask the patient to sit facing you and lightly palpate with your fingers the anterior contour of the chest wall for the upper ribs (figure 11.14a), looking for asymmetry. I suggest you use your index finger to ascertain motion/local tenderness at the costochondral junctions (figure 11.14b). From the sitting position you can also ascertain asymmetry and motion through the lateral aspect of the ribcage by placing your hands laterally onto the middle to lower outer ribs (figure 11.14c).

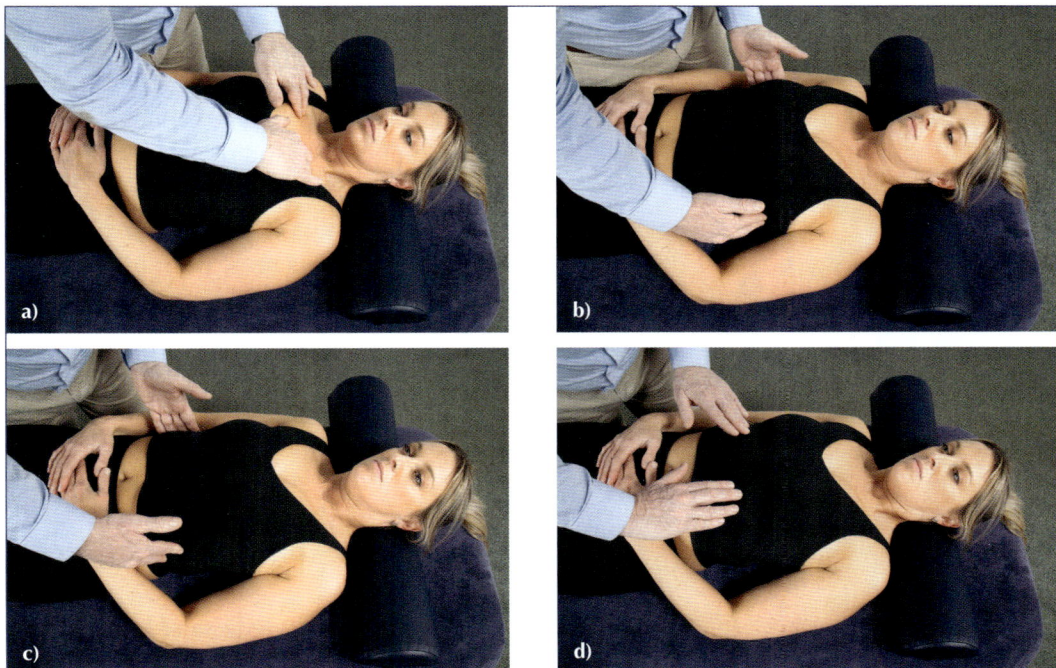

Figure 11.13. The therapist palpates (a) the upper ribs, (b) the middle ribs, (c) the lower lateral ribs, and (d) the lower anterior ribs.

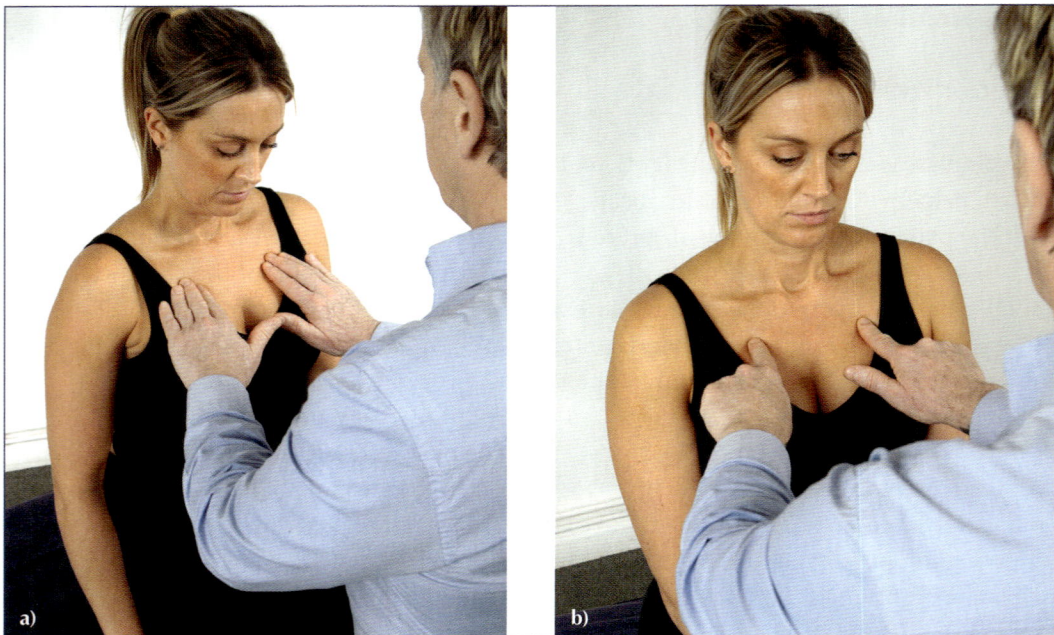

Figure 11.14. Palpation of the ribcage with patient sitting: (a) the upper ribs, (b) the costochondral junction.

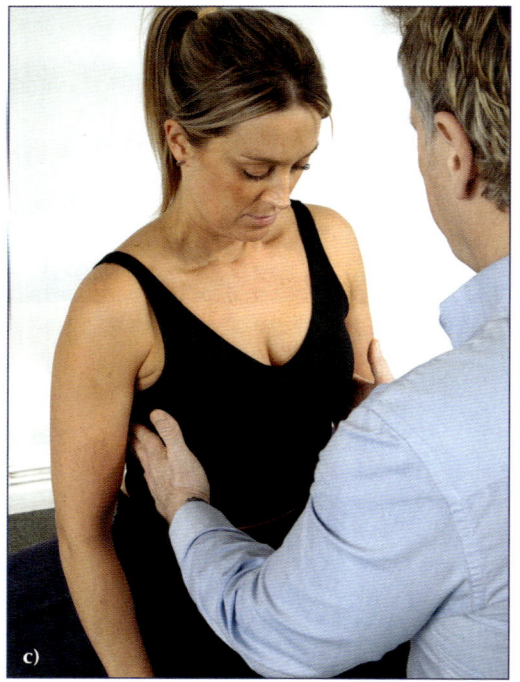

Figure 11.14. Palpation of the ribcage with patient sitting: (c) the middle to lower outer ribs.

Posterior Assessment

You can continue the assessment with the patient seated, and this time palpate the posterior convexity of the thorax. Continue to assess the angle of the ribs to determine if one is more prominent than on the other side. Also consider whether there is local tenderness at the rib angle or increased tonicity of the musculature, and assess the width of the intercostal space, and compare these findings for both sides.

First Rib Assessment

With the patient seated, stand behind them and place your fingers onto the trapezius (figure 11.15). To isolate the first rib, encourage the trapezius muscle to retract posteriorly, and then apply your index or middle finger caudally onto the posterior shaft of the first rib.

Ascertain whether your fingers are level—a difference of more than 4–6 mm is a positive finding. Typically a dysfunctional rib area is tender to palpate, and you will find the ipsilateral (same side as the dysfunction) scalene muscle has increased tonicity.

While palpating the first rib, ask the patient to take a deep breath in, and decide through the palpatory finger whether the first ribs rise equally on both sides during inspiration and whether they lower equally on exhalation. If one side palpates more cephalically and stays relatively high compared with the contralateral rib, you have found an inspirated first rib that requires treatment.

Rocking Motion Assessment

With the patient prone, place your right hand over the lumbosacral region and induce a natural rocking motion side to side, while your left hand is feeling for motion of the SPs of the thoracic spine. By simply moving your fingers laterally, you will be palpating motion of the ribcage (figures 11.16 and 11.17).

I suggest from this assessing position that you perform a basic soft-tissue treatment.

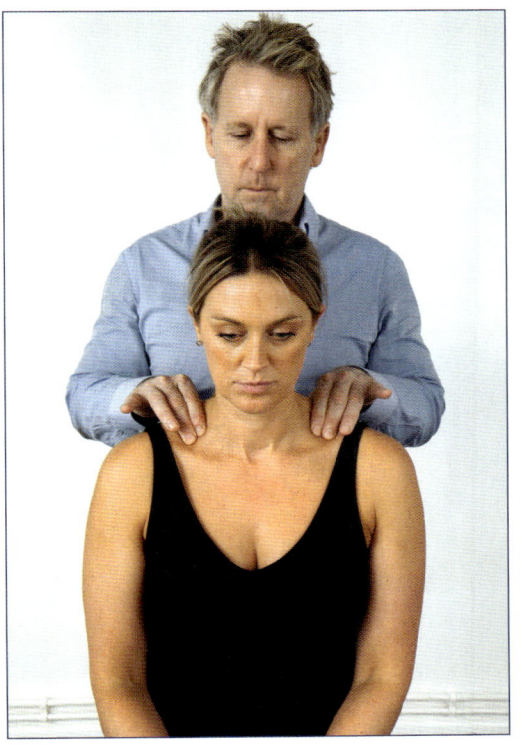

Figure 11.15. The therapist is palpating the first rib using their index and middle finger.

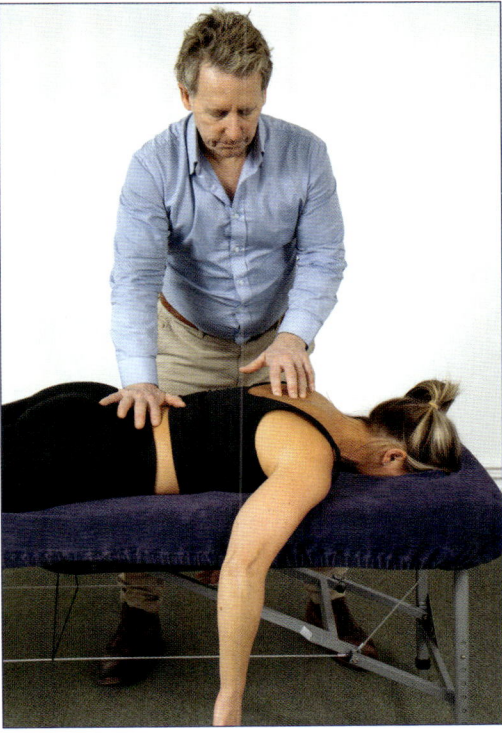

Figure 11.16. Palpation of the spinous processes while inducing motion of the lumbosacral region.

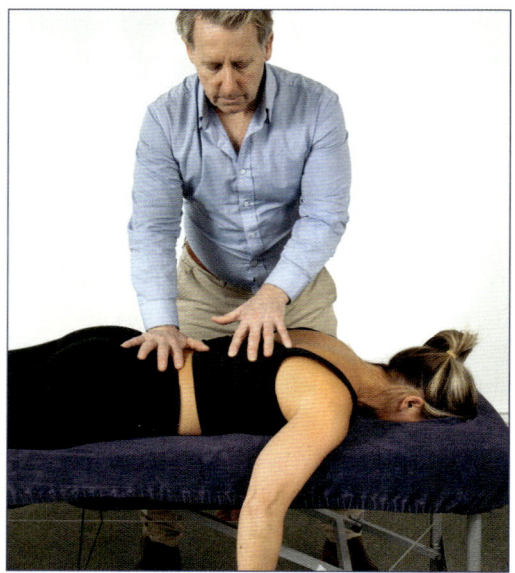

Figure 11.17. Palpation of the ribcage while inducing motion of the lumbosacral region.

This is done by using the heel of your hand to work up and down the contralateral erector muscles, while you maintain a rocking motion (figure 11.18).

Pelvis Rotational Technique (Soft Tissue)

With the patient prone, reach over with your right hand and (with permission) contact the patient's anterior superior iliac spine (ASIS) on their right side. This anatomical landmark is a good leverage point for when you come to mobilize the soft tissues and ribcage. The heel of your left hand is in contact

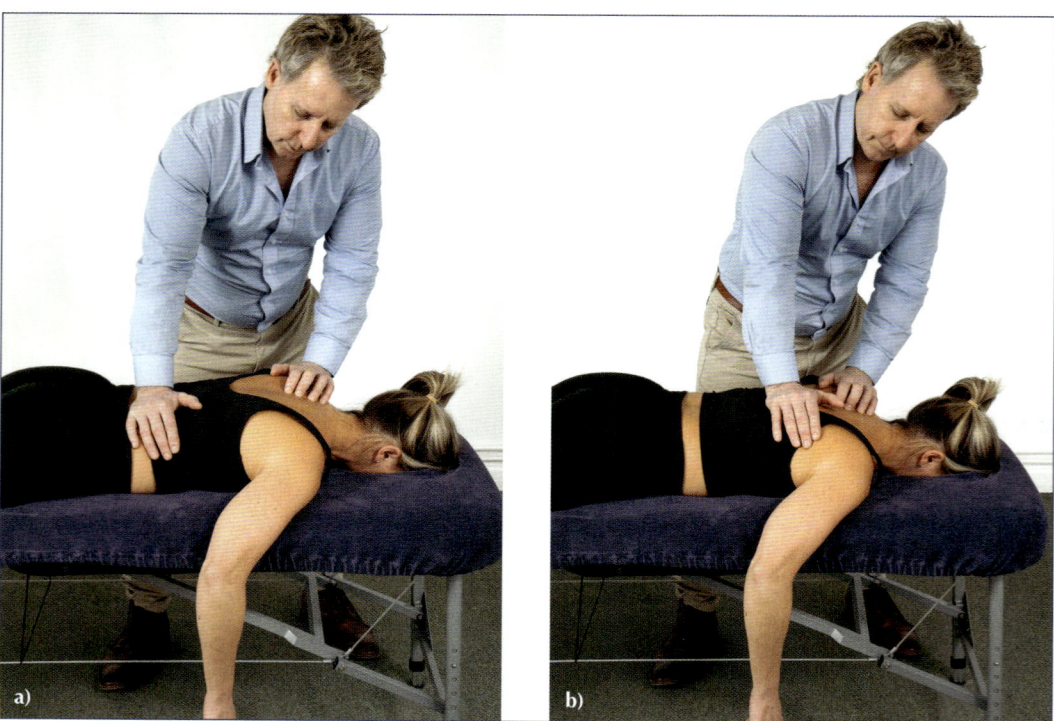

Figure 11.18. (a) Soft-tissue techniques of the contralateral lumbar spine erector muscles with a continuous rocking motion; (b) moving in a cephalad direction toward the thoracic erector muscles.

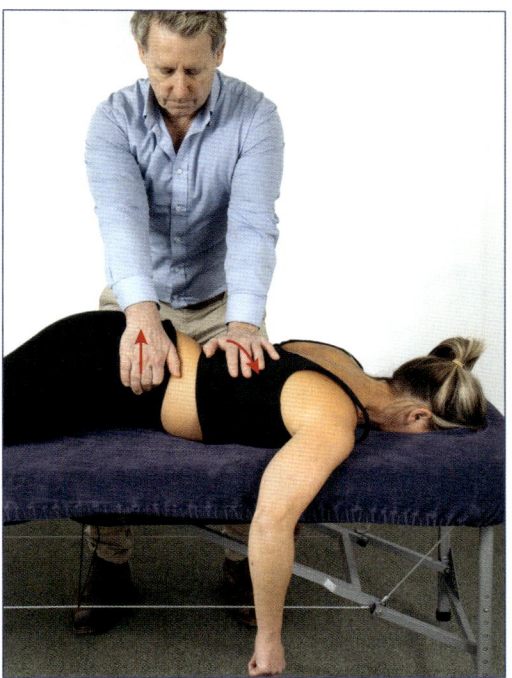

Figure 11.19. The therapist lifts the patient's pelvis toward them, simultaneously causing transverse pressure to the erector spinae muscles.

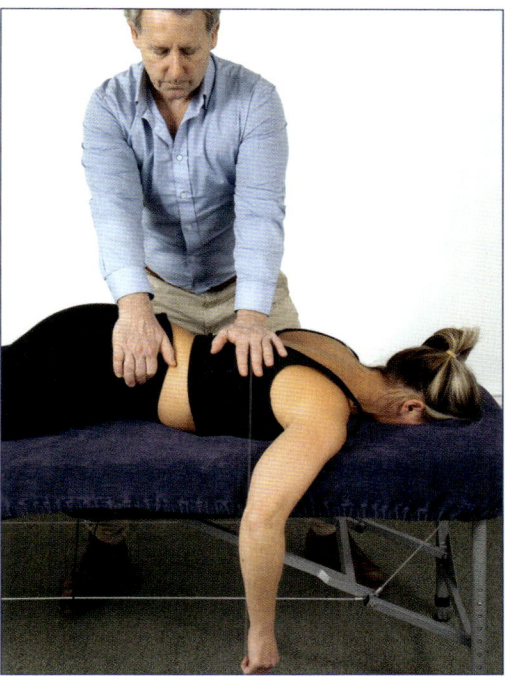

Figure 11.20. Hand placement is now toward the upper lumbar and lower thoracic spine.

with the erector spinae muscles of the lumbar spine, and the technique is applied by using your right hand to lift the patient's pelvis toward you while you apply transverse pressure laterally to the lumbar erector spinae muscles (figure 11.19).

This technique is very effective because it causes a stretching of the soft tissues of the erector spinae muscles, while at the same time promoting mobility of the pelvis and lumbar spine.

Next, continue this technique by slowly applying pressure to the soft tissues further up the lumbar spine and into the lower

thoracic region, while maintaining pelvis rotation (figure 11.20).

Pelvis Rotational Technique

Change your left hand placement so that the heel of the hand is now in contact with the angle of the patient's middle to lower right ribs, while at the same time maintaining contact with their ASIS with your right hand.

Ask the patient to take a breath in, and on the relaxation phase of the breath out, lift the pelvis toward you and simultaneously apply either a mobilization or a manipulative thrust to the angle of the affected rib. The direction of the

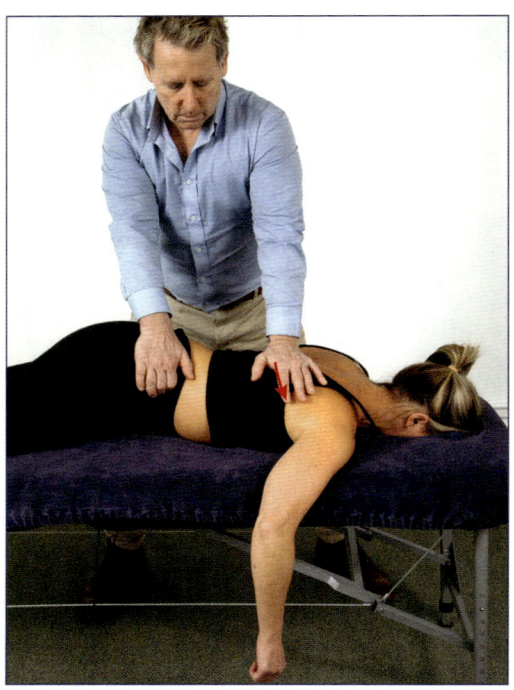

Figure 11.21. From this position, the therapist can apply either a mobilizing or a manipulative thrust toward the axilla.

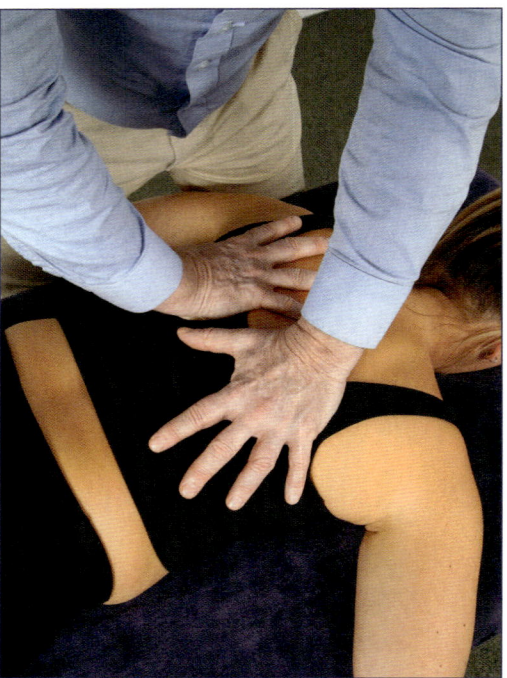

Figure 11.22. Hand placement number one for the butterfly spring technique over the ribcage.

technique is toward the patient's axilla (figure 11.21).

Mobilize ribcage using the pelvis

Butterfly Spring Technique

Similarly to earlier techniques, begin with the patient prone, spread your fingers and place your hands either side of the vertebrae to contact the angle of the ribs (regarding the hand position, the therapist can choose either position one [figure 11.22] or position two [figure 11.23], as it will be a personal preference).

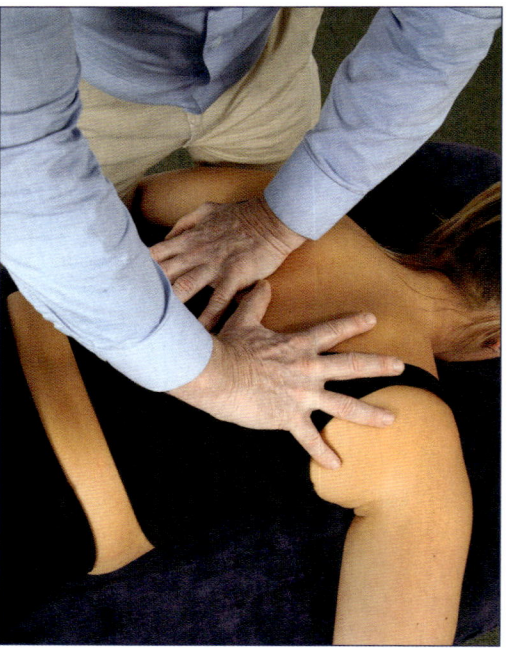

Figure 11.23. Hand placement number two for the butterfly spring technique over the ribcage.

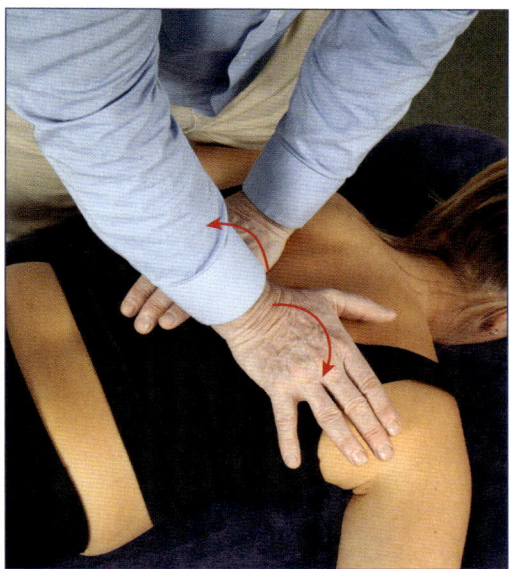

Figure 11.24. The therapist simultaneously applies a rotational motion of both hands and performs a mobilization or manipulation thrust toward the couch.

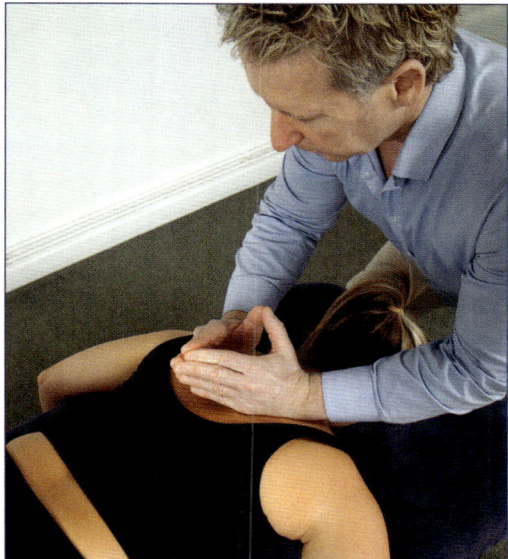

Figure 11.25. Hand placement for the triangular spring technique over the upper ribs.

Ask the patient to breathe in, and on the out breath apply a rotational pressure and at the same time a downward pressure toward the couch (figure 11.24). A gentle springing mobilization is recommended before any thrust is applied.

Mobilize ribcage using butterfly springing technique

Triangle Spring Technique—Caudal Direction

Stand at the head of the patient and apply pressure directly to the upper or middle ribs through contact of the pisiform bone of both hands (figure 11.25). Ask the patient to breathe in, and on the

out breath apply pressure until you feel a tension point within the ribcage. The mobilization or thrust is directed laterally and downward toward the couch.

Triangle Spring Technique—Cephalic Direction

Stand at the side of the patient and apply pressure directly to the middle or upper ribs through contact of the pisiform bone of both hands (figure 11.26a and b). Ask the patient to breathe in, and on the out breath apply pressure until you feel a tension point within the ribcage. The mobilization or thrust is directed laterally and downward toward the couch.

Mobilize ribcage using triangle technique

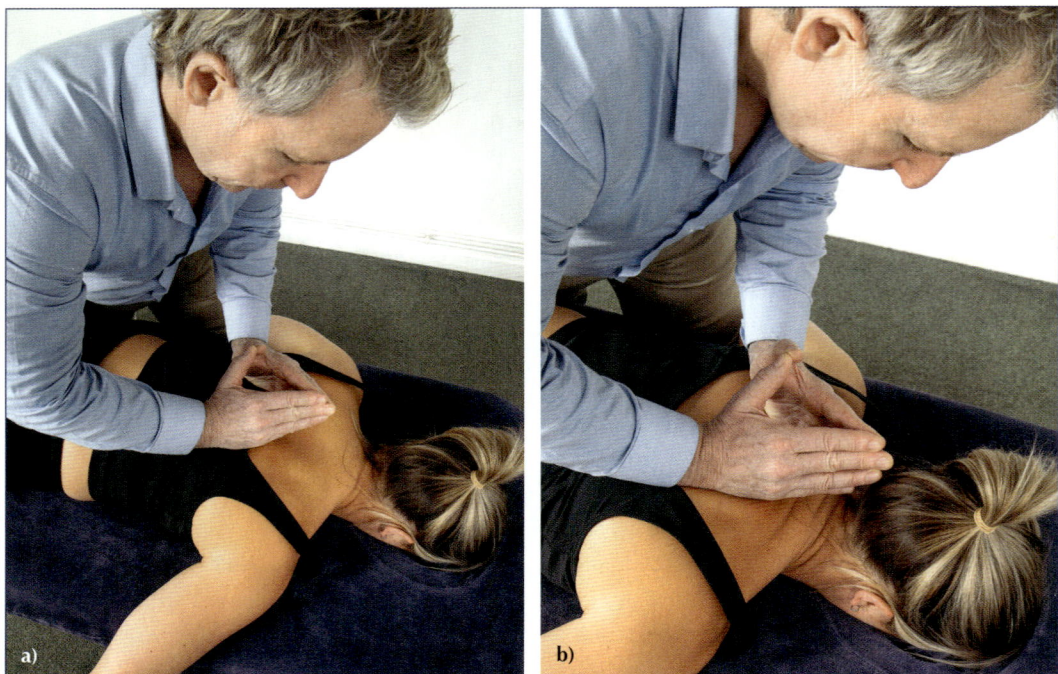

Figure 11.26. Hand placement for the triangular spring technique over (a) the middle ribs and (b) the upper ribs.

First Rib—MET

I suggest an MET is performed initially for the treatment of the first rib, mainly because of the anatomical structures located near this area—the brachial plexus and subclavian artery. One has to be very careful not to cause any direct trauma to these delicate structures. The technique demonstrated is for a left rib that is fixed in inhalation.

With the patient seated, stand directly behind them, place your right foot onto the chair, and place the patient's upper limb over your right thigh. Contact the patient's head and neck with your forearm, and place your right hand directly onto the patient's head. Using the second MCP joint, apply pressure to the patient's left first rib (figure 11.27).

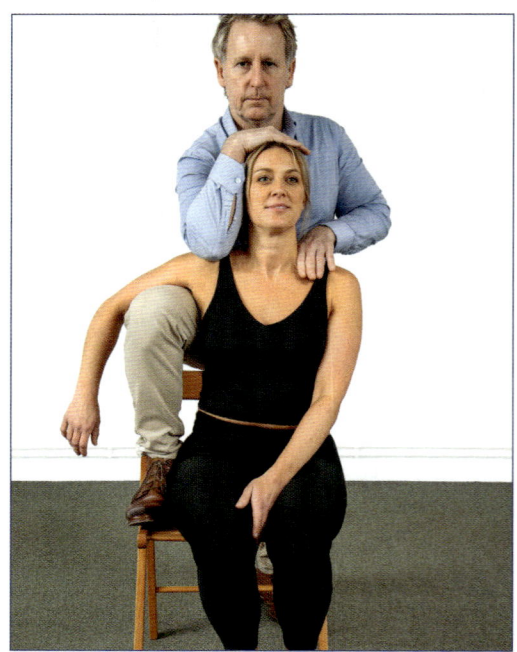

Figure 11.27. The patient's arm is placed over the therapist's leg and the therapist controls the head and neck with their forearm.

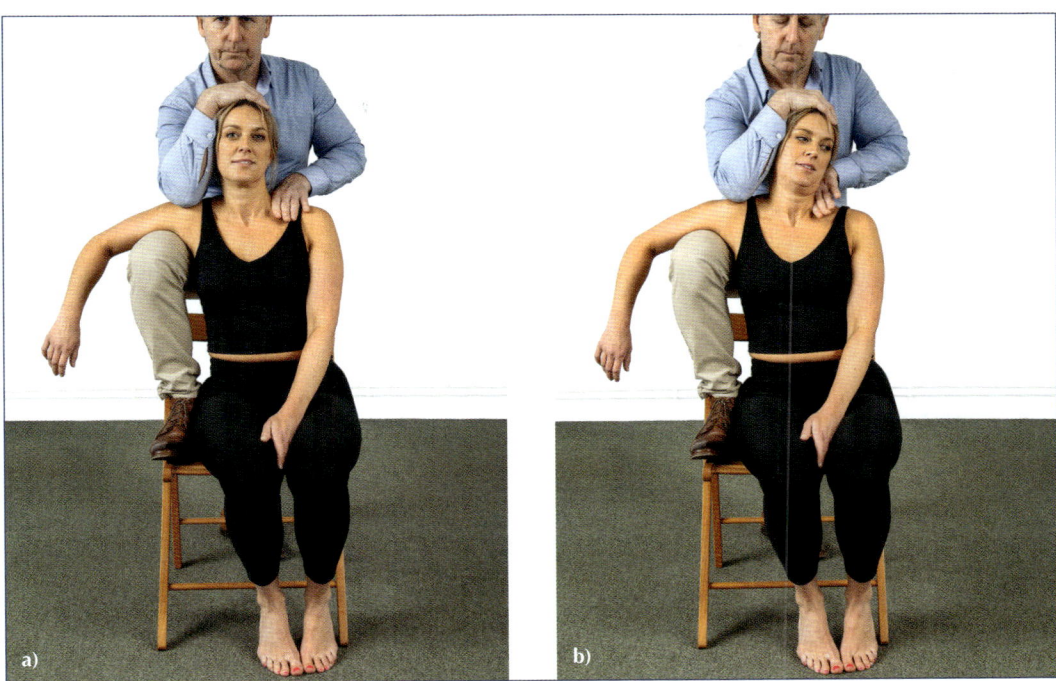

Figure 11.28. (a) After the contraction, the patient is guided into right translation, and (b) the head is taken into further left-side bending with combined right rotation.

Ask the patient to take a breath in and then to side bend their head to the right for approximately 10 seconds at 20% effort. After the contraction, and on an out breath, a few maneuvers are performed. Firstly, take the patient into right translation (side shift; figure 11.28a). Then guide the patient's head into further left-side bending with combined right rotation, while applying contact from the MCP joint directly onto the first rib (figure 11.28b). You apply gentle pressure to the first rib in the direction of their opposite axilla.

MET of the first rib

First or Second Rib—Mobilization

Ask the patient to adopt a prone position with their face located in a face hole (if you have one). Slowly position the patient's head into side bending (away) and rotation toward the same side as the rib being treated. Next, apply gentle pressure to the head to stabilize it, and place your pisiform bone directly to the rib of choice (first or second), as shown in figure 11.29.

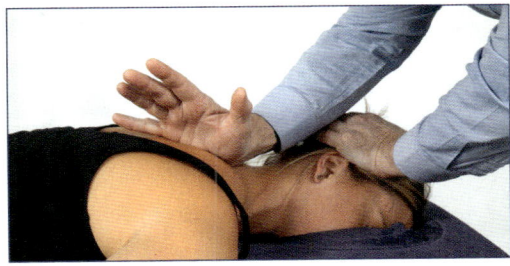

Figure 11.29. Hand placement for the first rib adjustment.

Ask the patient to take a breath in, and on the out breath, apply pressure laterally until you feel a tension point within the upper rib of choice. The thrust or mobilization technique is directed laterally toward the opposite axilla (figure 11.30). (Note that no directional force is applied to the cervical spine because this is a rib adjustment, not a cervical manipulation.)

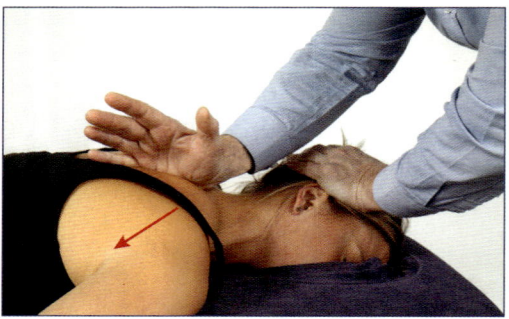

Figure 11.30. Direction of thrust toward the opposite axilla.

First rib manipulation

Techniques for the Lumbar Spine

12

This chapter gives the reader an insight into some of the techniques we can incorporate into a treatment protocol for the lumbar spine, as well as a brief introduction to some of the skeletal pathologies that can manifest within this area of the spinal column. However, in my opinion, it is logical to correct any pelvic dysfunctions (iliosacral, sacroiliac, and symphysis pubis) present before you assess, and subsequently treat, dysfunction of the lumbar spine (unless spinal rotation is the primary dysfunction).

It is essential to address any issues with an underpinning structure before tackling problems in other areas that depend on that structure. For example, I regard the pelvic girdle complex as similar to the foundations that are laid before building a house—we would not want to build on top of the foundations if they were not level. I use the same analogy when I look at and assess the lumbar spine. If the pelvis is not level, then the lumbar spine cannot be level either—this area of the spinal column will automatically compensate in some way by changing its natural spinal curvatures, which could result in functional/structural scoliosis. This unnatural positional change to the lumbar spine as a compensation mechanism can only lead to pain.

I am convinced that most of the spinal pathologies discussed in this chapter—and even throughout this book—are a direct or indirect consequence of the overall position and stability integration of the pelvic girdle. It is very difficult, however, to prove this, especially since I haven't been able to find any recent clinical research to support this claim. What I have stated has to be correct in one way or another, however, because the fundamental foundation (the pelvis) must be the main area of compensation for all of the various types of dysfunction that might be present within the body; this will have a direct knock-on effect on the entire kinetic chain, and the lumbar spine is clearly part of that compensatory chain mechanism.

However, by the time a patient presents with what might be diagnosed as a specific or nonspecific back pain, they probably already have some spinal pathology present. The patient might also have had confirmation of their spinal pathology by an MRI scan, X-ray, or some other diagnostic measures. Put simply, the patient's presenting spinal pathology already exists, even before they walk through your clinic door.

Out of thousands of patients, I can probably count on one hand those who have consulted me for an initial osteopathic assessment and treatment to prevent the onset of spinal and pelvic pathology, or indeed any other structural or soft-tissue ailment. Therefore, almost all patients who have visited my clinic already have a presentation of symptoms of pain/dysfunction somewhere in their body, and more than likely have some underlying form of spinal or pelvic dysfunction or pathology already present.

Anatomy of the Lumbar Spine

There are five individual spinal segments that make up the lumbar vertebrae, and each vertebra comprises the following structures (figure 12.1):

- Vertebral body
- Spinous process (SP)
- Transverse process (TP)
- Superior and inferior facets
- Intervertebral foramen
- Spinal canal

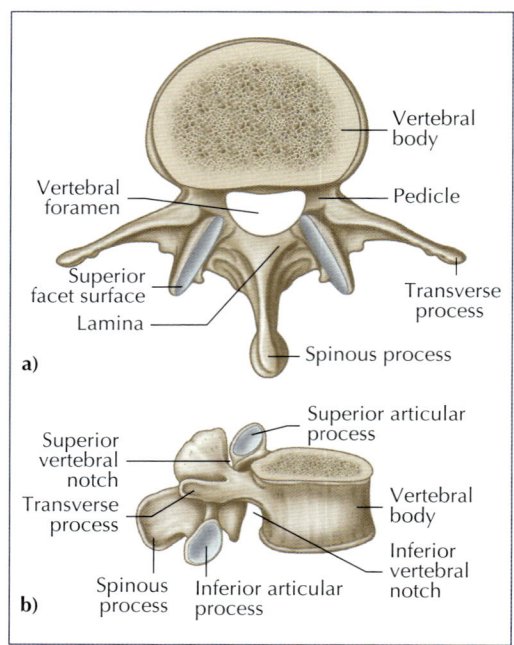

Figure 12.1. General anatomy of a lumbar vertebra (L3). (a) Superior view; (b) lateral view.

- Lamina
- Pedicle
- Intervertebral disc: nucleus pulposus/annulus fibrosus

The vertebral bodies of the lumbar spine are larger than the thoracic vertebral bodies and—because of their shape— they actually form a posterior vertebral body wedge, which in conjunction with the shape of the intervertebral disc assists to maintain the natural lumbar lordosis. The vertebral body, SP, and TPs all lie at the same level, unlike in the thoracic spine (rule of threes, p. 141). However, there is a slight variation within the lumbar spine. The vertebral body of L5 is larger, its SP is smaller, and its TPs are thicker but slightly shorter.

Between L5 and the first sacral segment, S1, there is a natural angle called the *lumbosacral angle*, which is typically 25°–35°. Lower back and pelvic pain can come from a change in this angle. Typically, if the lumbosacral angle is increased, it places extra shear forces on the lumbosacral joint and its associated soft-tissue structures (especially ligaments), directly increasing the lumbar lordosis.

Pathologies and underlying causes are numerous, encompassing conditions like spondylolisthesis, degenerative disc disease (DDD), pregnancy, obesity, and weakness of core musculature—such as the abdominals and gluteus maximus. Further, tightness of other muscles,

like the iliopsoas and erector spinae, can cause postural changes with a subsequent anterior pelvic tilt.

We briefly describe here the neurological anatomy of the lumbar and sacral spine: the manual therapy techniques described in this chapter will have a direct effect on the exiting nerve roots.

Lumbar Plexus

The lumbar plexus (figure 12.2) forms the upper part of the lumbosacral plexus and is formed by the anterior divisions of the first four lumbar nerves (L1–L4). The spinal roots divide into many cords

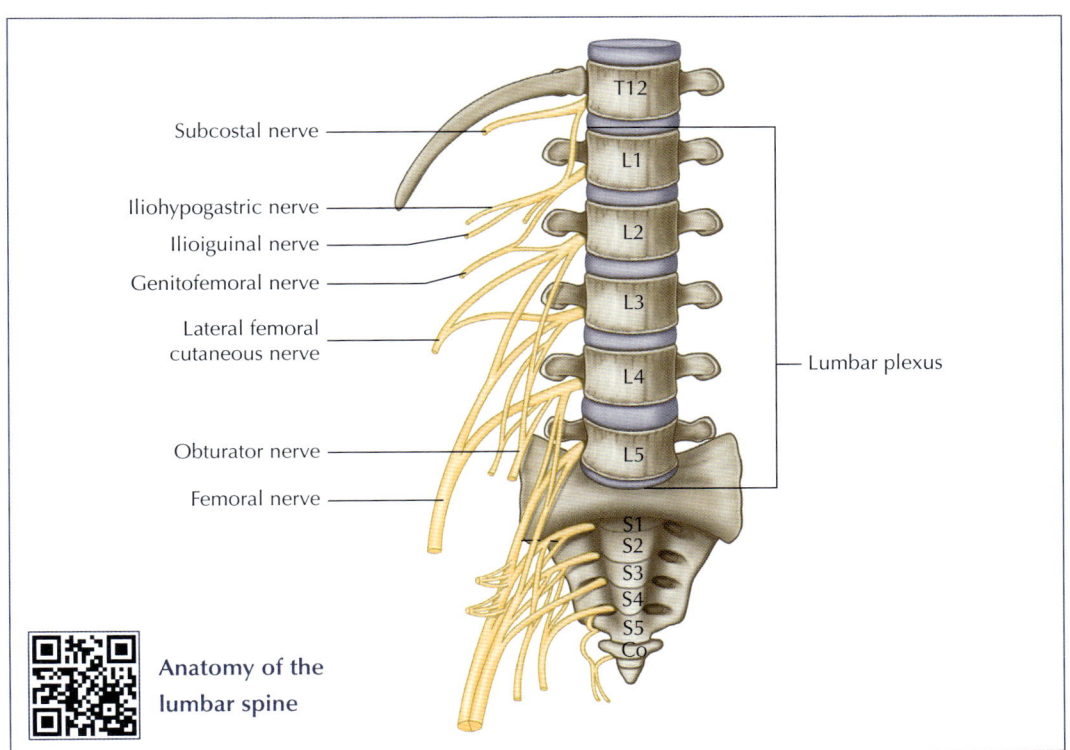

Anatomy of the lumbar spine

Figure 12.2. Lumbar plexus.

and then form the six major peripheral nerves to innervate the lower limb:

- Iliohypogastric nerve
- Ilioinguinal nerve
- Genitofemoral nerve
- Lateral femoral cutaneous nerve
- Femoral nerve
- Obturator nerve

Sacral Plexus

The sacral plexus (figure 12.3) is the lower part of the lumbosacral plexus and is a branching network of nerves that provide motor and sensory supply to part of the pelvis, the posterior thigh, most of the lower leg, and the entire foot. The sacral plexus is formed from the anterior rami of spinal nerves L4, L5, and S1–S4, and each of these anterior rami gives rise to anterior and posterior branches.

The anterior branches supply the flexor muscles of the lower limb, and the posterior branches supply the extensor and abductor muscles. All the nerve roots entering the sacral

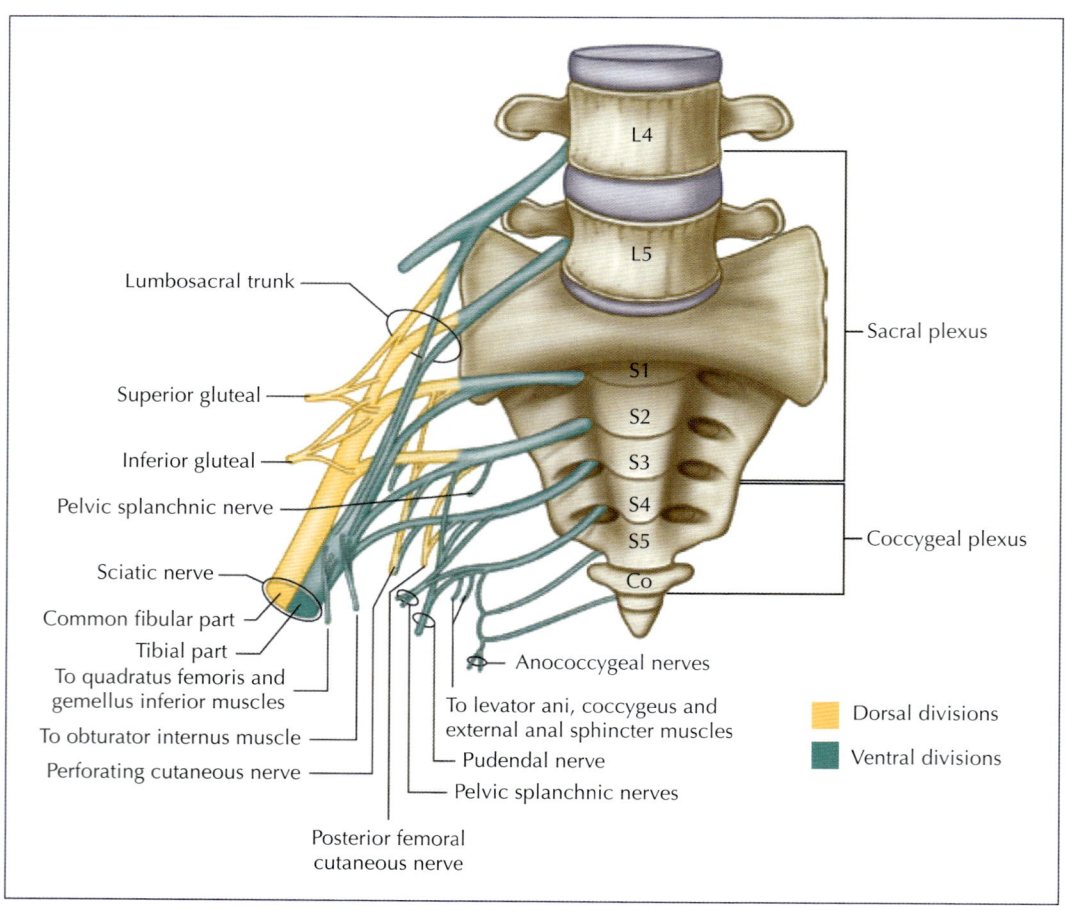

Figure 12.3. Sacral plexus.

plexus split into anterior and posterior divisions.

The nerves arising from these divisions are:

- Sciatic nerve
- Tibial nerve: L4–S3
- Common fibular nerve: L4–S2
- Superior gluteal nerve: L4–S1
- Inferior gluteal nerve: L5–S2
- Posterior femoral cutaneous nerve: S1–S3
- Pudendal nerve: S2–S4
- Nerve to quadratus femoris and gemellus inferior: L4–S1
- Nerve to obturator internus and gemellus superior: L5–S2
- Nerve to piriformis: S1–S2

Lumbar Intervertebral Discs

Between adjacent lumbar vertebrae there is an intervertebral disc, and the lower two discs in particular are susceptible to pathology.

A disc is made up of three components: a tough outer shell, the annulus fibrosus; an inner gel-like substance, the nucleus pulposus; and an attachment to the vertebral bodies, the vertebral end plate. As we age, the center of the disc starts to lose water content, a process that will make the disc less elastic and less effective to act as a cushion or shock absorber.

Nerve roots exit the spinal canal through small passageways between the vertebrae and the discs, known as intervertebral foramina. Pain and other symptoms can develop when a damaged disc pushes into the spinal canal or nerve roots—a condition referred to as a herniated disc.

Facet Joints

Located within the lumbar spine—like the rest of the spinal column—are the facet joints. These structures can be responsible for provoking great pain. The facet joints lie posterior to the vertebral body, and their role is to assist the spine in performing movements such as flexion, extension, side bending, and rotation. Depending on their location and orientation, these joints will allow certain types of motion but restrict others: for example, the lumbar spine is limited in rotation, but flexion and extension are freely permitted.

Each vertebra has two paired facet joints: The superior articular facet faces upward and creates a joint with the inferior facet of the vertebra above, which works similarly to a hinge. The inferior articular facet faces downward and creates a joint with the superior facet of the vertebra located below it. The L4 inferior facet, for example, articulates with the L5 superior facet.

Like all other synovial joints in the body, each facet joint is surrounded by a capsule of connective tissue and produces synovial fluid to nourish and lubricate the joint. The surfaces of the facets are coated with cartilage, which helps each joint to move (articulate) smoothly. The facet joint is highly innervated with pain receptors, making it susceptible to producing back pain.

Pathology of the Lumbar Spine

Disc Herniation

Herniated discs are often referred to as bulging discs, prolapsed discs, or even slipped discs. These terms are derived from the way the gel-like content of the nucleus pulposus is forced out of the center of the disc. As noted before, the disc itself does not slip; however, the nucleus pulposus tissue in the center of the disc can be placed under so much pressure that it can cause the annulus fibrosus to herniate or even rupture (figure 12.4).

In a severe disc herniation the bulging tissue may press against one or more of the spinal nerves, which can cause

local and referred pain, numbness, or weakness in the lower back, leg, or even ankle and foot. Approximately 85%–95% of lumbar disc herniations occur either at the L4–L5 or at L5–S1; the nerve compression caused by the contact with the disc contents can result in perceived pain along the L4, L5, or S1 nerve root pathways (figure 12.5).

Degenerative Disc Disease

Degenerative disc disease (DDD) tends to be linked to the aging process and is a syndrome in which a painful disc causes associated chronic lower back pain, which can also radiate symptoms to the hip region (figure 12.6). The condition generally occurs due to some form of injury to the lower back and the associated structures, such as the intervertebral discs.

An injury can trigger an inflammatory process and subsequent weakness of the annulus fibrosus, which will then have a pronounced effect on the inner nucleus pulposus. This reactive mechanism will lead to excessive movement, because the disc can no longer control the motion of the vertebral bodies located above and below. This excessive movement—combined with the natural inflammatory response—will produce chemicals that will irritate the local area, which will commonly produce symptoms of chronic lower back pain.

DDD has been shown to cause an increase in the number of clusters of chondrocytes (cells that form the cartilaginous matrix,

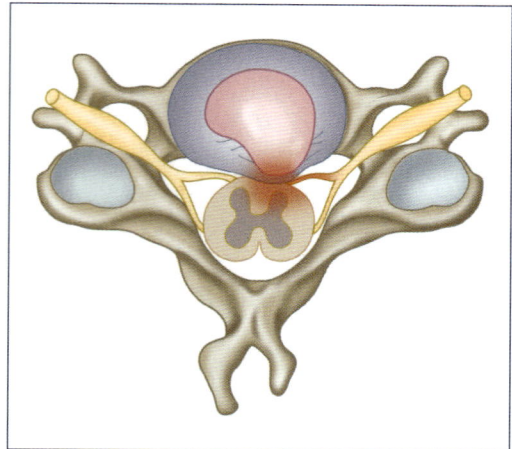

Figure 12.4. Disc herniation.

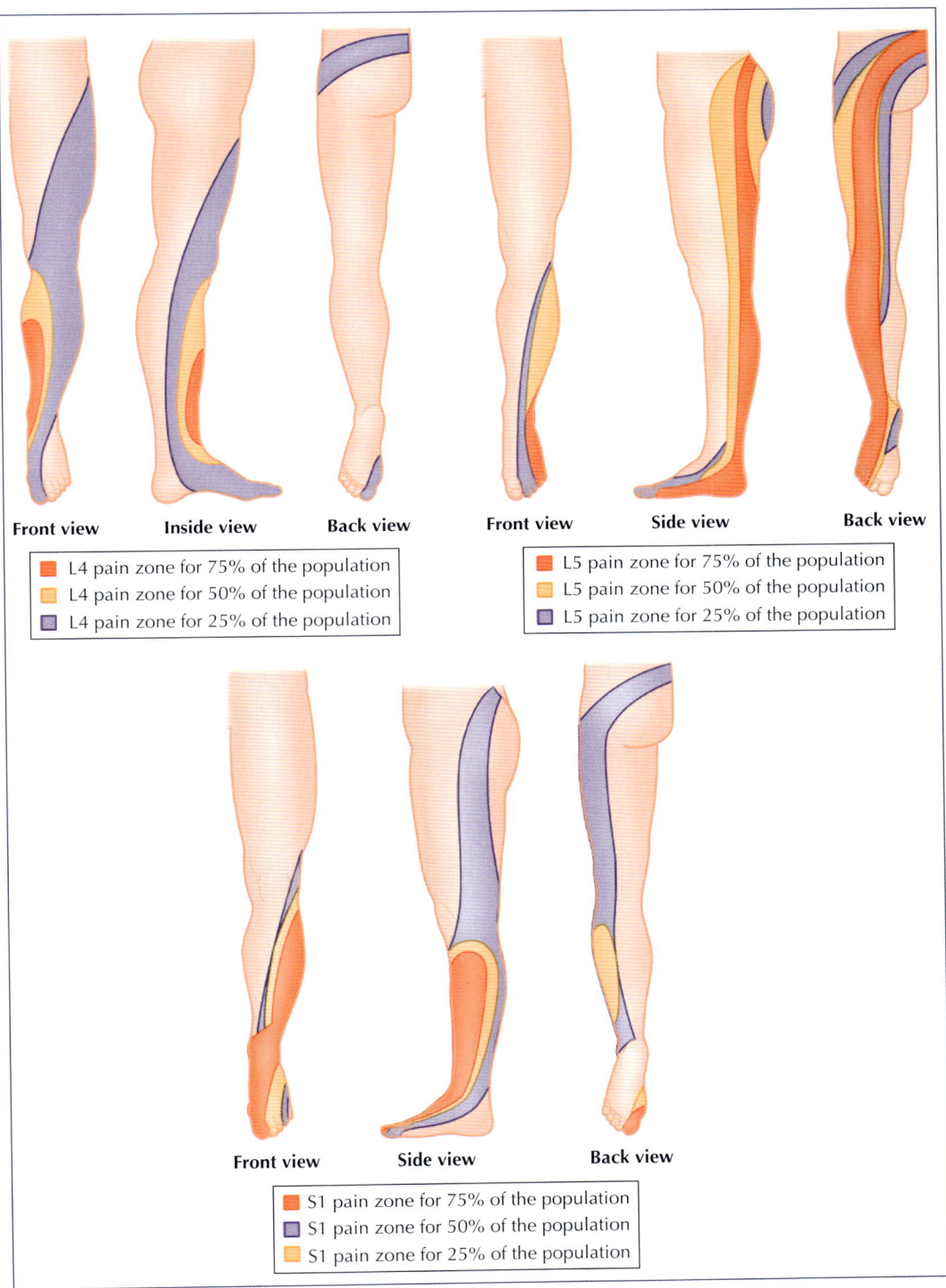

Front view   Inside view   Back view

■ L4 pain zone for 75% of the population
■ L4 pain zone for 50% of the population
■ L4 pain zone for 25% of the population

Front view   Side view   Back view

■ L5 pain zone for 75% of the population
■ L5 pain zone for 50% of the population
■ L5 pain zone for 25% of the population

Front view   Side view   Back view

■ S1 pain zone for 75% of the population
■ S1 pain zone for 50% of the population
■ S1 pain zone for 25% of the population

Figure 12.5. Dermatome pathway of pain for L4, L5, and S1 nerve roots.

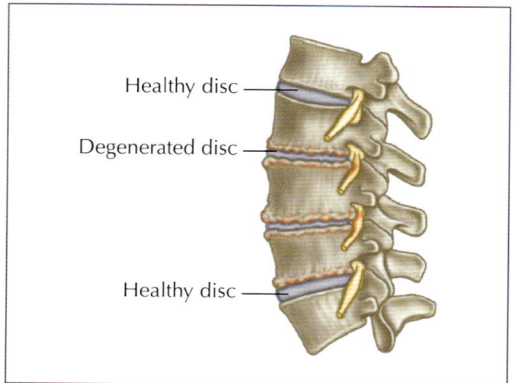

Figure 12.6. Degenerative disc disease.

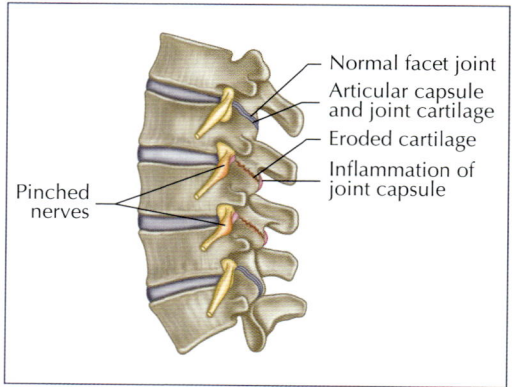

Figure 12.7. Facet joint syndrome and spondylosis.

which consists mainly of collagen) in the annulus fibrosus (consisting of fibrocartilage). Over a prolonged period, the nucleus pulposus can change to fibrocartilage, and it has been shown that the outer annulus fibrosus can become damaged in areas that allow some of the nucleus material to herniate through, causing the disc to shrink and eventually lead to the formation of bony spurs called osteophytes.

Unlike the muscles in the back, the discs of the lumbar spine do not have a natural blood supply and therefore cannot heal themselves; this means the painful symptoms of DDD can become chronic, eventually leading to further problems, such as discal herniation, facet joint pain, nerve root compression, spondylolysis (defect of the pars interarticularis), and spinal stenosis (narrowing of the spinal canal).

Facet Joint Syndrome/Disease

The articulating facets of facet joints tend to slide over each other, so are in constant motion with the spine. Like all types of

weight-bearing joint, they can simply wear out and start to degenerate over time.

When facet joints become irritated (the cartilage can even tear), this will cause the bone of the joint underneath the facet to start producing osteophytes, leading to facet joint hypertrophy, which is the precursor of facet joint syndrome/disease (figure 12.7) and eventually leads to spondylosis. This type of disease process is very common in patients presenting with chronic back pain.

Lumbar Spine as a Cause of Pelvis Dysfunctions

I have mentioned the idea that the pelvis and possibly the hip joint are the key areas responsible for the presentation of pain in the lumbar spine and pelvic girdle regions. However, there will be times when other structures need to be incorporated into the bigger picture to solve the problem. These structures might play an even greater role. Once you understand the next concept, I hope it will help you place the jigsaw puzzle pieces in the correct sequence so that a clearer picture will begin to appear.

It could be that the underlying issue is hidden and dormant and not showing itself as a dysfunction: the musculoskeletal problem is lying quietly in the grass and minding its own business. Let's consider for a moment the possibility that the problem is within the lumbar spine. This structure could be the key to solving the mystery, and the main factor perpetuating the pelvic dysfunctions.

For example, a patient has ongoing, recurrent pelvic dysfunctions that you have been correcting repeatedly without success. Frustratingly, what you are doing in terms of treatment does not seem to be solving the problem, despite it being effective for previous patients. It may be that the problem lies within the lumbar spine, and this skeletal structure is the underlying causative factor maintaining and controlling the chronic dysfunctional pelvic pattern. A rotational component at the lumbosacral junction (L5/S1) has been recognized as one cause of recurrent pelvic malalignment.

Let's look at an example. If we have a clockwise rotation—that is, to the right of L5—the right-sided TP will rotate backward (posteriorly). There are soft-tissue attachments onto the L4 and L5 TPs for the iliolumbar ligament, and this ligamentous tissue attaches directly to the iliac crest. The induced rotation increases the tension within the iliolumbar ligament, and the L5 rotation to the right will force the right innominate to rotate posteriorly;

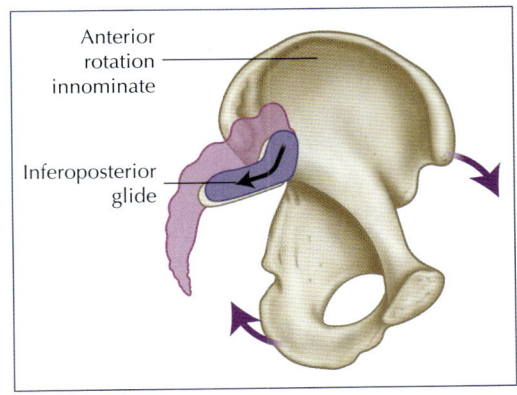

Figure 12.8. Anterior position of the left innominate.

the left TP of L5 is rotating anteriorly, and this creates an anterior position (anterior rotation) of the left innominate (figure 12.8).

Farfan (1973) reasoned that the shorter the TP, the longer the iliolumbar ligament and the greater the torsional force.

The L5 right inferior facet will be in a relatively open position on the superior facet of S1; the left inferior facet, however, will be in a closed position on the superior facet of S1. If the left facet joint is compressed, and the position is maintained and continued, it can now become a pivot point (fulcrum). This fixation (left) of the L5/S1 facet joint will now start to encourage the sacrum to rotate to the right axis (right on right), which will eventually force the whole pelvis into a right rotated position (figure 12.9).

So how do we go about correcting a dysfunction of the lumbar spine? The treatment of the pelvis in chapter 13 contains snippets of valuable information

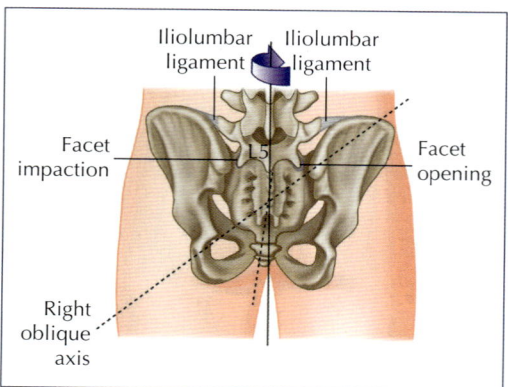

Figure 12.9. Rotational effect of L5 on the sacrum and on the innominate (via the attachment to the iliolumbar ligament).

that will help you ascertain if a lumbar dysfunction exists. Once you have read and understood how to determine a lumbar dysfunction, you will then need to read the appropriate text located within this and the next chapter, which explains in detail how to correct any possible dysfunctions that may be found within the lumbar spine complex.

Note: I would still recommend that you first treat any pelvic dysfunctions before embarking on realigning specific dysfunctions that you find within the lumbar spine complex.

Assessment and Treatment of the Lumbar Spine

I mentioned earlier that I consider lumbar spine dysfunctions to be caused by a compensatory mechanism associated with underlying malalignments of the pelvis. In my opinion, dysfunctions of the lumbar spine are a secondary type of dysfunction resulting from a primary dysfunction within the pelvic girdle complex; this is

the main reason why I leave treating the lumbar spine until last.

There are exceptions to these rules, of course, where the lumbar spine is the primary cause rather than the compensatory secondary cause. Either way, the realignment techniques I will demonstrate shortly will be of value because they will assist you in correcting the presentations that are commonly found within the lumbar spine.

I would like to keep things simple to start with, although this subject matter is by no means simple to understand. For the first example, when I say that the facet joint is fixed in a *closed position*, this refers to the specific position of the inferior facet being closed in extension, side bending, and rotation (normally to one side) on the superior facet of the vertebra immediately below. Think back to chapter 6 where I talked about this situation as an ERS, a type 2 dysfunction (non-neutral mechanics), because the rotation and side bending are coupled to the same side but in an extended position, either to the left (ERS[l]) or to the right (ERS[r]).

The opposite motion, and the second example, is where the facet joint is now fixed in an *open position*; in this case the motion is related to the specific position of the inferior facet being open in flexion, side bending, and rotation (normally to one side) on the superior facet of the vertebra immediately below. This type of spinal dysfunction is referred to as an FRS, which is also a type 2 dysfunction (non-neutral mechanics), because the rotation and side bending are coupled to the same side but this time in a flexed position, either to the left (FRS[l]) or to the right (FRS[r]).

Note: Regarding the position of a facet joint that is fixed in an open position, remember from chapter 6 that the joint will be open on the opposite side. For example, an FRS(l)—flexion, rotation, and side bending left—indicates that the facet joint is fixed *open* on the *right* (opposite) side.

The following lumbar spine dysfunctions are discussed:

- L5 ERS(l)
- L4 ERS(r)
- L5 FRS(l)

Assess and mobilize the lumbar spine

Diagnosis L5 ERS(l)

Treatment: MET

Position: Side lying

This spinal dysfunction relates to the inferior facet of L5 being fixed in a position of extension, rotation, and side bending to the left side on the superior facet of the S1 vertebra. This basically means that the left facet joint of L5/S1 is fixed in a closed position (figure 12.10). The subsequent motion restriction will affect movements on the side opposite the fixation—namely, flexion, right rotation, and right-side bending.

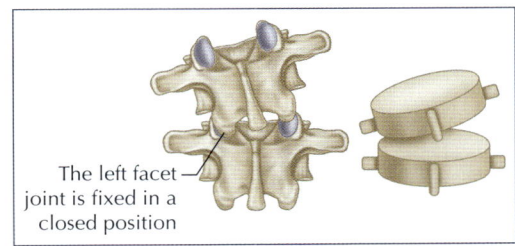

The left facet joint is fixed in a closed position

Figure 12.10. L5 ERS(l) on S1.

Ask the patient to adopt a side-lying position facing you, with the posterior TP of the dysfunctional L5 toward the couch (i.e., dysfunction side down—in this case, left side down). Palpate the interspinous space of L4/5 with your left hand and at the same time cradle the patient's left arm and introduce flexion and right rotation of the patient's trunk down to the relevant lumbar level (figure 12.11).

Cradle the patient's legs and introduce the hips into flexion, while at the same time palpating with your right hand the L5/S1 interspinous space for motion (figure 12.12).

From this position, ask the patient to push both their feet toward the floor

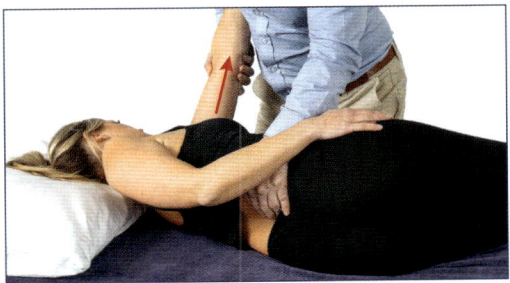

Figure 12.11. The therapist palpates the interspinous space of L4/5 and introduces flexion and right rotation of the lumbar spine down to that level, to prevent over-locking of L5/S1.

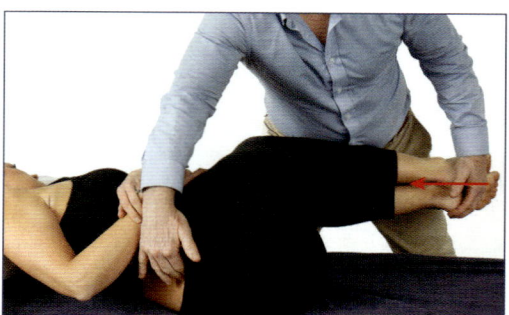

Figure 12.12. The therapist introduces hip flexion to both legs while they palpate the L5/S1 interspinous space for motion.

(side bending left), as indicated by the arrow in figure 12.13, for 10 seconds at a contraction of between 10% and 20% of maximum.

After the contraction, and during the relaxation phase, encourage the patient's legs toward the ceiling, as this motion introduces right-side bending of the lumbar spine (figure 12.14). This movement subsequently opens the left L5/S1 facet joint, which is fixed in a closed position.

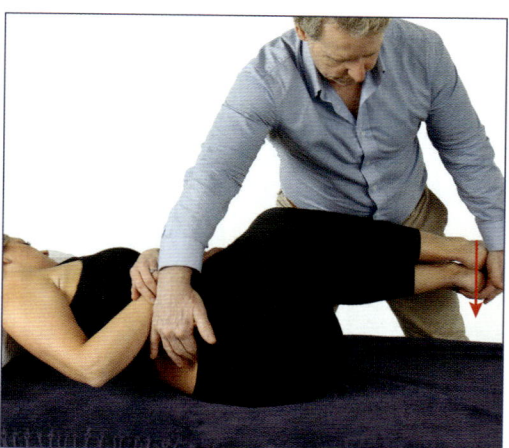

Figure 12.13. The patient pushes both feet toward the floor for 10 seconds.

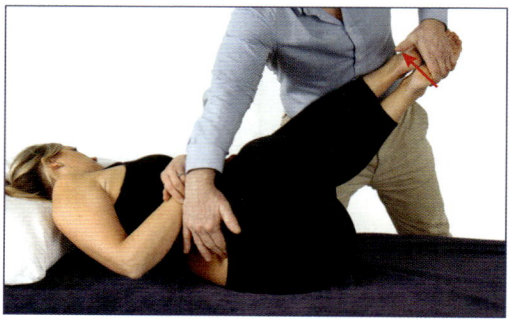

Figure 12.14. After the contraction the therapist introduces right-side bending by using the motion from the legs toward the ceiling to open the left facet joint.

Diagnosis L4 ERS(r)

Treatment: MET, thrust technique (HVT)

Position: Side lying

This spinal dysfunction relates to the inferior facet of L4 being fixed in a position of extension, right rotation, and right-side bending on the superior facet of L5. This basically means that the right facet joint of L4/5 is fixed in a closed position (figure 12.15). The subsequent motion restriction will affect movements on the side opposite the fixation—namely, flexion, left rotation, and left-side bending.

Ask the patient to adopt a side-lying position facing you, with the posterior TP

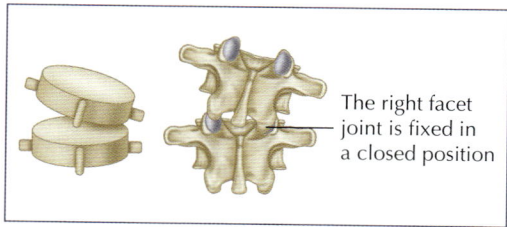

The right facet joint is fixed in a closed position

Figure 12.15. L4 ERS(r) on L5.

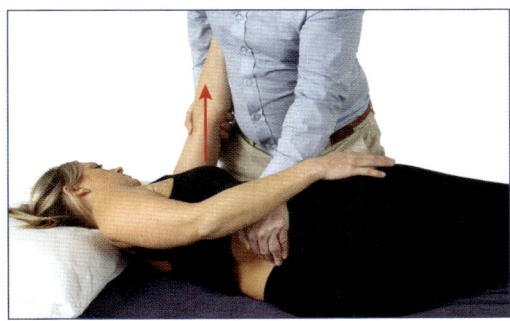

Figure 12.16. The therapist palpates the interspinous space of L3/4 and introduces flexion and right rotation of the lumbar spine down to L4.

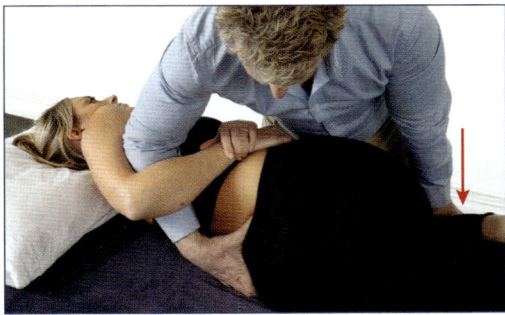

Figure 12.17. The therapist palpates L4 and fine-tunes the position by using the patient's top leg.

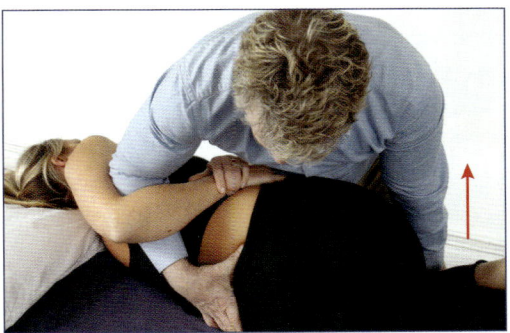

Figure 12.18. The patient abducts their right hip for 10 seconds.

of L4 toward the ceiling (i.e., dysfunction side up—in this case, right side up). While palpating the interspinous space of L3/4 with your left hand, introduce flexion and right rotation of the lumbar spine down to L4 with your right hand (figure 12.16).

Next, place the patient's right hand onto their right hip to stabilize the position. Palpate the L4/5 interspinous space with your right hand and feel for specific motion as you take the patient's bottom leg into flexion.

The patient's top leg should then be flexed, with the foot in the crease of the left knee. Place your right hand through the natural gap formed by the patient's hand on their hip and palpate the L4/5 interspinous space. Guide the patient's trunk gently toward the floor using your left hand, placed on the patient's right knee and controlling the motion (figure 12.17).

Once you have fine-tuned the position, ask the patient to abduct their right hip against your resistance for 10 seconds (figure 12.18).

After the contraction, and during the relaxation phase, encourage motion of the top leg toward the floor, as this type of movement introduces left-side bending of the lumbar spine (figure 12.19). This movement subsequently opens the right L4/5 facet joint, which is fixed in a closed position.

If you are suitably qualified, from the fine-tuned position (as above), you can apply a thrust technique (HVT) in the direction through the long lever of the femur toward the floor (figure 12.20). This quick motion will cause a left-side bending motion to L4/5, and a cavitation may be elicited from the joint.

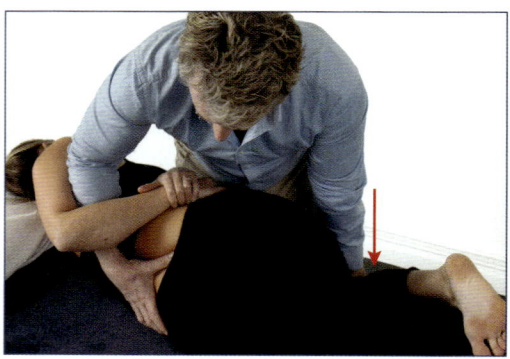

Figure 12.19. After the contraction the therapist introduces left-side bending of the lumbar spine to open the right L4/5 facet joint.

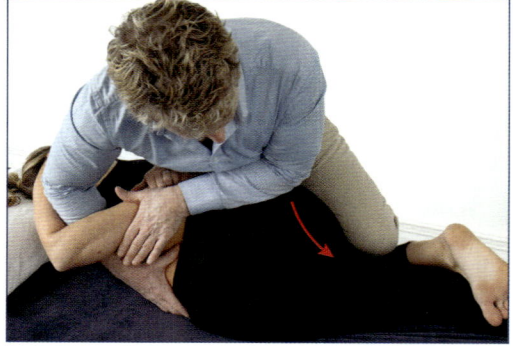

Figure 12.21. The therapist uses their knee in the kick-start technique.

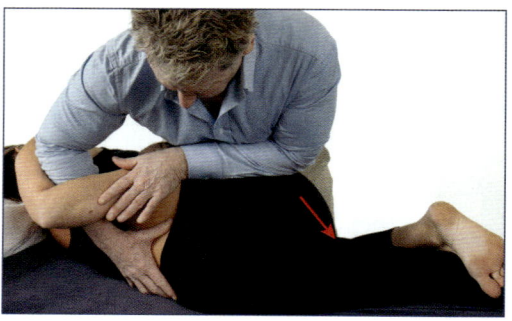

Figure 12.20. From the fine-tuned position, the therapist applies a quick thrust technique to encourage left-side bending of the lumbar spine, which may elicit a cavitation from the right L4/5 facet joint.

Kick-Start Technique

An alternative to the standard lumbar roll technique is the "kick-start" technique—so-called because of its similarity to kick-starting a motorbike—where you place your knee over the top leg of the patient (figure 12.21), and then use your leg, combined with your forearm and bodyweight dropping through the patient's hip region, to execute the thrust maneuver.

 Manipulation of lumbar spine using kickstart technique

 Mobilization of lumbar spine

 Manipulation of lumbar spine (female)

 Manipulation of lumbar spine (male)

Diagnosis L5 FRS(l)

Treatment: Soft-tissue technique

Position: Prone

This spinal dysfunction relates to the inferior facet of the L5 vertebra having become fixed in a position of flexion, left rotation, and left-side bending on the

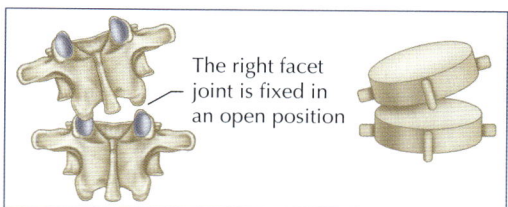

The right facet joint is fixed in an open position

Figure 12.22. L5 FRS(l) on S1.

superior facet of S1. This basically means that the right facet joint of L5/S1 is fixed in an open position (figure 12.22). The subsequent motion restriction will affect movements on the side opposite the fixation—namely, extension, right rotation, and right-side bending.

With the patient lying prone, confirm using your thumbs that the left TP of L5 is shallow and the right TP is deep, indicating a left rotation. When the patient backward bends, the left TP appearing shallower and the right TP becoming deeper confirms the presence of an FRS(l), where the right facet joint is fixed in an open position (figure 12.23).

The correction of this spinal dysfunction is very simple in some respects, as it can be treated from the backward-bent position.

Apply between 5 and 10 lb (2–4 kg) of direct pressure onto the right L5 TP, either with a reinforced thumb (figure 12.24) or with your elbow (figure 12.25). Then wait for the tissues to soften, before retesting the position to see if there has been any change.

In the case of an FRS(r), the opposite procedure would be performed.

Treatment of an FRS(L) of L5/S1

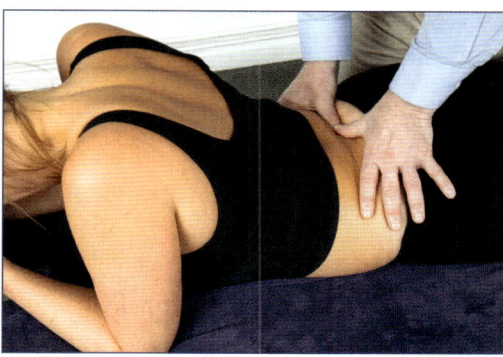

Figure 12.24. With the patient in a backward-bent position, the therapist applies pressure with a reinforced thumb directly onto the right L5 TP, to encourage closure of the right facet joint.

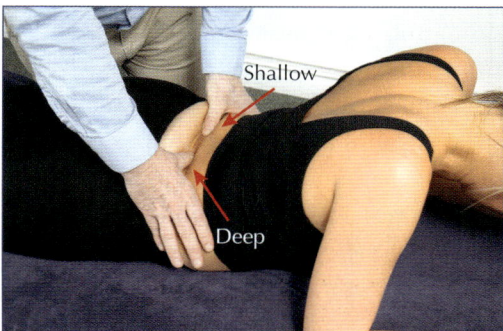

Shallow

Deep

Figure 12.23. With the patient in a backward-bent position, the therapist's left thumb palpates shallow and the right thumb palpates deep, indicating an FRS(l).

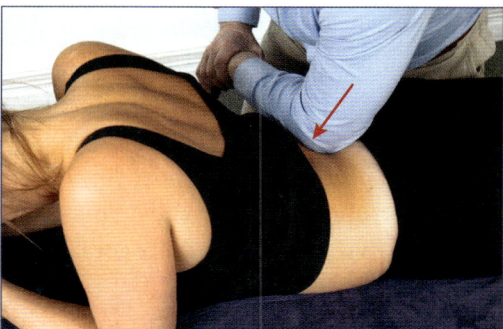

Figure 12.25. With the patient in a backward-bent position, the therapist applies pressure with their elbow directly onto the right L5 TP, to encourage closure of the right facet joint.

CHAPTER

Techniques for the Pelvic Girdle

13

Anatomy of the pelvis and SIJ

Treatment Strategy for the Pelvic Girdle Complex

Other experts in this complex field of manual medicine start their treatment of the vertebral column by initially correcting the position of the lumbar spine. They then move on to dysfunctions found within the iliosacral area, followed by the region of the sacroiliac, and finish off with treatment of the symphysis pubis joint.

In DeStefano's (2011) article, Greenman's suggestion of the treatment sequence is symphysis pubis, hipbone shear (upslip is considered a hipbone shear) dysfunction, sacroiliac dysfunction, and iliosacral dysfunction.

My preference is to start the corrective treatment with the symphysis pubis joint, followed by treatment of iliosacral

dysfunctions (upslip first), and then move on to sacroiliac dysfunctions. I would finish the treatment, if I felt it necessary, with any compensatory dysfunctions present within the region of the lumbar spine, as described in chapter 12.

Greenman recommends treating the symphysis pubis joint early on during the assessment process. The reason for this is that SIJ dysfunctions are typically found in a patient in the prone position; if a symphysis pubis dysfunction is present at the front of the body, the patient is not symmetric in the prone position, resting on the tripod formed by the two ASISs and the symphysis pubis.

Greenman also suggests treating superior shear (upslip) after the symphysis pubis, because he found that the presence of shear restricts all other motions within that SIJ; therefore, he says, shear deserves attention early in the treatment process. He mentions that you need to have two symmetric hipbones available to assess the position of the sacrum between them.

Treatment Protocol for Symphysis Pubis Dysfunctions

Symphysis pubis dysfunctions (SPDs) are very common, but are often neglected in terms of treatment by physical therapists, which is probably because of the lack of symptomatic pain within the symphysis pubis joint (SPJ). The pubic bone in SPDs tends to be either superior or inferior (although other types of dysfunction are discussed by some authors). For this text, we will focus on:

- Superior/inferior SPD
- Left superior SPD
- Right inferior SPD

Diagnosis: Superior/Inferior SPD

Treatment: MET/thrust technique (shotgun technique)

Position: Supine

Ask the patient to lie supine with their knees and hips bent and feet flat. Stand at the side of the couch and place your hands on the outsides of the patient's knees.

Ask the patient to abduct their hips against your resistance for 10 seconds (figure 13.1), which causes an RI effect in the adductors; this isometric contraction is repeated about three times. Then place a clenched fist between the patient's knees, and ask the patient to squeeze the fist tightly (adduction), as in figure 13.2. This motion of adduction is generally enough to cause a realignment of the symphysis pubis joint—it is very common for a noise (due to cavitation) to be heard from the

joint, indicating a release. There is no direct thrust involved with this technique, so it is very safe to perform.

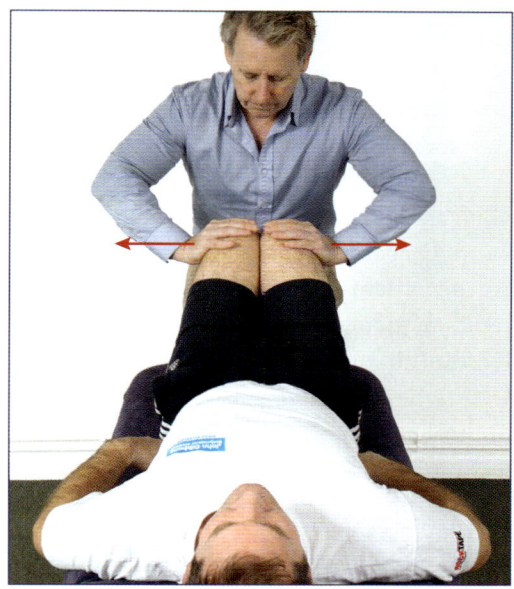

Figure 13.1. The patient abducts their hips against a resistance applied by the therapist.

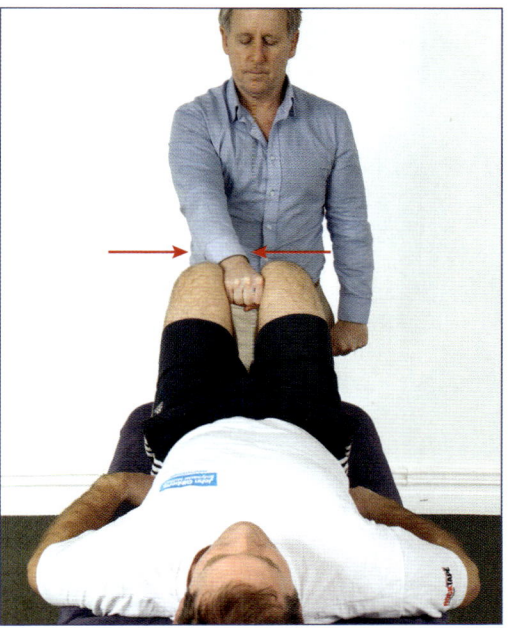

Figure 13.2. The therapist places a clenched fist between the patient's knees as the patient adducts firmly.

If there is no sound of cavitation using the above technique—and you still consider the joint to be dysfunctional—a thrust/HVT technique is appropriate. After the patient has abducted the hip three times (figure 13.1), place your hands on the insides of the patient's knees (figure 13.3), or you could use your forearms if easier (figure 13.4).

Then ask the patient to adduct quickly and strongly against the applied resistance. As the patient adducts, you can apply a rapid abduction motion (figure 13.5). If a dysfunction is present, this technique will often cause a cavitation of the symphysis pubis joint; hence this technique is known as the shotgun.

 MET of symphysis pubis using shotgun technique

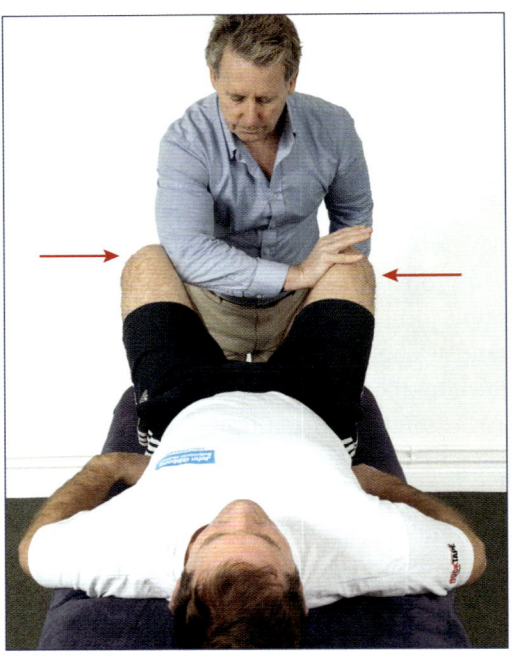

Figure 13.4. The therapist places their forearm between the patient's knees as the patient adducts firmly.

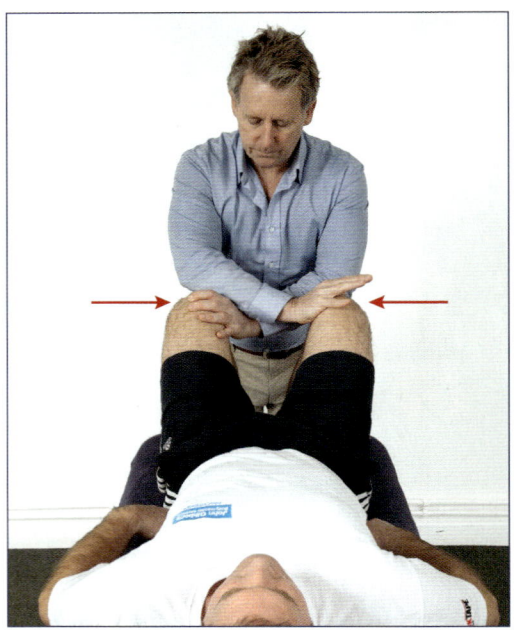

Figure 13.3. The therapist places their hands between the patient's knees as the patient adducts firmly.

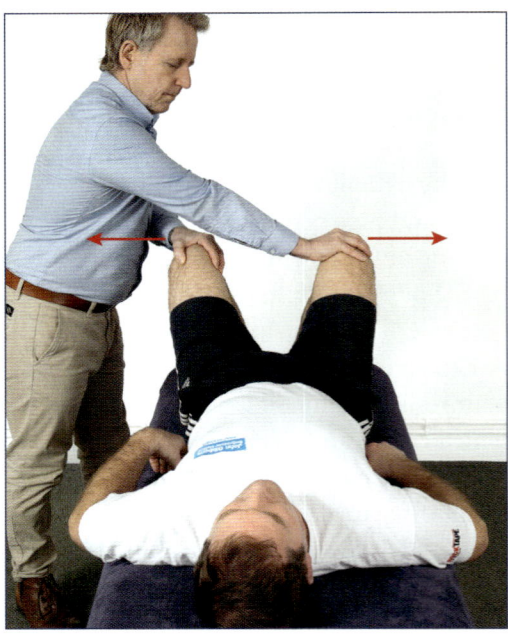

Figure 13.5. The therapist quickly separates the patient's knees while they are still adducting; a noise is sometimes heard as the symphysis pubis joint undergoes cavitation.

Diagnosis: Left Superior SPD

Treatment: MET

Position: Supine

Ask the patient to lie supine at the edge of the couch with their arms placed across their body for extra support. Stand on the same side as the dysfunction, and place the patient's left leg so that it hangs off the couch. Stabilize the right side of the patient's pelvis with your left hand, and place your right hand above the left patella to stabilize the patient's left leg (figure 13.6).

From this position, ask the patient to flex their left hip against your resistance for 10 seconds (figure 13.7). On the relaxation phase, guide the patient's left leg into further extension, which will encourage the left side of the symphysis pubis joint to move inferiorly (figure 13.8).

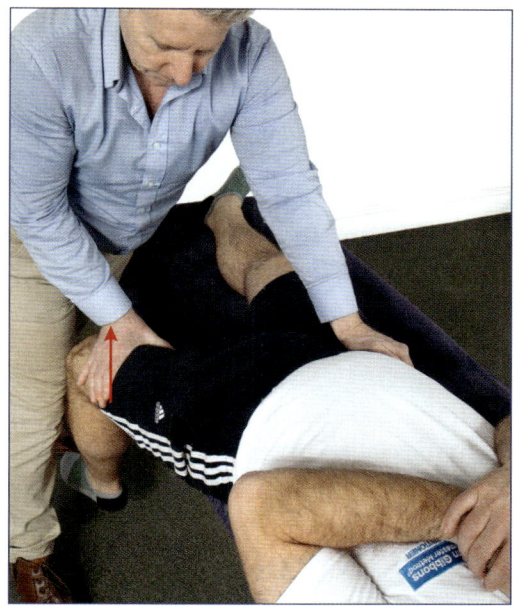

Figure 13.7. The patient lifts their left hip into flexion against a resistance applied by the therapist.

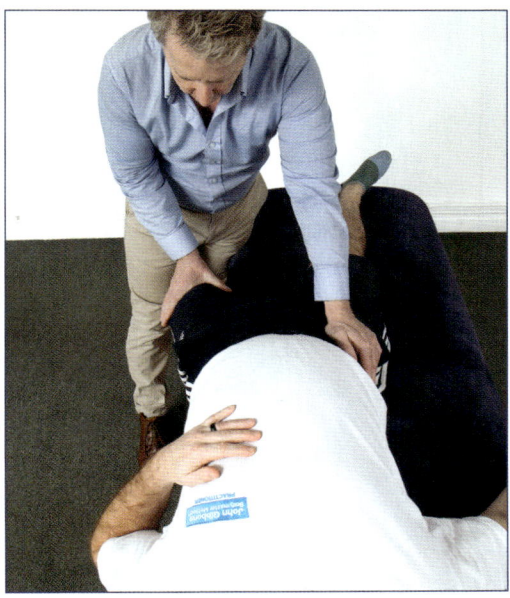

Figure 13.6. The therapist supports the patient, whose left leg hangs off the couch.

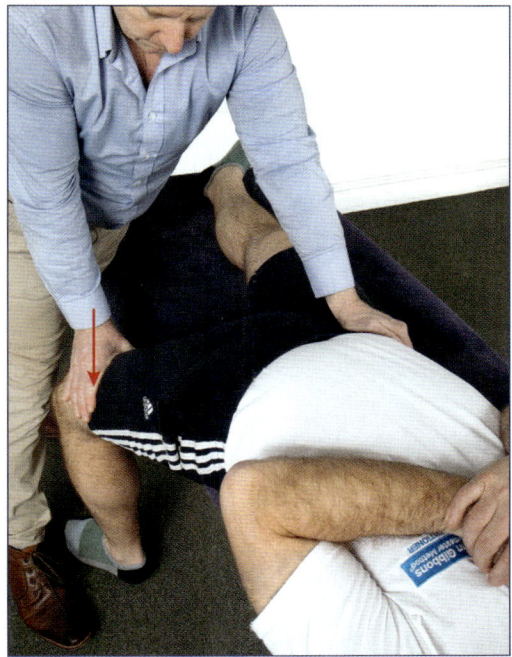

Figure 13.8. After the 10-second contraction, the therapist takes the leg into further extension, which encourages the left side of symphysis pubis to move inferiorly.

Diagnosis: Right Inferior SPD

Treatment: MET

Position: Supine

Ask the patient to lie supine at the edge of the couch with their arms placed across their body for extra support. Stand on the side opposite to the dysfunction.

Then flex and adduct, with a slight internal rotation, the patient's right leg, to encourage superior motion of the right side of the symphysis pubis.

Using the patient's leg as a lever, lift the right side of the patient's pelvis off the couch, so that you can place your left hand on the patient's right PSIS while putting the heel of the same hand onto the ischial tuberosity (figure 13.9).

Lower the patient's pelvis down onto your hand; from this position, ask the patient to extend their left hip

against your resistance for 10 seconds (figure 13.10). On the relaxation phase, encourage the patient's left leg into further flexion, while at the same time applying pressure to the ischial tuberosity (figure 13.11); this will encourage the

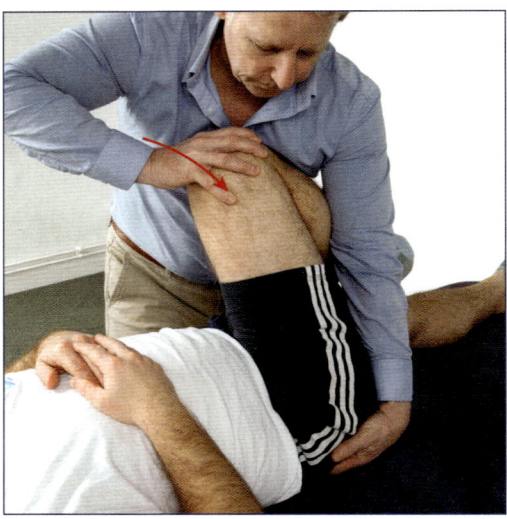

Figure 13.10. The patient extends their hip against a resistance applied by the therapist.

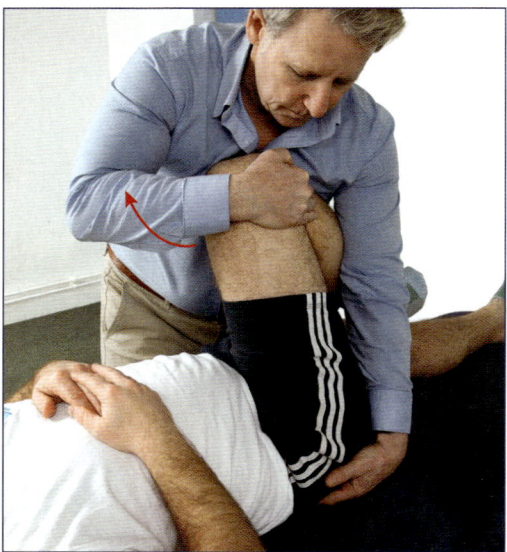

Figure 13.11. The therapist guides the patient's leg into further flexion while applying pressure to the ischial tuberosity.

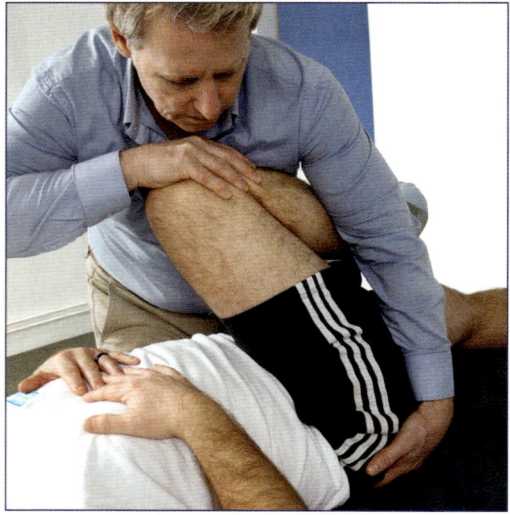

Figure 13.9. The patient's right hip is guided into flexion, adduction, and internal rotation.

right side of the symphysis pubis joint to move superiorly.

Treatment Protocol for Iliosacral Dysfunctions

The following iliosacral dysfunctions are possible within the pelvic girdle:

- Anteriorly rotated innominate
- Posteriorly rotated innominate
- Superior shear (cephalic)—upslip

Diagnosis: Right Anteriorly Rotated Innominate

This is the most common iliosacral dysfunction.

Treatment: MET

Position: Side lying

Ask the patient to adopt a side-lying position, and stand on the same side as the dysfunction. Flex the patient's hip and knee to approximately 90° and bring them over the edge of the couch. Fine-tune this position by palpating the PSIS with your right hand as you flex the patient's hip until you feel a point of bind at the level of the PSIS (figure 13.12).

From this position, ask the patient to extend their hip (Gmax and hamstrings) against your resistance for 10 seconds using approximately 20% effort (figure 13.13).

After the contraction, and on complete relaxation, guide the right

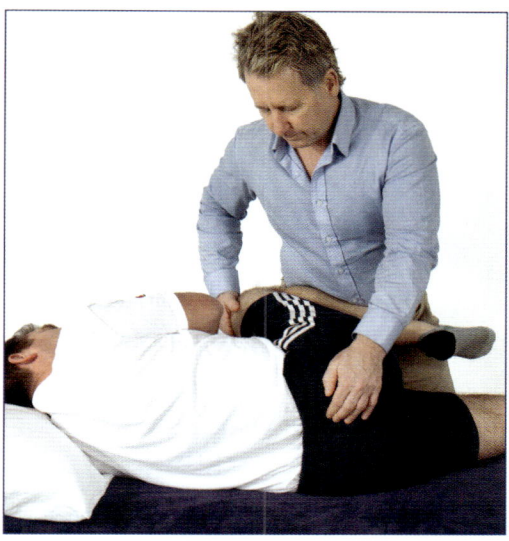

Figure 13.12. The therapist cradles the patient's knee and hip at 90° whilst palpating the PSIS.

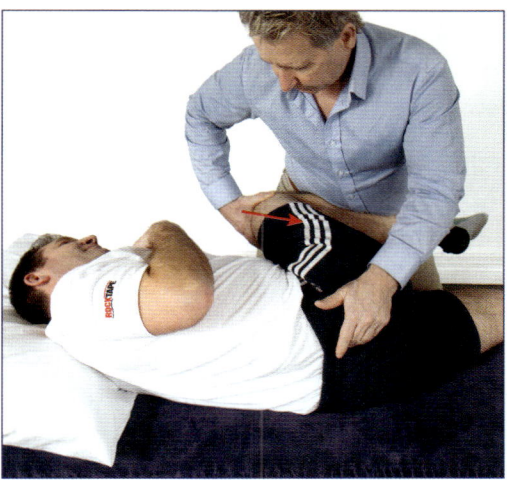

Figure 13.13. The patient extends their hip against a resistance applied by the therapist.

innominate bone using your left hand (figure 13.14a) or an alternative cradle hold (figure 13.14b) into a posteriorly rotated position, while flexing the hip and knee. Repeat this (normally three times) until a new point of bind has been achieved.

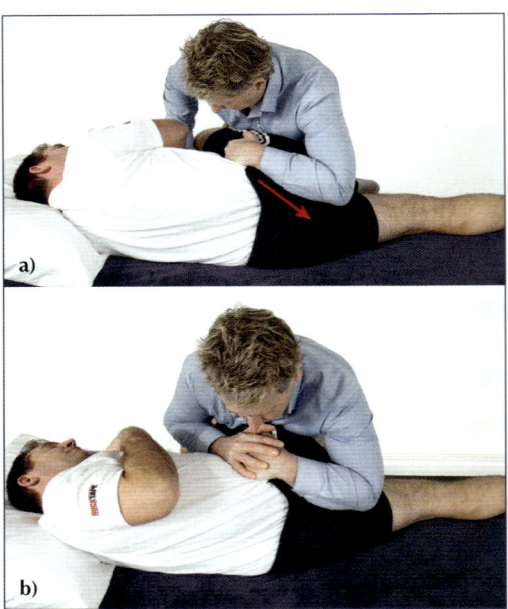

Figure 13.14. (a) The therapist guides the patient's innominate bone into a posteriorly rotated position as the knee and hip are being flexed; (b) an alternative cradle hold technique.

MET treatment of anterior rotation of innominate

Diagnosis: Left Anteriorly Rotated Innominate

Treatment: MET

Position: Side lying

To correct a left anterior innominate rotation, this is an alternative technique to the one above, but with a few modifications. This time the dysfunction relates to a left anterior innominate rather than a right anterior innominate.

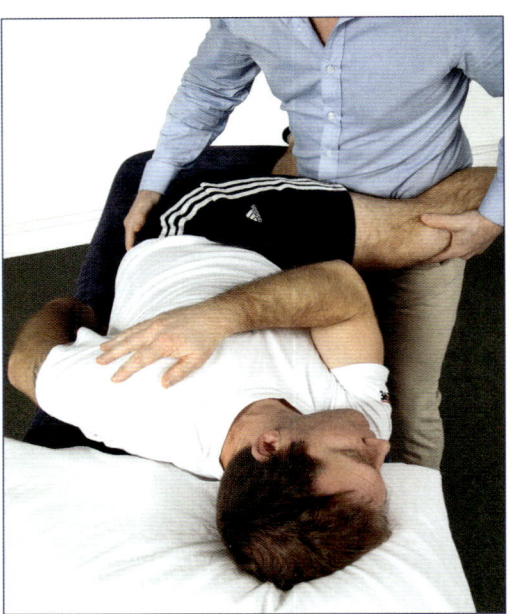

Figure 13.15. The patient's torso is placed in a left rotation, and the therapist cradles the patient's hip at 90° while palpating the left PSIS.

Ask the patient to adopt a side-lying position, and stand on the same side as the dysfunction. Place the patient's upper torso in a left rotation to induce tension down to the lumbosacral junction and prevent unnecessary motion of the lumbar spine. Next, place the patient's left hip into flexion, with their posterior thigh resting against your hip (the patient hooks their left leg around the therapist), as in figure 13.15. Place the patient's right lower leg in an extended position. Palpate the PSIS and encourage flexion of the hip until you feel a point of bind.

From this position, ask the patient to extend their hip (Gmax and hamstrings) against your resistance for 10 seconds using approximately 20% effort (figure 13.16). On complete relaxation, guide the left innominate bone into a

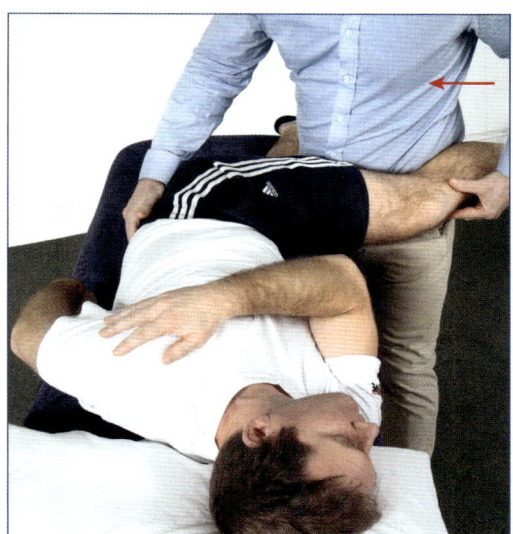

Figure 13.16. The patient extends their hip for 10 seconds while the therapist palpates the left PSIS.

posteriorly rotated position using your right hand, while at the same time flexing the hip and knee (figure 13.17). Repeat this (normally three times) until a new barrier has been achieved.

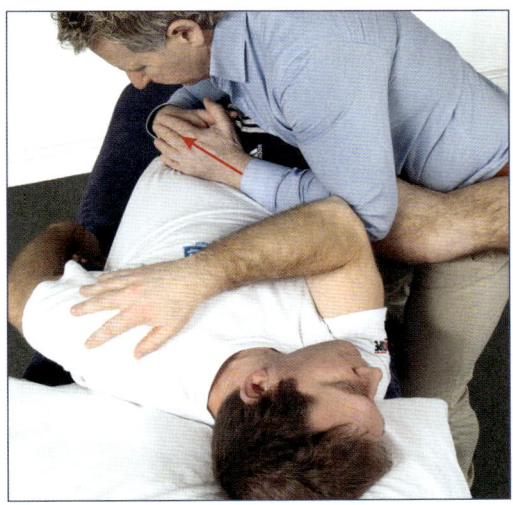

Figure 13.17. The therapist guides the patient's innominate bone into a posteriorly rotated position as the knee and hip are being flexed.

Diagnosis: Right Posteriorly Rotated Innominate

Treatment: MET

Position: Prone

Ask the patient to adopt a prone position, and stand on the side opposite to the dysfunction (the left side; the right side is fixed posteriorly). Ask the patient to lift their left leg a few inches, so that you can place your right hand under the patient's right knee, while your left hand rests just at the level of the patient's right PSIS. (Some patients' legs are extremely heavy, and in those cases this technique is a little easier to perform compared to some other techniques).

Fine-tune this position by slowly extending and adducting the right hip until you feel a barrier. From this barrier, ask the patient to gently flex the right hip against your resistance for 10 seconds (figure 13.18).

On complete relaxation, take the right leg further into hip extension and adduction, while applying pressure with your left hand to the patient's right PSIS. This combined movement induces an anterior rotation of the right innominate bone (figure 13.19). Repeat this (normally three times) until a new barrier has been achieved.

If the rectus femoris muscle is particularly tight, it might be easier and more effective to perform the same technique with a straight leg, as this motion of straightening the leg will take the tension off the muscle (figure 13.20).

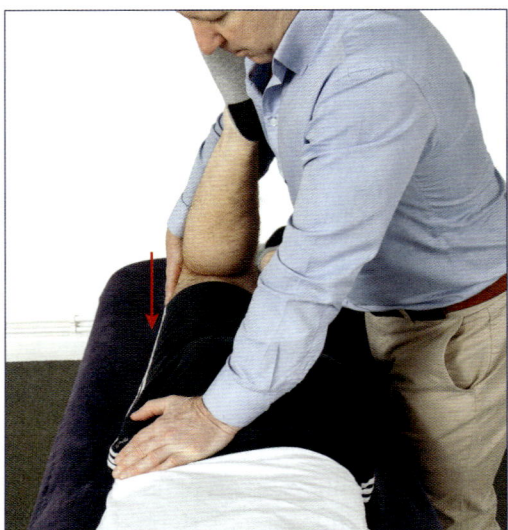

Figure 13.18. The therapist supports the patient's leg, while controlling the innominate bone with their hand, then the patient flexes their hip against a resistance applied by the therapist.

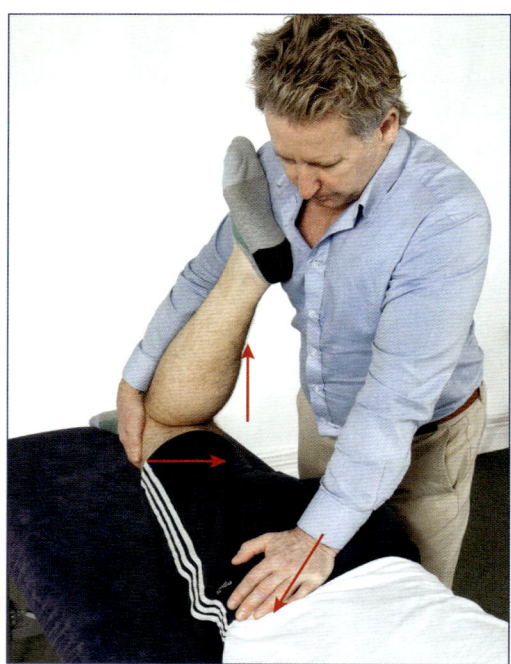

Figure 13.19. The therapist guides the patient's innominate in an anterior rotation direction, while at the same time the hip is extended and adducted.

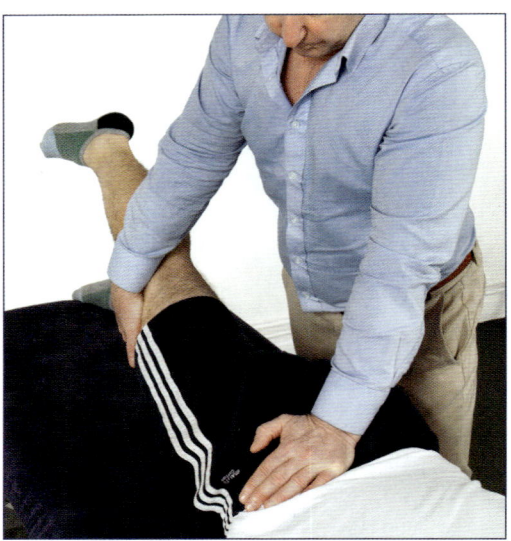

Figure 13.20. The same technique is performed but this time the leg is straight, which will take the tension off the rectus femoris muscle.

MET treatment of posterior rotation of innominate

Diagnosis: Right Superior Shear (Cephalic)—Upslip

Treatment: MET/mobilization/thrust technique

Position: Prone

Ask the patient to lie prone as you stand on the same side as the dysfunction. Ask the patient to slide down the couch until their knees are just off the edge and to look to one side (either) without holding on to anything. Straddle the patient's right leg and internally rotate the patient's thigh to cause a close-packed position of the hip joint (figure 13.21).

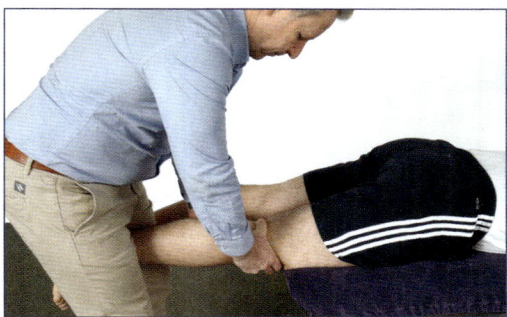

Figure 13.21. The therapist straddles the patient's right leg and internally rotates their hip to establish a close-packed position of the hip joint.

Palpate the patient's right PSIS with your right hand, while your left hand stabilizes either the sacrum or the left thigh.
With your thigh, slowly start to grip the patient's right leg, while applying some traction to the leg by inducing a caudal pull to the right leg until you reach a barrier.

At the barrier, apply an MET by asking the patient to hitch their pelvis up by activating their quadratus lumborum muscle for 10 seconds against a resistance applied by the straddling of your legs (figure 13.22).

After the contraction, and during the relaxation phase, find a new point of bind by gently applying a caudal/inferior

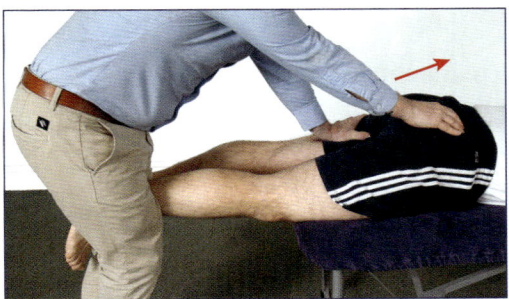

Figure 13.22. Using their quadratus lumborum muscle, the patient hitches the pelvis up in a cephalic/superior direction for 10 seconds.

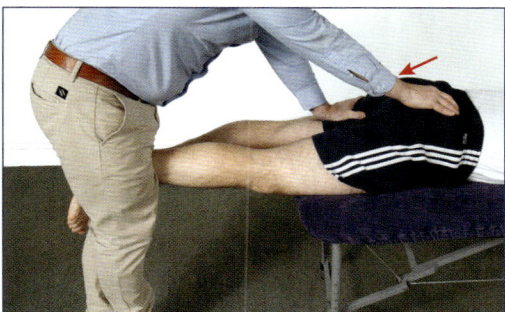

Figure 13.23. The therapist performs a traction/ mobilization or a manipulation (thrust) technique to the leg in a caudal direction after the initial MET contraction/treatment.

traction to the leg. Repeat this three times. A mobilization or a manipulation (thrust) technique can also be performed from this position to encourage a caudal/downward movement of the right innominate bone (figure 13.23).

 Treatment of an upslip

Diagnosis: Left Superior Shear (Cephalic)—Upslip

Treatment: MET/mobilization/thrust technique

Position: Supine

Ask the patient to lie supine, with their right knee bent at 90° (this prevents unnecessary motion of the right innominate bone). Stand on the same side as the dysfunction, and internally rotate the patient's thigh to introduce a close-packed position of the left hip joint (figure 13.24).

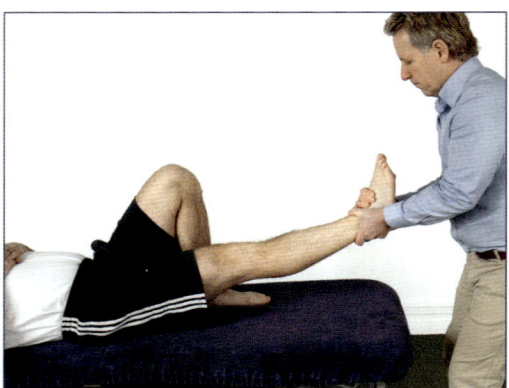

Figure 13.24. The therapist stabilizes the patient's left leg and internally rotates their hip to establish a close-packed position of the hip joint.

Gently grip the patient's lower leg with your hands and start to apply light traction to the left leg by inducing a caudal pull to engage the point of bind. At the point of bind, you can perform a mobilizing technique, MET, or HVT to encourage a caudal/downward movement of the innominate bone (figure 13.25).

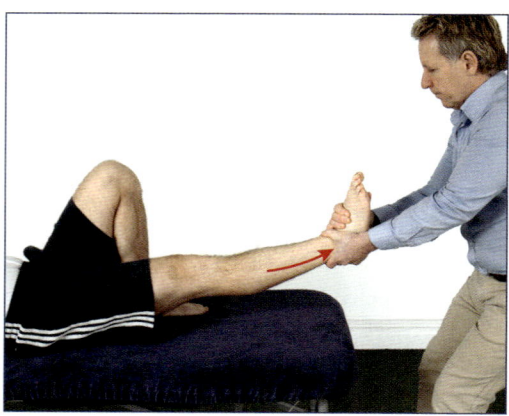

Figure 13.25. The therapist has the choice of performing an MET, a mobilization, or a manipulation technique from this position.

Treatment Protocol for Sacroiliac Dysfunctions

The two sacroiliac dysfunctions discussed here are relatively common. These are what they call a forward sacral torsion, which simply implies that the sacrum can potentially be fixated either to the right side or the left side. In a right-side fixation, known as an R-on-R sacral torsion, the sacrum has rotated to the right on the right oblique axis. If the sacrum gets fixated to the left side, known as an L-on-L sacral torsion, the sacrum has rotated to the left on the left oblique axis.

However, there are many other, less common, sacroiliac dysfunctions that can present within the pelvic girdle, known as posterior sacral torsions. These dysfunctions are rare and relatively complex to assess and treat (see Gibbons 2016). Here I will discuss:

- Left-on-left (L-on-L) anterior (forward) sacral torsion
- Right-on-right (R-on-R) anterior (forward) sacral torsion

Diagnosis: L-on-L Anterior (Forward) Sacral Torsion

Treatment: MET

Position: Sims

In this dysfunction, the sacrum has rotated left (side bent right) on the left oblique axis, and the right sacral base has anteriorly nutated (figure 13.26).

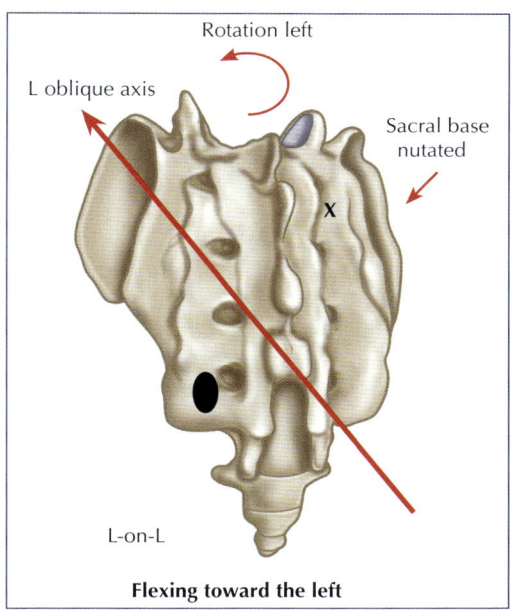

Figure 13.26. L-on-L sacral motion/torsion; X = anterior or deep, black circle = posterior or shallow.

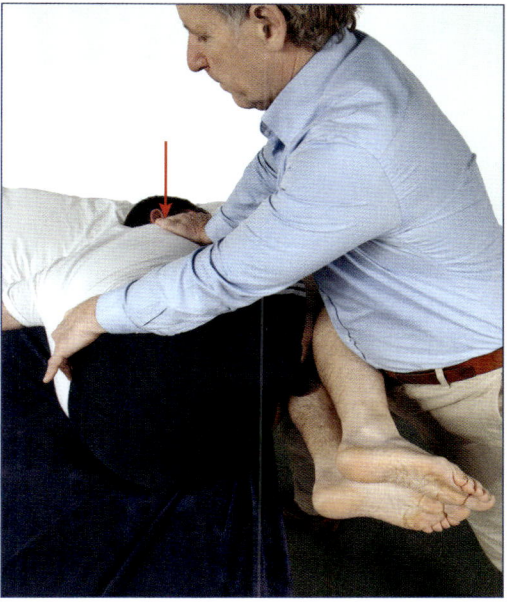

Figure 13.27. The therapist fine-tunes the position and introduces a rotation of L5 to the left.

Ask the patient to lie prone on the couch, while you stand on the right side of the couch and flex the patient's knees to 90°. Turn the patient onto their left hip to achieve the Sims position. (Note that the patient's left arm is held back, and the right arm is held forward.)

With the patient's knees placed on your left thigh, palpate the lumbosacral junction using your left hand, while you introduce a left rotation of the patient's trunk until you feel L5 rotate to the left (figure 13.27).

From this position, palpate the lumbosacral junction and the right sacral base with your right hand, and then, using the patient's legs as a lever, introduce a flexion motion to the trunk until you feel a barrier (figure 13.28).

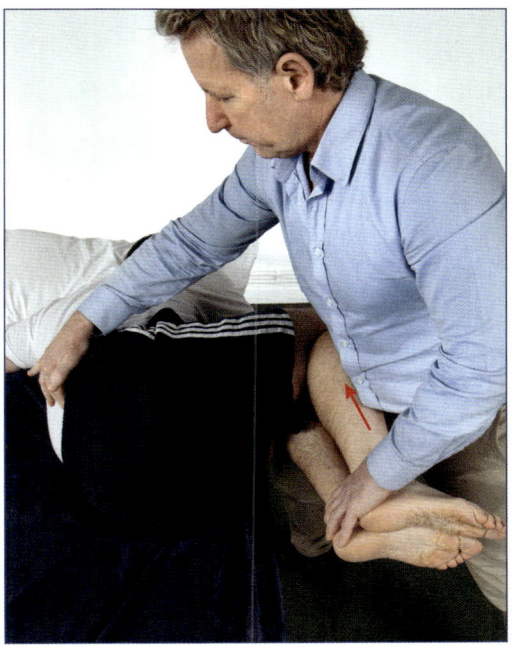

Figure 13.28. Using the patient's legs as a lever, the therapist flexes the patient's trunk until a barrier is felt at the lumbosacral junction.

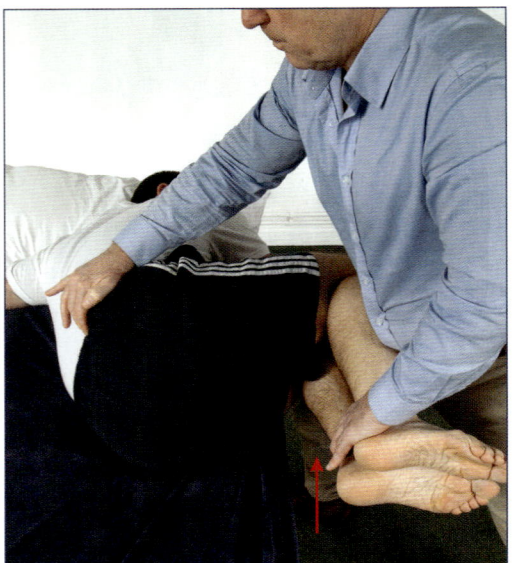

Figure 13.29. The patient pushes their legs toward the ceiling, which activates the right piriformis muscle.

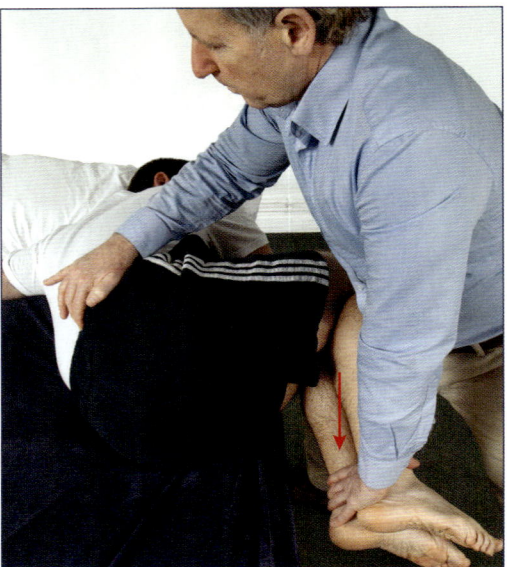

Figure 13.30. The therapist palpates the right sacral base and feels for posterior motion as the patient's legs are directed toward the floor.

Ask the patient to push their legs toward the ceiling against your resistance for 10 seconds (which activates the right piriformis muscle), as in figure 13.29.

On the relaxation phase, take the patient's legs toward the floor until you feel movement posterior to the right sacral base (figure 13.30).

Note: The Sims technique works well because it challenges the sacral position to correct itself by using the motion of the lumbar spine and motion from the lower limbs to facilitate the correction.

For example, with an L-on-L type of dysfunction, we know that the right sacral base has migrated forward into a fixed position of nutation, so the restriction is due to the right sacral base being unable to counter-nutate. The first process in the technique is flexion of the lumbar spine,

which encourages an extension of the sacrum. Second, left rotation is introduced to the lumbar spine, which encourages right rotation of the sacrum (a movement it cannot perform). The third phase is the combination of the motion and MET of the legs, which introduces the right piriformis muscle to assist in restoring the sacral position.

 Sims for sacral torsion, L-on-L

Diagnosis: R-on-R Anterior (Forward) Sacral Torsion

Treatment: MET

Position: Sims

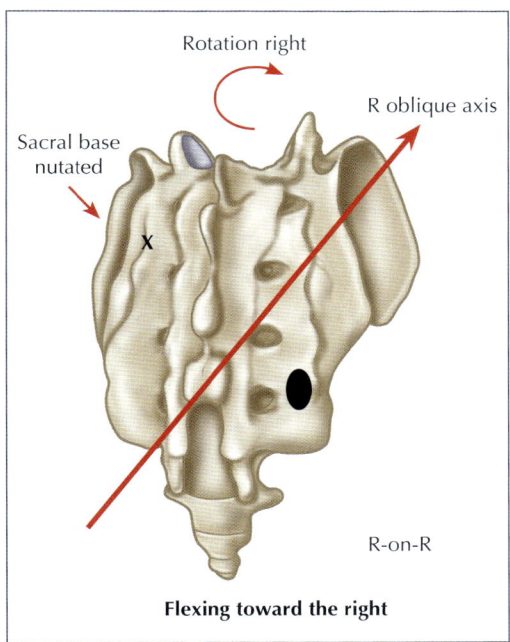

Figure 13.31. R-on-R sacral motion/torsion; X = anterior or deep, black circle = posterior or shallow.

In this dysfunction the sacrum has rotated right (side bent left) on the right oblique axis, and the left sacral base has anteriorly nutated (figure 13.31).

Ask the patient to adopt a prone position on the couch, while you stand on the left side of the couch and flex the patient's knees to 90°. Turn the patient onto their right hip into the Sims position (left arm forward, right arm back).

With the patient's knees placed on your right thigh, palpate the lumbosacral junction using your right hand, while you introduce a right rotation of the patient's trunk until you feel L5 rotate to the right (figure 13.32).

From this position, palpate the lumbosacral junction and the left sacral

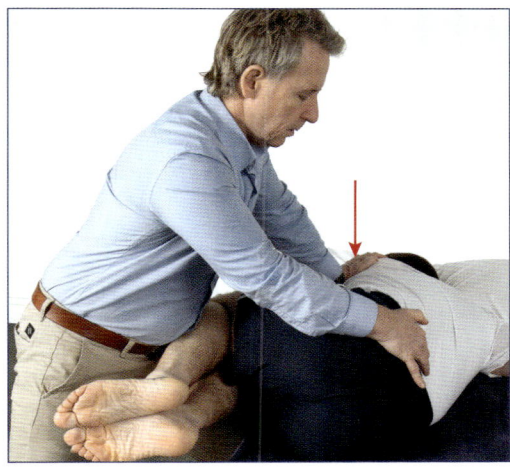

Figure 13.32. The therapist fine-tunes the position and introduces a rotation of L5 to the right.

base with your left hand, then, using the patient's legs as a lever, introduce a flexion motion to the trunk until you feel a barrier (figure 13.33).

Ask the patient to push their legs toward the ceiling against your resistance for 10 seconds (which activates the left piriformis muscle), as in figure 13.34.

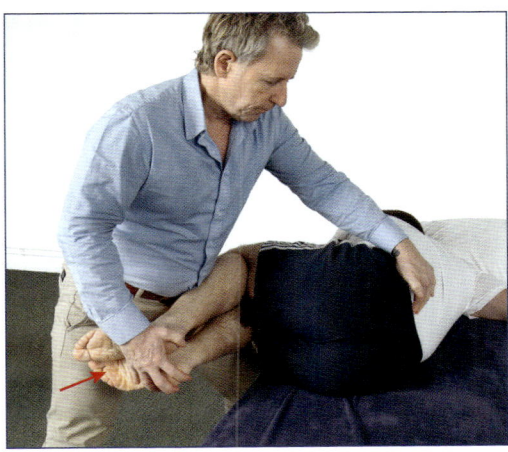

Figure 13.33. Using the patient's legs as a lever, the therapist flexes the patient's trunk until a barrier is felt at the lumbosacral junction.

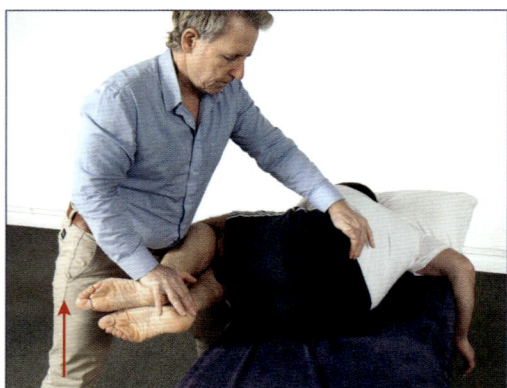

Figure 13.34. The patient pushes their legs toward the ceiling, as this activates the left piriformis muscle.

On the relaxation phase, take the patient's legs toward the floor until you feel movement posterior to the left sacral base (figure 13.35).

Note: The R-on-R sacral torsion is the same concept as the L-on-L sacral torsion. The Sims technique again works well, because it challenges the sacral position to correct itself by using the motion of the lumbar spine as well as the motion from the lower limbs.

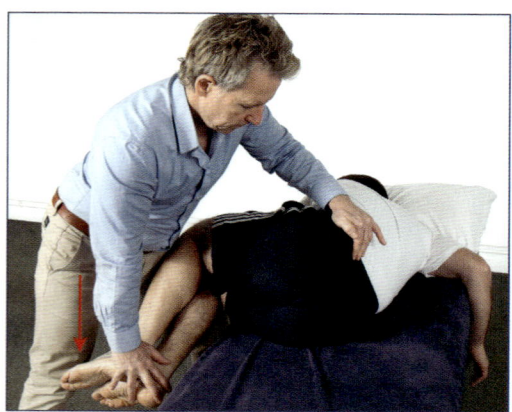

Figure 13.35. The therapist palpates the left sacral base and feels for posterior motion as the patient's legs are directed toward the floor.

For example, with an R-on-R type of dysfunction, we know that this time the left sacral base is fixed forward in a position of nutation, so the restriction is due to the sacral base being unable to counter-nutate on the left side. The first process is to induce flexion of the lumbar spine, which encourages an extension of the sacrum. Second, right rotation is introduced to the lumbar spine, which encourages left rotation of the sacrum (remember, this is a movement it cannot perform). The third phase is the combined effect of the motion and the MET of the lower legs; this introduces the left piriformis muscle to assist in restoring the sacral position.

 Sims for sacral torsion, R-on-R

Chicago Roll Technique—Diagnosis: Right Anterior Rotation of the Innominate

Treatment: Thrust technique

Position: Supine

This technique is used to correct an anterior rotation of the innominate. There are a few versions, and I will show a couple of alternatives. When this technique was taught to me during my osteopathy studies, the tutor mentioned that it could also correct a posterior sacral torsion on the right side (known as R-on-L, where the right side of the sacral base is fixed in counter nutation) as well as an anterior rotation of the innominate.

Place the patient's right leg over their left leg to induce a posterior rotation of the right innominate (figure 13.36).

Then place the patient into a banana (smile away) position (figure 13.37). Ask the patient to interlock their fingers behind their head and to bring their elbows together, place your left hand through the patients right arm, and place the back of your hand onto their sternum (figure 13.38).

Next, rotate the patient's torso toward you, and at the same time, place your left hand directly onto the ASIS (a towel or small pillow can be used to make it more comfortable). When you feel the appropriate tension down to the innominate, apply a thrust directly to the couch (figure 13.39).

For a female patient, I suggest you ask them to cross their arms over their chest rather than to interlock their fingers

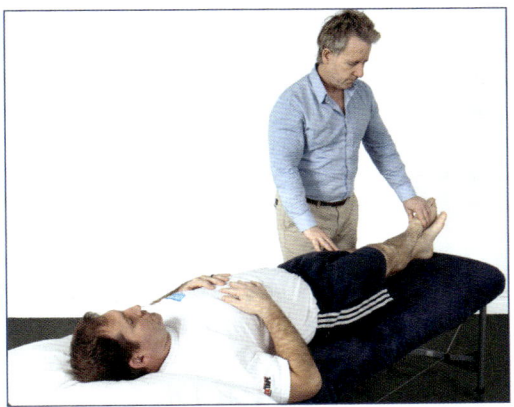

Figure 13.36. The patient's right leg is crossed over the left leg.

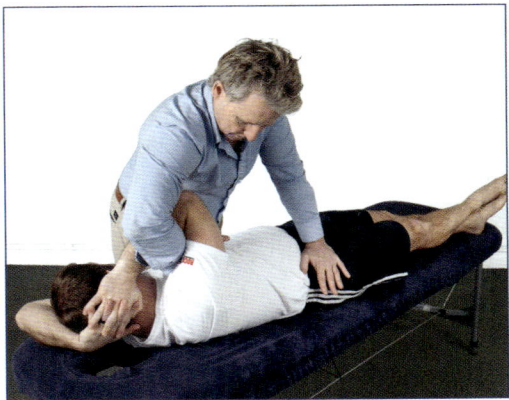

Figure 13.38. The therapist places their hand through the patient's right arm and contacts their sternum.

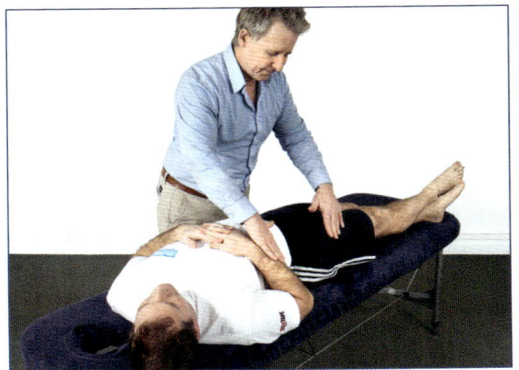

Figure 13.37. Patient is placed in a smile away position.

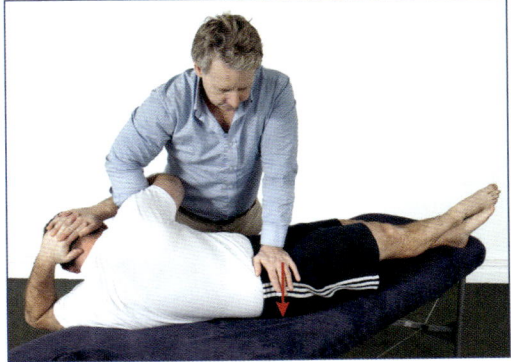

Figure 13.39. The therapist rotates the patient toward them, pressure is applied directly to the ASIS, and a thrust is administered.

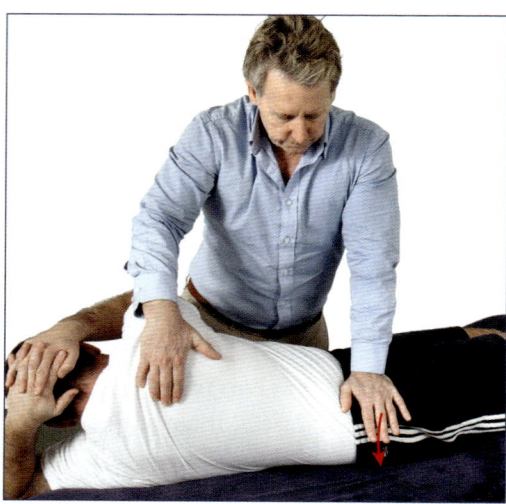

Figure 13.40. The alternative technique applied for a female patient.

behind their neck, while you place your hand onto the scapular region of their body, and induce the rotation of the torso from this position (figure 13.40).

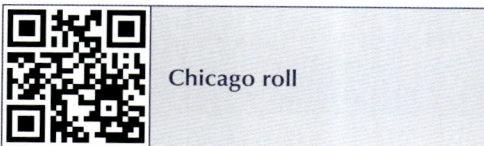

Chicago roll

SIJ Manipulation—Diagnosis: Posterior or Anterior Rotation of the Innominate

Treatment: Thrust technique

Position: Side lying

This technique is used to correct either a posterior or an anterior rotation of the innominate, as the position can be modified accordingly, or it can be used to simply "gap" the sacroiliac joint.

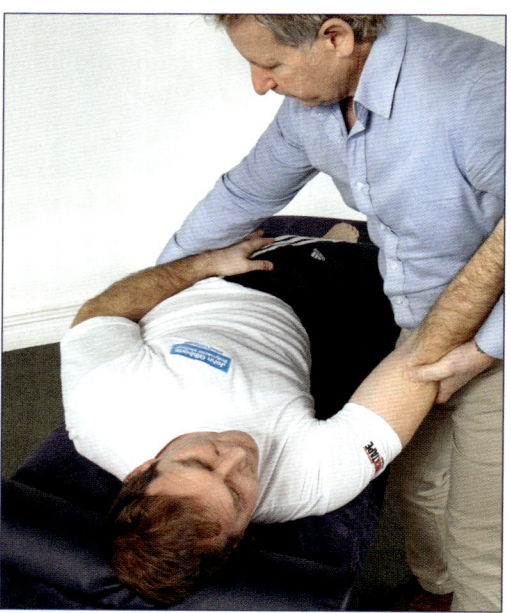

Figure 13.41. With the couch as low as possible, the patient is fully rotated down to L5 with their top leg fully flexed at hip and knee.

Lower the couch as far as possible. The technique is modified from the lumbar roll; the only difference is that you place the patient into full spinal rotation to lock down to the LS junction (L5/S1) as the focus is the sacroiliac joint and not the lumbar spine (figure 13.41). The patient's top leg is also fully flexed at the hip and knee joints and then is stabilized by your leg to prevent it from moving.

Place one of your hands on the patient's shoulder, with the other on top of their innominate bone. Encourage the patient—through guided motion—to roll toward you until they are almost falling off the couch (figure 13.42). When you feel the appropriate tension, apply a thrust in the direction through the femoral bone (figure 13.43).

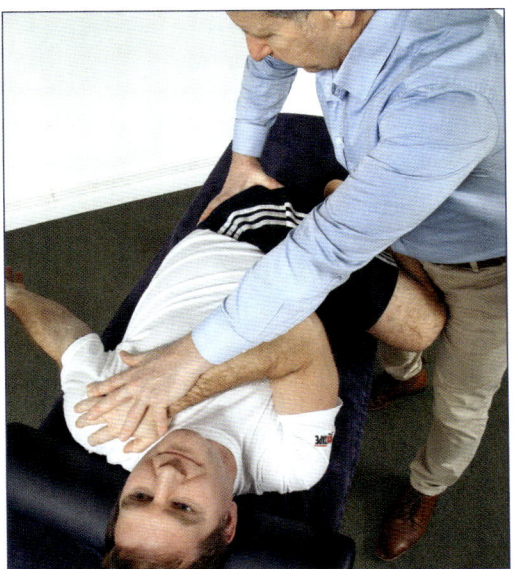

Figure 13.42. The patient is rolled toward the therapist, while the therapist maintains contact to the patient's shoulder and innominate bone.

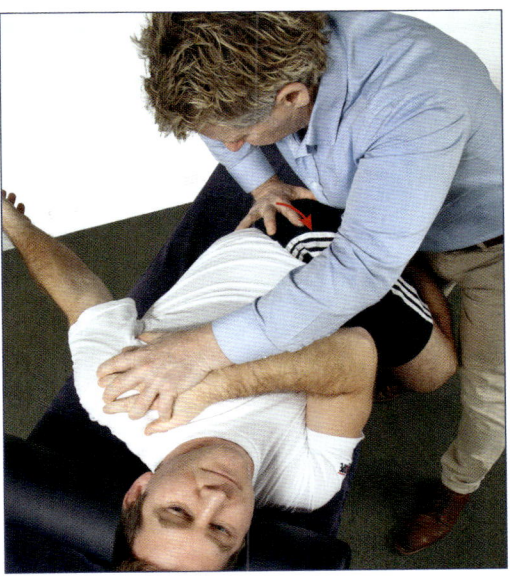

Figure 13.43. Direction of thrust through the long bone of the femur.

SIJ manipulation

Abbreviations

AAJ	atlanto-axial joint	**Gmax**	gluteus maximus
AIIS	anterior inferior iliac spine	**HID**	herniated intervertebral disc
AOJ	atlanto-occipital joint	**HVLA**	high velocity with low amplitude
AP	anterior–posterior	**HVT**	high velocity thrust
AROM	active range of motion	**LS**	lumbosacral
ASIS	anterior superior iliac spine	**LSp**	lumbar spine
CES	cauda equina syndrome	**MCP**	metacarpophalangeal
CSp	cervical spine	**MET**	muscle energy technique
CT	cervicothoracic	**NSAID**	nonsteroidal anti-inflammatory drug
CTJ	cervicothoracic junction	**OA**	osteoarthritis
DDD	degenerative disc disease	**PA**	posterior–anterior
DRG	dorsal root ganglion	**PID**	prolapsed intervertebral disc
DTR	deep tendon reflex	**PIR**	post-isometric relaxation
FAI	femoral-acetabular impingement		

PROM	passive range of motion	**SPD**	symphysis pubis dysfunction
PSIS	posterior superior iliac spine	**SPJ**	symphysis pubis joint
RI	reciprocal inhibition	**TFL**	tensor fasciae latae
SCM	sternocleidomastoid	**TLJ**	thoracolumbar junction
SIJ	sacroiliac joint	**TP**	transverse process
SLR	straight leg raise	**TSp**	thoracic spine
SP	spinous process	**VBI**	vertebral basilar insufficiency

References

Anekstein, Y., Blecher, R., Smorgick, Y., and Mirovsky, Y. 2012. "What is the best way to apply the Spurling test for cervical radiculopathy?" *Clin. Orthop. Relat. Res.* 470 (9): 2566–72.

DeStefano, L. 2011. *Greenman's Principles of Manual Medicine*, 4th ed. Baltimore, MD: Lippincott, Williams, and Wilkins.

Edmondston, S. J., and Singer, K. P. 1997. "Thoracic spine: Anatomical and biomechanical considerations for manual therapy." *Man. Ther.* 2 (3): 132–43.

Egund, N., Olsson, T. H., Schmid, H., and Selvik, G. 1978. "Movements in the sacroiliac joints demonstrated with roentgen stereophotogrammetry." *Acta Radiol. Diagn. (Stockh.)* 19 (5): 833–46.

Farfan, H. F. 1973. *Mechanical Disorders of the Back*. Philadelphia, PA: Lea and Febiger.

Gibbons, J. 2016. *Functional Anatomy of the Pelvis and Sacroiliac Joint: A Practical Guide*. Chichester, UK: Lotus.

Gibbons, J. 2020. *The Vital Nerves: A Practical Guide for Physical Therapists*. Chichester, UK: Lotus.

Gibbons, J. 2022. *Muscle Energy Techniques: A Practical Guide for Physical Therapists*, 2nd ed. Chichester, UK: Lotus.

Harrison, D. E., Cailliet, R., Harrison, D. D., and Janik, T. J. 2002. "How do anterior/posterior translations of the thoracic cage affect the sagittal lumbar spine, pelvic tilt, and thoracic kyphosis?" *Eur. Spine J.* 11 (3): 287–93.

Kampen, W. U., and Tillmann, B. 1998. "Age-related changes in the articular cartilage of human sacroiliac joint." *Anat. Embryol.* 198: 505–13.

Lee, D. G. 2004. *The Pelvic Girdle: An Approach to the Examination and Treatment of the Lumbopelvic-Hip Region*. Edinburgh: Churchill Livingstone.

Mitchell, F. L., Moran, P. S., and Pruzzo, N. A. 1979. *An Evaluation and Treatment Manual of Osteopathic Muscle Energy Procedures*. Valley Park, MO: Mitchell, Moran, and Pruzzo.

Sturesson, B., Selvik, G., and Uden, A. 1989. "Movements of the sacroiliac joints: A roentgen stereophotogrammetric analysis." *Spine* 14 (2): 162–65.

Sturesson, B., Uden, A., and Vleeming, A. 2000a. "A radiostereometric analysis of the movements of the sacroiliac joint in the reciprocal straddle position." *Spine* 25 (2): 214–17.

Sturesson, B., Uden, A., and Vleeming, A. 2000b. "A radiostereometric analysis of the movements of the sacroiliac during the standing hip flexion test." *Spine* 25 (3): 364–68.

Vleeming, A., Mooney, V., and Stoeckart, R. (eds.). 2007. *Movement, Stability and Lumbopelvic Pain: Integration of Research and Therapy*. Edinburgh: Churchill Livingstone.

Vleeming, A., Stoeckart, R., and Snijders, D. J. 1989. "The sacrotuberous ligament: A conceptual approach to its dynamic role in stabilizing the sacroiliac joint." *Clin. Biomech.* 4: 200–203.

Index